Ken Terry has produced a *tour de force* analysis of the current s
health care. In a world filled with "alternative facts," Ken's ency
research evidence, instructive interviews, and clear writing ma
reading, whether or not you agree with his prescriptions for reform. An essential
resource.

Robert Berenson, MD, Institute Fellow, Urban Institute

Mr. Terry has again dissected the health care industry and all of its faults with an
eye toward finding solutions rather than merely pointing out defects. This is a
timely book which should be required reading for any public figure who wants
to talk intelligently about real-life situations and practical solutions to the most
problematic social issue facing our political structure today.

A. Michael La Penna, Principal, The La Penna Group, Inc.

Ken Terry's book, *Physician-Led Healthcare Reform: A New Approach to Medicare for
All*, offers an encyclopedia of knowledge on the U.S. healthcare system, written in
an engaging, popular style. Up-to-date as of 2020, the information will be timely for
years to come.

**Tom Bodenheimer, MD, MPH, Founding Director of the Center for
Excellence in Primary Care**

Every country on the planet struggles to control their healthcare costs. Nowhere
else is this struggle so palpable nor the consequences of inaction so clear as in
America. Healthcare rationing occurs in some form in every wealthy country;
however, in those countries rationing takes the form of limiting low value care that
hasn't been demonstrated to improve the health of its population. On the other
hand, in America, where over 30% of the care we provide is low value care, we
instead ration care by leaving 44 million Americans uninsured and taxing those
with insurance through high premiums and high out-of-pocket costs. Set against
this backdrop is Ken Terry's comprehensive treatise on Medicare for All (MFA).
The solution to our healthcare crisis lies in the elimination of low value care and
redirection of those resources towards improved health outcomes and reduced
cost of care. Ken elegantly outlines the potential of a single-payor model to achieve
these goals. He applies his quarter century of health economic experience to
help readers understand this complex calculus, including the political, economic,
and societal changes that would occur as a result of this change. He also analyzes
current care models within the U.S. that align with MFA and would therefore
contribute to its success. The unanswered question is at what point the financial
pain of the average American will create enough influence to counterbalance
the lobbying forces of big pharma, hospitals, physician groups, and insurance
companies to tip the scale in favor of a sustainable healthcare model.

**Ken Cohen MD, CMO, FACP, Chief Medical Officer at New West Physicians
and Senior Medical Director OptumCare**

PHYSICIAN-LED HEALTHCARE REFORM

A New Approach to Medicare For All

BY KEN TERRY

Foreword by David B. Nash, MD, MBA

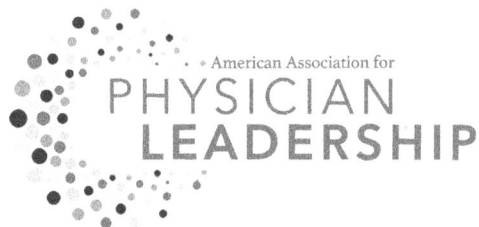

American Association for
PHYSICIAN
LEADERSHIP

Copyright © 2020 by **American Association for Physician Leadership**®

978-0-9848310-5-0 Print

978-0-9848310-6-7 eBook

Published by **American Association for Physician Leadership, Inc.**

PO Box 96503 | BMB 97493 | Washington, DC 20090-6503

Website: www.physicianleaders.org

All rights reserved. No part of this publication may be reproduced, stored in a retrieval system, or transmitted in any form or by any means, electronic, mechanical, photocopying, recording or otherwise, without prior written permission of the American Association for Physician Leadership. Routine photocopying or electronic distribution to others is a copyright violation.

AAPL books are available at special quantity discounts to use as premiums and sales promotions, or for use in corporate training programs. For more information, please write to Special Sales at journal@physicianleaders.org

This publication is designed to provide general information and is sold with the understanding that neither the author nor the publisher is engaged in rendering legal, accounting, ethical, or clinical advice. If legal or other expert advice is required, the services of a competent professional person should be sought.

13   8 7 6 5 4 3 2 1

Copyedited, typeset, indexed, and printed in the United States of America

PUBLISHER
Nancy Collins

EDITORIAL ASSISTANT
Jennifer Weiss

DESIGN & LAYOUT
Carter Publishing Studio

COPYEDITOR
Pat George

To my father Morris Terry, who showed me how to be a mensch.

Table of Contents

Acknowledgments

First and foremost, I'd like to thank my editor Nancy Collins, who believed in the value of my book from the outset and persuaded the AAPL to publish it. I'm also grateful to Grace Terrell, who steered me to the AAPL and vouched for me.

Many industry sources and experts—including friends whom I've known for years—helped me shape this book. Some of them encouraged me to pursue my vision when it was still in the formative stages. Among those I leaned on especially while writing the book were David Nash, Grace Terrell, Kenneth Cohen, Farzad Mostashari, Robert Berenson, Michael La Penna, Lawrence Casalino, Thomas Bodenheimer, Gregg Bloche, Amitabh Chandra, Karen Handmaker, Steven Waldren, Peter Basch, Jonathan Weiner, David Blumenthal, and Donald Berwick.

Among the other experts and group leaders who gave unselfishly of their time to help me out were Bo Bobbitt, Gerald Friedman, Jacob Hacker, Travis Singleton, Victoria Farias, Mark Wagar, Paul Keckley, Paul Grundy, Ashok Rai, Anas Daghestani, Melinda Abrams, Mickey Tripathi, Richard Isaacs, Joseph Kvedar, and Joe Selby.

A number of primary care physicians also informed my views on the challenges that practicing doctors face and how they're coping with those difficulties. Thanks to David Boles, Kenneth Kubitschek, Jeffrey Kagan, Robert Lambert, Jeffrey Pearson, Jennifer Brull, and many other physicians I've interviewed and gotten to know over the years.

I'd also like to acknowledge some former colleagues at *Medical Economics*, where I got my start as a healthcare reporter. Jeff Burger, who has been my best friend since college, persuaded *Medical Economics* to hire me when I was transitioning out of entertainment journalism in the early 1990s. The magazine's then-editor in chief, Steve Murata, who was somewhat skeptical that I could cut it, threw the hardest assignments he could think of at me. The fact that I survived lends credence to the old saw, "Whatever doesn't kill you makes you stronger." Finally, Leslie Kane, who rose to become editor in chief at the same publication, encouraged me to pen my first book, *Rx for Health Care Reform*. If I hadn't written that book, I wouldn't have had the courage to tackle this one.

I'm also grateful to Charley Paikert, another old friend and fellow journalist, who always encouraged me to push myself further as a writer and to tackle big subjects.

Finally, I want to thank my family. Besides my wife Lisa Lucas, who has been beside me every step of the way, I wrote this book for my children, Selene, Alycia, Justin, and Adam, and my grandchildren, Dylan and Mia. My father Morris, who recently died at 99, taught me to stand up for what I believe in, and my late mother Laurette imbued me with a love of literature, which taught me how to write. I thank them above all.

About the Author

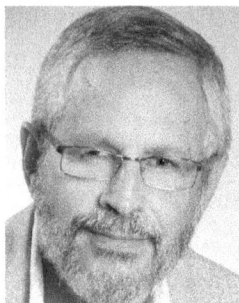

Ken Terry, the author of a previous book on health care policy and practice, has been writing about the health care field for more than 25 years. As a senior editor at *Medical Economics* magazine from 1993–2007, he covered all aspects of medical practice business, focusing especially on managed care and health information technology. Among the topics that his writing brought to life for *Medical Economics* readers were technology costs, financial risk contracting, electronic health records, and evidence-based medicine. While at *Medical Economics*, Terry received journalism awards from the American Society of Business Publication Editors (2000), the American Society of Healthcare Publication Editors (2001–2002), and American Business Media, which gave him a Neal award in 2007.

Since 2008, Terry has contributed freelance articles to a wide variety of publications, ranging from *Medical Economics*, *Medscape Medical News*, and *cio.com* to *InformationWeek* and *FierceHealthIT*. He has written for many other consumer and business publications, and he blogged for CBS Interactive's BNET Healthcare from 2008 to 2011. He has also undertaken a variety of writing projects for business clients such as IBM Watson Health, Phytel, AT&T, Microsoft, McKesson, Allscripts, and the Institute for Health Technology Transformation.

Terry's first book, *Rx for Health Care Reform* (Vanderbilt University Press, 2007), won acclaim from a number of health policy experts. Joseph E. Scherger, MD, then a professor at the University of California, San Diego, and a thought leader in primary care, called the book "just the kind of bold analysis needed today to put reason and common sense back into health policy." The book was also reviewed favorably in the Journal of the American Medical Association.

kenjterry@gmail.com

Lead or Abrogate

I've had the privilege of knowing Ken Terry for more than two decades. So, when he invited me to write the foreword to his new book, I jumped at the opportunity. In addition, when I learned that the American Association of Physician Leaders (AAPL) was to be his publisher, this really sealed the deal for me!

Having taught for the AAPL for nearly 30 years, I have had the great privilege of meeting literally thousands of AAPL members. My career at Thomas Jefferson University in Philadelphia paralleled my involvement with AAPL. In both organizations, I strove to recognize, nurture, and prepare a new type of physician leader for the future.

The reason Ken Terry's book is so compelling is that it is written by the right person and at the right time. As a non-physician, he evidently has the courage to call it as he sees it, and in so doing, he makes a number of important contributions to our collective understanding about what we really mean when we say "a New Approach to Medicare for All." Let me give you some examples.

Most experts agree waste consumes somewhere between one-quarter and one-third of all spending in our system. I think this is the only book that makes the explicit connection between the need for clinicians to reduce this waste and the ability to reallocate these resources to improve health. Terry makes the important point that only clinicians, acting with the best available evidence to reduce unexplained clinical variation, can reduce said waste. I've been proselytizing this position in my entire teaching career with AAPL, so to see it in a brand new book really warms my heart.

The second major take home from this amazing book is the fact that Terry recognizes the primacy of primary care. He analyzes and promotes the unheralded role that primary care has played in previous attempts to reform our broken system, and he notes unequivocally that primary care expansion must be at the heart of any system level reform. He makes clear sense out of the veritable alphabet soup of acronyms that emanate from places like the Center for Medicare and Medicaid Services and the Center for Medicare and Medicaid Innovation. Who among us can honestly say that he or she has a complete grasp of all of the proposals coming from these organizations? Terry not only has a tight grasp on the details, but he can explain them in everyday prose.

Finally, and most importantly, Terry makes the deep connection between the economic consequences of reform and the outcome of said reform. To put it bluntly, healthcare is America's job engine. Nearly 40 companies in the Fortune 500 are related to healthcare, including two in the Fortune 10. Do you want to mess with this incredibly important connection between the economic engine of healthcare and its contribution to our capitalist society?

Whatever your politics, Terry has the political courage, the knowhow, and the smarts to put it all together in the final portion of this important book. He knows that haphazard reform might have dire economic consequences, given the size and scope of the healthcare economic engine. That's why he calls for a 10-year, level-headed and pragmatic transition plan.

In sum, I found this book very easy to read and I found myself vigorously nodding in agreement with most of the well-organized chapters. The table of contents is comprehensive and the flow is smooth.

Kudos to Terry as a non-doctor for laying out the issues that every clinician ought to be familiar with. His timing is pretty darn good too, as I bet this book will be dog-eared by many members of the policy community as they try to decipher what "Medicare for All" really means and then try to teach these concepts to the vast number of politicians who have no concept as to what it means to be at the bedside of an ill individual.

As a long-time AAPL member, I'm especially proud that our organization has agreed to publish this important piece of work, and I hope that every AAPL member will read this book and share it with a colleague.

Only clinicians can reduce waste because it's easy for politicians to reduce cost. Only physicians can reduce unexplained clinical variation and follow appropriate economic incentives. Only clinicians have the visceral understanding of how important improving health really is to the future of our nation.

In closing, whatever your politics, this important book by my long-time friend, Ken Terry, is going to make a critical contribution to the national conversation that we must have about the future of our largest, and of course, in my view, our most important industry.

DAVID B. NASH, MD, MBA
Founding Dean Emeritus
Jefferson College of Population Health

CHAPTER 1

Medicare for All Lives

T he last time political support for Medicare for All was as strong as it is today, Richard Nixon was president and impeachment was in the air.

From 1960 to 1970, per capita health spending had more than doubled, and the advent of Medicare and Medicaid in 1965 had greatly accelerated that cost growth. Many people on the left viewed national health insurance as the best way to control costs while guaranteeing universal coverage. In 1970, Sen. Edward Kennedy (D-MA) issued his first call for "Medicare for All." Labor unions and some corporate leaders backed the idea of national health insurance, which had been proposed by President Truman in the late 1940s.

Recognizing the popular appeal of Medicare for All, Nixon proposed a free-enterprise plan to subsidize and promote HMOs instead. His program also would have required all employers to cover their workers. In the shadow of Watergate, however, many Democrats saw no reason to give up on Medicare for All. After the upcoming midterm elections, they thought, they'd stand a better chance of enacting their universal coverage plan. So, Nixon's plan died in Congress. The Democrats did win a commanding Congressional majority in 1974, but a severe recession and runaway inflation in the mid-1970s blocked further efforts to adopt national health insurance.[1]

Since then, healthcare reform efforts have hewed closer to the Nixon model than to Medicare for All. The Clinton Health Plan relied on "managed competition" among "accountable health plans." Similarly, the Affordable Care Act (ACA) established government-sponsored health insurance "markets" on which private health plans compete to provide individual coverage. A "public option" provision, which would have included a public plan in the insurance exchanges, did not make it into the final legislation.

Medicare for All Lives

Nevertheless, the idea of Medicare for All never went away. Sen. Kennedy kept pushing for it while he was alive, and in 2003, the late Rep. John Conyers (D.-MI) introduced a single-payer bill (HR 676) that, with modifications, he and his cosponsors continued to reintroduce through the 2017–2018 session of Congress.[2] Sen. Bernie Sanders (I-VT) backed HR 676, and his sequential Medicare for All bills are patterned after that legislation.

When Sanders proposed Medicare for All during his 2016 campaign for president, he offered a sharp contrast to Hillary Clinton, who favored reinforcing and building on the Affordable Care Act. At that time, Medicare for All was still regarded as a fringe position in policy circles.[3] The centrist Democratic position on healthcare had more mainstream support, but Sanders came close to defeating Clinton for the nomination.[4]

As of this writing, Sanders has dropped out of the race for the 2020 Democratic nomination for president, and former Vice President Joe Biden is the presumptive nominee. Sen. Elizabeth Warren (D-MA), who has a single-payer proposal similar to Sanders', halted her bid for the nomination earlier.

While Sanders and Warren were the only presidential hopefuls who advocated for Medicare for All, Biden favors a public option plan that could lead to Medicare for All over time. Sen. Amy Klobuchar (D-MN) and South Bend, Indiana Mayor Pete Buttigieg, both of whom have left the Democratic presidential race and now endorse Biden, support similar public options.

Meanwhile, Medicare for All legislation introduced by Reps. Pramila Jayapal (D-WA) and Debbie Dingell (D-MI) has more than 100 cosponsors in the House. While this bill is not going anywhere in the foreseeable future, the fact remains that for the first time in decades, the Democratic party is taking a single-payer system seriously. After many years in the political wilderness, Medicare for All has become mainstream.

This astonishing reversal is reflected in public opinion surveys. A Reuters poll conducted in August 2018, for example, showed that 70% of Americans supported Medicare for All. That included 85% of Democrats and 52% of Republicans.[5] A February 2020 poll by the Kaiser Family Foundation (KFF) found less support for Medicare for All, but 52% all of respondents still endorsed it, down from 59% in March 2018. The reasons for this majority support are not hard to discern: With insurance premiums, deductibles, and drug prices continuing to rise, 70% of respondents in a 2019 Gallup poll said the U.S. healthcare system had major problems or was in a state of crisis.[6]

Before the coronavirus pandemic came along, some experts cautioned that the public did not really understand the implications of Medicare for All and that many people were less favorably disposed toward it after they learned more about it. Support for the idea dropped from 62% to 34% in one poll, for example, when respondents were informed that Medicare for All would require a big tax increase and that they'd have to give up their employer-sponsored health plans. A national health insurance law would cancel more than 175 million private policies; Obamacare was harshly criticized when just 2.5 million people had to replace their individual plans with new ones that met ACA requirements.[7]

The pandemic, which is still in its early stages as I write this, is likely to increase public support for Medicare for All in the long run. Although national legislation to make COVID-19 testing free was signed into law on March 22, 2020,[8] treatments for the virus are not free (although some insurers have temporarily waived cost-sharing), and the majority of Americans could not afford even one day of treatment in an intensive-care unit. If we had Medicare for All, that would not be a concern for anyone in this country. Because so many people cannot afford treatment, however, many Americans infected with COVID-19 are likely to avoid going to the hospital even after they become very sick. As a result, they'll continue infecting others, including their own families, and many of them will die.[9]

Cracks in the Dam

If President Trump is reelected, Medicare for All will not be adopted, regardless of the toll that COVID-19 takes on our country. Nevertheless, it's likely that, sooner or later, the United States will have a single-payer healthcare system. The turnaround in public attitudes toward Medicare for All shows that cracks are beginning to appear in the dam holding back this epochal shift. When enough voters are fed up with the current system and are concerned about their own or their families' access to healthcare, the dam will break. At that point, neither politicians nor healthcare lobbyists will be able to hold back the flood that will carry us to Medicare for All.

There are many reasons Americans are increasingly concerned about the failure of our healthcare financing system. To start with, 28 million people remain uninsured—a number that has begun to rise again after falling substantially during the rollout of Obamacare.[10]

Meanwhile, insurance premiums and out-of-pocket costs are rising rapidly for those who have coverage. The average cost of a family policy sponsored by an employer exceeded $20,000 in 2019, of which, according to the Kaiser Family Foundation (KFF), workers contributed about $6,000, on average. Since 2009, family insurance premiums have increased by 54% and employees' contribution by 71%.[11] Many low-wage workers can't afford these policies even if their companies offer them.[12]

"The single biggest issue in health care for most Americans is that their health costs are growing much faster than their wages are," KFF President and CEO Drew Altman said in a news release. "Costs are prohibitive when workers making $25,000 a year have to shell out $7,000 a year just for their share of family premiums."

Out-of-pocket expenses are also soaring. More than one in four workers now have deductibles of over $2,000 a year, four times the number in 2009.[13] These high deductibles often reduce access to care. In one survey, 40% of people with high deductibles said they hadn't visited a doctor when sick or had skipped tests because of the deductible.[14] In another poll, 40% of respondents with employer-based plans said they had trouble paying medical bills, whether or not they had a high deductible.[15] Twenty-nine percent of Americans are considered to be underinsured, up from 12% in 2003.[16] According to Elizabeth Warren, the primary reason American families declared bankruptcy from 2013-2016 was because of healthcare—although 91% had health insurance in 2016.[17]

This is why real healthcare reform is so badly needed in the United States, and why the majority of people will support it, sooner or later. How we'll get there is still far from clear.

CURRENT REFORM PROPOSALS

Among the Democrats who view the ACA as a jumping-off point rather than as a permanent feature of the landscape, the debate over healthcare reform revolves around whether to go directly to Medicare for All or to expand public insurance more gradually. The latter group of proposals are variations on the public option missing from Obamacare. They would allow people to buy into Medicare or a Medicare-like public plan, but wouldn't require the elimination of private insurance.

Although Biden is regarded as a centrist on healthcare, the public option he favors would allow anyone to buy into a plan patterned after Medicare.[18] Millions of people could potentially enroll in this plan, including the uninsured, the individually insured, workers dissatisfied with their employer-sponsored plans, and low-income people not covered by Medicaid in states that chose not to expand Medicaid eligibility under the Affordable Care Act (ACA). This government plan would use its purchasing power to negotiate prices with healthcare providers. As a result, the plan's premiums would be lower than those of private insurers, potentially luring many people away from employer-provided insurance. Small businesses could give workers money to enroll in this lower-priced public plan, which could pave the way toward Medicare for All.

Biden's public option has a couple of serious flaws. First, it doesn't include Medicare and doesn't require hospitals and physicians to participate in the public option as a condition of Medicare participation. As a result, providers would be less disposed to accept patients in the public plan if it paid less than private insurance. Second, Ezra Klein of Vox has pointed out, larger employers would not be allowed to buy into the public plan on behalf of their workers.[19]

Nevertheless, the Biden scheme does provide a starting point for a more expansive public option—perhaps one similar to the Medicare for America plan described in the sidebar.

Biden's platform also expands Obamacare in two ways. First, government subsidies on the ACA insurance exchanges would be pegged to plans with more generous benefits, lowering their deductibles and copayments. Second, he'd remove the current cap on ACA subsidies, which phase out when family income exceeds 400% of the federal poverty level. Instead, his plan would limit spending for nongroup health insurance to 8.5% of household income.[20]

Biden says his plan would cost $750 billion over 10 years. He'd pay for it by eliminating capital gains tax loopholes and rolling back the Trump tax cut for the wealthy. Unlike Sanders, he has rigorously avoided any discussion of a middle-class tax increase.

In April 2020, Biden also proposed lowering the age for Medicare eligibility from 65 to 60. If that idea became law, it would accelerate the move toward a single-payer system.[21]

Under Sanders' latest bill, which was also part of his campaign platform, all U.S. residents would be covered by Medicare within four years of passage. Private insurers would be able to sell insurance only for benefits not covered by Medicare. The government program would offer expanded benefits, including vision, dental, hearing, and non-institutional long-term-care coverage. Medicare would negotiate payments to drug and medical device companies. There would be no cost-sharing with individuals, beyond small copayments for drugs. Payments to hospitals, doctors, and other providers would be cut to unspecified levels under a global national health budget. The plan would be financed through payroll taxes, higher taxes on the wealthy and corporations, and the increase in Treasury revenue that would result from ending employers' tax exclusion for health insurance.[22]

Elizabeth Warren offered a two-part proposal. She would have started off with an expansive public option and other reforms, and in the third year of her presidency, if she'd been elected, would have tried to pass a Medicare for All bill.[23] That legislation would have provided benefits as rich or richer than Sanders, if her proposed coverage of all long-term care were included. The government would have negotiated lower drug prices to bring them down to international levels. If overall cost growth had exceeded gross domestic product (GDP) growth, she would have used global budgets or automatic rate reductions to bring it down.[24]

Warren estimated the cost of her plan at $20.5 trillion over 10 years, which she said would be about the same as current spending projections after adding government healthcare spending on Medicare, Medicaid, and other programs.[25] In her view, that would be a good deal, considering that everyone would be covered with much better benefits than Medicare or private insurance now provides. She would have paid for it all with huge tax increases on the wealthy. Middle-class taxes would not have gone up under her plan. In effect, this would have represented a tax cut for most people, since they'd no longer have had the cost of insurance premiums or out-of-pocket expenses.

Other Reform Ideas

In addition to these proposals, several healthcare reform bills are bouncing around Congress. Some would create public plans of various types; others would expand Medicare gradually by letting people buy into Medicare at age 50 or by allowing small companies to buy in. One measure would let people at all income levels buy into Medicaid.[26]

The most advanced of these proposals, Medicare for America, could enable the United States to achieve universal coverage fairly quickly, its proponents say (see the accompanying sidebar). Other experts offer different ideas on how to achieve universal coverage without going to a single-payer system.[27] Universal coverage, however, doesn't necessarily provide universal access to comprehensive healthcare. Medicare for All advocates guarantee their system would do that.

On the other hand, Medicare for All has serious flaws of its own. By eliminating private health insurance, it would subtract administrative costs that represent about 10% of overall spending. But, after that one-time reduction, healthcare costs would continue to rise. To control costs, the Medicare for All proposals would greatly reduce provider payments; however, as the next section explains, there are limits to what can be done in that regard. Also, if physician incomes dropped significantly, doctors would be unhappy. In fact, many of them criticized Warren's plan for this reason.[28] And unhappy physicians spell doom for any healthcare reform plan.

Underlying cost growth can't be controlled without reducing the waste in the system, which is estimated to be around a third of total spending, and physicians are best positioned to do that. They're the only ones, in fact, who know which healthcare services can be eliminated without harming patient care. So, to be successful, any Medicare for All proposal must include provisions to engage doctors in eliminating waste.

MEDICARE FOR AMERICA

Of the non-single-payer reform bills now in Congress, the most comprehensive and fully thought-out measure is the Medicare for America Act. Based on proposals from the left-leaning Center for American Progress and Yale health policy expert Jacob Hacker, the measure was introduced in May 2019 by Reps. Rosa DeLauro (D-CT) and Jan Schakowsky (D-IL).

Medicare for America would achieve universal coverage by enrolling the uninsured, people who purchase individual insurance, and those currently in Medicare, Medicaid, and the Children's Health Insurance Program (CHIP). People would be enrolled automatically at birth. Large companies could continue to provide private insurance if it met certain requirements. These firms also could enroll some or all of their employees in Medicare for America. If they did so, they'd pay 8% of their annual payroll for those workers to the Medicare Trust Fund. They'd also have to pay into the fund if they didn't cover their workers. Companies with fewer than 100 workers could enroll their workers in Medicare, as well, but would have not have to pay the employer contribution.[29]

Alternatively, employees could opt out of their employer-sponsored plans and enroll in Medicare. Whether they did that on their own or their employer enrolled them, they would be eligible for government insurance subsidies if their incomes fell between 200% and 600% of the federal poverty level (FPL). The premiums would be limited to no more than 9.69% of an individual's or a household's monthly income. Those earning less than 200% of the FPL would pay nothing. Annual out-of-pocket costs would be capped at $3,500 for an individual and $5,000 for a family on a sliding scale.[30]

The benefits under Medicare for America would be nearly as comprehensive as those under Medicare for All. Because of those enhanced benefits, the coverage expansion and the premium subsidies, the plan's financing would require rolling back the 2017 income tax cuts. In addition, there would be new wealth and investment taxes, higher Medicare payroll taxes, and new excise taxes on tobacco, alcohol, and sugary drinks.[31-32]

Computer modeling shows that over time, Medicare for America would grow as more privately insured people joined it, Hacker said in an interview. Some large employers and companies with highly paid employees, he added, would continue to offer private plans to generate loyalty and/or attract the best workers. But in a *New York Times* op-ed, he wrote, "The idea is that the system would evolve toward universal Medicare if employers and individuals saw the expanded Medicare program as a better deal than private insurance."

More and more employees might opt out of employer-sponsored plans and enroll in Medicare because of lower premiums and cost-sharing and greater provider choice. If the goal was to gradually move toward a single-payer system—say, over 10 years—tweaks in Medicare enrollees' out-of-pocket costs and the share of household income they had to pay for coverage might accelerate the move away from private insurance. As some employees deserted their companies' plans, their companies might find it more cost-effective to subsidize their workers' Medicare coverage than to continue buying private insurance for a shrinking population. Eventually, nearly everyone would be covered by Medicare.

FINANCING MEDICARE FOR ALL

The current debate among Democrats revolves around how far and how fast we should go to achieve universal coverage and how much private insurance we should keep. None of the bills includes a formal financial plan with costs and revenues; however, several independent experts and think tanks have analyzed Sanders' Medicare for All plan. Their evaluations provide the starting point for our discussion.

The first thing to know about the Sanders Medicare for All model is that it would provide comprehensive coverage for all U.S. residents, including undocumented immigrants. This means that the 10.4% of Americans under 65 who are now uninsured would be covered. The underinsured would also receive full benefits. And the benefits guaranteed to everyone would be much more comprehensive than Medicare's current benefits.

Second, unlike in today's Medicare, there would be little cost-sharing under Sanders' plan. Drew Altman, president and CEO of the Kaiser Family Foundation, has pointed out that this would make Medicare for All more generous than the system of any other developed nation. Consumers in other high-income countries, he notes, pay an average of $857 per person annually out of pocket.[33]

Based on these three factors—universal coverage, comprehensive benefits, and no cost-sharing—financing Medicare for All is not as simple as replacing private insurance premiums with payroll taxes. More revenues must be found somewhere. To do that, various Medicare for All proposals have included some combination of payroll, income, sales, and investment taxes.

An Urban Institute analysis of Sanders' 2016 Medicare for All bill found that it would add about $32 trillion to current federal healthcare spending over 10 years. Sanders' revenue-increasing proposals, the researchers said, would raise just $15.3 trillion of that amount from 2017 to 2026. Moreover, they noted, their estimate of program cost assumed provider payment reductions that would be difficult to achieve.[34]

In a recent comparison of eight models of healthcare reform, the Urban Institute estimated the cost of the new Sanders Medicare for All plan at about $34 trillion for the period from 2020 to 2029. While many of the Urban Institute model's assumptions have changed, it still presumes providers would be paid at approximately Medicare rates. After subtracting $2 trillion for income tax gains that were not included in the previous analysis, the final tally comes to $32 trillion—the same as in 2016.[35]

Cost Savings

Sanders' Medicare for All proposal would save money in several ways. First, there would be a significant drop in administrative costs for providers and payers. Instead of many different insurance companies processing claims, making payments, and managing networks, there would be a single payer: the U.S. government. Estimates of how much billing and insurance-related activities would cost in a Medicare for All system range from 2% to 6% of total costs. By comparison, the average private health plan spends 12% on administration and profits.[36]

Medicare for All advocates assume that administration would cost only 2%, because that's about what traditional Medicare spends on paying claims. However, the Urban Institute analysis of Sanders' proposal assumes that Medicare for All administration would cost upwards of 6%. The think tank estimate includes the cost of administration in Medicare Advantage plans, which would go away under Medicare for All. But it also encompasses the administrative costs of care management, utilization control, and fraud and abuse policing.[37]

Hospitals, doctors, and other healthcare providers also spend a great deal on billing and collections. Gerald Friedman, an economics professor at the University of

Massachusetts at Amherst who crunched the numbers for Sanders' 2016 plan, says that about 10% of physicians' and hospitals' revenues are allocated to these activities. Billing Medicare under Medicare for All, in contrast, would cost providers very little, Friedman maintains. These savings would not be directly captured by the government but would counterbalance lower payments to providers.

A government-run single-payer system also would be able to negotiate favorable rates with pharmaceutical companies and device manufacturers. If the United States brought drug prices down to world levels, Friedman says, those prices would be 37% lower than they are today. (This is a very optimistic assumption, as Chapter 12 explains.)

The most important factor in determining the magnitude of potential savings under Medicare for All is how much providers would be paid. While Sanders' latest bill doesn't specify how the payment rates would be set, his previous bill said they'd be consistent with Medicare rates, and the expert analyses assume that payments would be close to those levels. Friedman's latest report qualifies that slightly by assuming that hospitals would be paid 110% of Medicare rates.[38]

Advocates' Numbers

In Sanders' summary of his current Medicare for All bill, he refers to a study of his proposal by a group of liberal economists and single-payer proponents at the Political Economy Research Institute (PERI) of UMass Amherst. According to PERI's paper, about $1 trillion a year would be required to cover the gap between the cost of existing public programs such as Medicare and Medicaid and the cost of Medicare for All from 2017 to 2026. PERI calculates that Medicare for All would reduce healthcare costs by about 19% through lower administrative, drug, and provider payment costs and increased efficiency. Over the 10-year period, Medicare for All would cover everyone, improve benefits, and cost $5 trillion less than the government's projection of national healthcare spending under the current system, the PERI researchers say.[39]

In his 2018 paper, Friedman calculates even bigger savings during the first decade of Medicare for All. Using a range of assumptions about cost-sharing and the percentage of potential administrative and hospital cost savings that might be achieved, he estimates that the program would save between $5.5 trillion and $12.5 trillion from 2019 to 2028, compared to the government's projection of national healthcare expenditures during that period.[40]

Conservative Analysis

At the other end of the political spectrum, Charles Blahous of the conservative Mercatus Institute at George Mason University estimates that from 2022 to 2031, Sanders' Medicare for All proposal would add $32.6 trillion to the federal budget.[41]

Blahous uses different assumptions than PERI's and Friedman's for administrative cost savings, increased utilization of services, prescription drug costs, and the cost of expanding benefits. For example, Blahous estimates that lower administrative and prescription drug costs would save $2 trillion over the 10-year period. By comparison, Friedman expects that administrative savings alone would total $4.5 trillion.

After factoring in all of the costs and savings under Medicare for All, Blahous figures that total personal healthcare spending would drop slightly from the current Centers for Medicaid and Medicare Services (CMS) estimate of $3.86 trillion in 2022. ("Personal health care," a component of national health expenditures, comprises all of the medical goods and services used to treat or prevent diseases or medical conditions.) Over the 10-year period from 2022 to 2031, Blahous estimates, personal healthcare spending under Medicare for All would be $50.1 trillion, nearly identical to the total projected under current law. However, because of the shift of individual and state healthcare spending to the federal ledger, there would be a huge increase in federal spending.

In contrast, the UMass Amherst experts assume that the states would be required to maintain their contributions. How big a difference would that make? If the states contributed an amount equal to what they would have otherwise spent on Medicaid and the Children's Health Insurance Program, the Urban Institute estimates, the cost of the Sanders Medicare for All plan would be $3 trillion lower from 2020 to 2029.[42]

PROVIDER PAYMENTS

The cornerstone of all these scenarios is massive cuts in provider payments. Under Medicare for All, several analysts assume, average payment rates would range from 100% to 110% of what Medicare pays—far below commercial insurance rates.[43] Insurance companies pay physicians an average of 128% of Medicare, according to the Medicare Payment Advisory Commission,[44] and estimates of how much private insurers pay hospitals, on average, range up to 189% of Medicare.[45] Employer-sponsored plans paid hospitals an average of 241% of Medicare in 2017, a RAND study found.[46] So Medicare for All rates of 100%–110% of Medicare would represent a steep drop in income for the portion of their revenues that providers now receive from private payers.

On average, Medicaid pays physicians considerably less than Medicare, with estimates ranging from 66% to 72% of Medicare rates.[47-48] So, depending on how much of a physician's practice comes from Medicaid, he or she could see a significant bump in payment from that source under Medicare for All.

In contrast, Medicaid payment rates to hospitals are not very different from Medicare rates. According to a recent Stanford University study, Medicare and Medicaid now pay hospitals 87% and 88% of their average costs of providing care, respectively, while private payers pay hospitals 144% of their average costs. This cost shifting would go away under Medicare for All.[49]

For hospitals, the study authors observe, Medicare for All would lead to "a marked decline in revenue from formerly privately insured patients and a small increase in revenue from formerly Medicaid-covered patients . . . The estimated net effect on hospitals would be a 15.9% decline in revenue, equal to a loss of $151 billion nationally incurred by over 5,262 U.S. community hospitals."

The average profit margin of acute care hospitals, the paper notes, is currently 7%. Under Medicare for All, hospitals could face a "negative" margin of 9%, equal to an $85.6 billion annual loss, unless they rapidly reduced waste and became more efficient.

Because labor costs are the most flexible part of a hospital cost structure, an estimated 1.5 million hospital jobs could be lost if hospitals reduced labor costs to compensate for the entire revenue shortfall, the study says. About 856,000 jobs would be lost if hospitals sacrificed their current operating margin and just broke even.

Access to Healthcare

Across-the-board Medicare rates might threaten the survival of some hospitals and physician practices. Blahous, for instance, cites a CMS estimate that more than 80% of hospitals lose money treating Medicare patients. At Medicare payment rates, this would be true for every patient under Medicare for All. Blahous comments:

> Perhaps some facilities and physicians would be able to generate heretofore unachieved cost savings that would enable their continued functioning without significant disruptions. However, at least some undoubtedly would not be, thereby reducing the supply of healthcare services at the same time as Medicare for All sharply increases healthcare demand. It is impossible to say how much the confluence of these factors would reduce individuals' timely access to healthcare services, but some such access problems almost certainly must arise.[50]

The Urban Institute's researchers, similarly, say that providers would be "seriously affected" if they were paid at Medicare rates. "Payment rates may in fact have to be higher, at least initially and perhaps indefinitely, to be acceptable to providers," they state.

While hospitals would be less impacted than physicians, the Urban Institute says, "different types of hospitals would be advantaged and disadvantaged, depending on their patient mix . . . Physician incomes would be squeezed by the new payment rates because such rates would be considerably below what physicians are paid by private insurers."[51]

Financial Impact Would Vary

Michael La Penna, a healthcare consultant based in Grand Rapids, Mich., says that the effect of Medicare for All on hospitals would vary a great deal, depending on their current payer mix. Some facilities might see only a 5% drop in revenue, while others would lose 40%–50% of their volume. Inner-city hospitals that depend largely on Medicare and Medicaid would be least affected, while suburban facilities that depend more on commercial insurance would be hit hard.

Going to Medicare rates across the board, he adds, "is going to affect some hospitals in a very severe fashion," and some will go out of business. "Right now, some hospitals are technically bankrupt. Those hospitals that are on the edge will go completely over."

In La Penna's view, physicians would experience less hardship, because the differential between what Medicare and commercial insurers pay is less for them. But independent physicians would feel the crunch first, while those employed by hospitals probably wouldn't see decreased earnings until their contracts came up for renewal.

Patient access, he says, "will absolutely worsen" if providers are paid Medicare rates. "Private physicians will have to adjust the size of their practice to maintain their income levels. That means limitations on staffing. And some doctors may just retire."

Physicians' Attitudes

According to a poll conducted in late 2018, about two-thirds of U.S. physicians support moving to a single-payer system.[52] That makes sense, considering how much doctors dislike insurance companies. But the survey didn't ask how many doctors would favor Medicare for All if it led to a substantial drop in their incomes. One indication of their likely response was the vigorous resistance of physicians to Medicare's Sustainable Growth Rate (SGR) program, which was supposed to lower their fees when their aggregate utilization of services increased. In the course of this program, which lasted from 1997 until it was replaced by "value-based" payments in 2015, doctors repeatedly pressured Congress not to let the statutory payment reductions go into effect, and they didn't from 2002 onward.[53]

There is evidence that doctors would push back equally hard against fee cuts under Medicare for All. For example, after Sen. Elizabeth Warren unveiled her single-payer plan, there was an overwhelmingly negative reaction from physicians. A common response was that many doctors would retire or leave the field. One internist told *Medscape Medical News*, "Suddenly I'm afraid of a future in which we won't be able to attract the best talent into the medical field because salaries will be too low to cover the growing astronomical burden of our student loans."[54]

In an interview, David Boles, DO, a family physician in Clarksville, Tenn., said that private insurers pay him and the other eight providers in his practice about 125% of the Medicare fee schedule. Currently, they get about half of their revenue from commercial health plans and the other half from Medicare and Medicaid. If they were paid across the board at the Medicare rate, he says, "I don't think we'd be here. It would not be worth the pain."

Barbara McAneny, MD, a former president of the American Medical Association (AMA) and a practicing oncologist/hematologist in New Mexico, said the same thing about her practice. If she were paid at Medicare rates across the board, she told reporters, "my doors would be closed. I would no longer be able to make payroll."[55]

In contrast to the AMA, which opposes Medicare for All, the American College of Physicians (ACP)—the second largest medical association in the United States—announced in January 2020 that it supported a move to either a single-payer system or a public option model. However, the ACP stressed that under either plan, "payments to physicians and other health professionals, hospitals, and others delivering healthcare services must be sufficient to ensure access and not perpetuate existing inequities, including the undervaluation of primary and cognitive care."

The ACP wasn't too specific about how it would control costs. But it did refer to "global budgets and all-payer rate setting," both of which have been proposed to lower hospital spending. The association also mentioned "increasing investment in primary care, reducing administrative costs, promoting high-value care, and incorporating comparative effectiveness and cost into clinical guidelines and coverage decisions."[56]

Reduced Provider Supply

With fewer hospitals and fewer or downsized physician practices, there would be less provider supply to meet the demand for services, which would rise significantly with more people covered, greater benefits, and little or no cost-sharing. Currently, the American Association of Medical Colleges (AAMC) estimates the United States could see a physician shortage of up to 120,000 physicians by 2030.[57] Rural and inner-city hospitals have been also been closing in greater numbers in recent years.[58-59] Cutting provider compensation to Medicare levels could accelerate that trend.

The Congressional Budget Office (CBO) in May 2019 released a report on policy choices related to switching to a single-payer system. "Setting payment rates equal to Medicare fee-for-service rates under a single-payer system would reduce the average payment rates most providers receive—often substantially," the CBO predicted. "Such a reduction in provider payment rates would probably reduce the amount of care supplied and could also reduce the quality of care."

In the long term, if payment rates were significantly reduced, fewer people might become doctors, a number of hospitals would close, and there would be less investment in new and existing facilities, the CBO stated. "That decline [in provider supply] could lead to a shortage of providers, longer wait times, and changes in the quality of care, especially if patient demand increased substantially because many previously uninsured people received coverage and if previously insured people received more generous benefits."[60]

Robert Berenson, MD, a senior fellow at the Urban Institute and a former CMS and White House official, says, "If you immediately went to Medicare rates, there would be huge dislocations. But Medicare for All would probably wind up somewhere above Medicare rates. If you phased that in over five to eight years, I don't think you'd cause dislocations."

Berenson emphasizes that it would be impractical to pay physicians at Medicare levels across the board. "I don't think U.S. physicians, who are the highest-paid in the world, are going to live with the average salaries in other advanced countries. And Medicare is already above that. But the politics of this is that physician incomes are always going to be pretty good."

He makes a similar point about hospital payments. "Bernie Sanders wants to pay everybody the Medicare rate. I don't think that's politically sustainable. You have to tolerate variations across hospitals initially, and then over many years, try to even that out."

"Gigantic Political Issue"

The problem with this approach, some observers note, is that paying providers substantially above Medicare rates would greatly increase the cost of Medicare for All. Just the difference between paying providers at Medicare rates or at 110% of Medicare, Blahous points out, would be hundreds of billions of dollars a year.[61] If provider payments were set too high, the government would have to face the political cost of raising taxes, cutting benefits, and/or requiring cost-sharing from patients.

Friedman argues that providers would not be as severely impacted by lower payments as other observers claim. First, he points out, hospitals and doctors would reduce their billing and insurance-related costs if they were dealing with a single payer rather than many payers. If this expense equaled 10% of revenues, and they could eliminate most of it, that would cushion the impact of being paid at Medicare rates.

Despite that consideration, he admits, paying hospitals at 110% of Medicare rates probably wouldn't be enough, at least initially. The problem, Friedman says, is that many hospitals have created cost structures that are bigger than they have to be. They've built beautiful facilities with lots of amenities to lure patients in. They spend a lot of money on unnecessary marketing. And they pay lavish salaries to their top executives, even if they're not-for-profit institutions. According to a study published in the *Wall Street Journal*, he says, two-thirds of the 3,500 Americans who are paid over $1 million a year by nonprofit companies are in healthcare.

Friedman concedes that the massive reduction in hospital payments proposed by Medicare for All advocates "is going to be a gigantic political issue." But he predicts that if Medicare for All is adopted, the new pricing structure will be phased in gradually. "The hospitals will have to be given time to adjust their cost structure."

Sanders' bill, however, would provide only four years to phase in his Medicare for All plan. Jayapal and Dingell allow just two years for this huge transition. In Friedman's view, that's not enough time. "Realistically, there's going to have to be a longer phase-in period," he says.

ROOTING OUT WASTE

It has been estimated that between 30% and 34% of all healthcare services are unnecessary and don't improve health.[62-63] This is the central challenge that private health insurers, accountable care organizations, and the government have been grappling with for years. If the waste could be substantially reduced, health costs would drop dramatically. But the Medicare for All proposals downplay this issue.

For example, Sanders' Medicare for All legislation would establish regional Medicare offices that would devise a mechanism "to minimize both under-utilization and over-utilization and to ensure that all providers meet high quality standards." Medicare also would establish national quality and performance measures and medical review criteria.[64] The Centers for Medicare and Medicaid Services (CMS), however, has had such programs for many years and still hasn't been able to improve quality or reduce costs significantly.

Jayapal's and Dingell's position on performance improvement is similar to Sanders'. However, their bill undercuts cost control by prohibiting "bonuses, incentive payments, or compensation based on utilization of services or the financial results of any healthcare provider."[65] In other words, they'd remove any incentive to make healthcare more efficient. Under a volume-based payment system, in fact, physicians would be motivated to provide more services to make up for lower payment rates.

Cracking Down on Waste

PERI takes on the problem of waste more directly. It's possible, the PERI paper concedes, that providers will order more tests, procedures and expensive tests when these services are fully covered by insurance. Physicians may also influence patient demand for their own self-interest, the researchers say. But "physician-induced demand" will diminish within a single-payer system that establishes price controls and "effective regulation over the level of service provision," the PERI report maintains.[66]

Following the taxonomy of a 2010 Institute of Medicine (IOM) Report, the PERI experts say that the four main areas of wasteful expenditures are unnecessary services, inefficiently delivered services, missed prevention opportunities, and fraud. They estimate that achievable cost savings in these areas through Medicare for All would total about 1.5% of system costs in the first year and 1% a year for the following decade. But they don't explain how they would cut these costs.[67]

Although the main cost containment mechanism in Medicare for All is price controls, Friedman sees no evidence that price controls reduce waste, and he doesn't believe that switching to a single-payer system is going to root out the waste in the system. On the other hand, he notes that with Medicare paying all the bills, it will be able to assemble comprehensive data sets that will cover the entire population. With that data in hand, he says, Medicare could inform physicians when their use of certain services is excessive.

Of course, insurance companies have been doing this since the dawn of HMOs, but the majority of physicians have not changed how they practice. For some reason, however, Friedman believes the government will be more credible to doctors than health plans are.

Physician Engagement

David Boles, the Tennessee family doctor, says that his practice's best payer is Cigna HealthSpring, a Medicare Advantage plan. About a third of Medicare beneficiaries have enrolled in similar private plans, which receive a risk-adjusted, monthly payment from Medicare for each of their members. These insurers pay Medicare fee-for-service rates to providers, but they also offer managed care contracts to selected physician groups.

Under Boles' contract with HealthSpring, his group is capitated—that is, they receive a set amount per member per month—and they also have bonus opportunities for superior performance. While it takes much longer to provide coordinated, in-depth care to HealthSpring members than it does to treat other patients, Boles estimates that he and his colleagues earn about twice as much per patient from HealthSpring as they do from traditional Medicare.

"Profit" may be a dirty word to some Medicare for All advocates. But the profit motive springs from a basic human instinct, and physicians are no different from most other people in that regard. This is not to say that doctors are greedy. In my quarter century of covering healthcare as a journalist, I've interviewed many physicians about their business activities, and they all say that their first concern is the welfare of their patients. While that may be more or less true for some doctors, it's still the reason most of them went into medicine.

What's missing from Bernie Sanders' Medicare for All plan and other MFA proposals is the concept of physician engagement. If the system included financial incentives for doctors—and they also believed that what they were doing could improve care for their patients—they would be much more inclined to cooperate with Medicare for All. Boles, for example, says he'd gladly accept Medicare rates if he had the opportunity to earn more by providing better care.

Medicare and private payers already have shared savings programs; however, as detailed in Chapter 2, this approach has not moved the dial on healthcare costs significantly. To turn this dial up enough to have a real impact, the care delivery system must be restructured completely. Hospitals can no longer be allowed to dominate the care delivery system, and physicians must be reorganized so that they have strong incentives to increase their effectiveness and efficiency. All of this requires a government-managed single-payer system. Conversely, a single-payer system cannot be effective in reducing costs without getting providers involved.

THE PATH FORWARD

Healthcare reform seems to be stuck between a rock and a hard place, but there is a rational way forward. This approach, which I call "physician-led healthcare reform," would engage doctors in building a system that was safe, effective, patient-centered, timely, efficient, and equitable, to use the Institute of Medicine's set of foundational goals.[68] Primary care physicians, rather than hospitals, would be in charge of the system, and they'd work closely with specialists and other healthcare professionals to produce the best patient outcomes at the lowest cost.

It would take a decade or more to restructure the healthcare system so that this goal could be achieved. Similarly, the transition to a single-payer system needs to be accomplished gradually. Most people are not yet ready to abandon employer-sponsored insurance, and there's still a lot of distrust of the government. Providers are more likely to accept changes in how they're paid over time than all of a sudden. Additional benefits can also be brought online slowly. Ideally, we could transform healthcare financing over a 10-year period while rebuilding the care delivery system at the same time.

That is why implementing Medicare for America makes more sense than going directly to Medicare for All: it changes the system incrementally while achieving universal coverage fairly quickly. Friedman objects to Medicare for America because it includes a major role for private health plans; however, an approach like this could gradually move us away from private insurance and could morph into a single-payer system over time. If so, the taxes required to support the system would have to be raised. Nevertheless, private insurance premiums would go away and insurance costs (or health taxes) for individuals would become income-related, greatly increasing affordability. Whatever gap that left in healthcare financing could be filled by raising taxes on the wealthy and corporations.

The big debate would be over how much to increase benefits. Should they be limited to the "essential" health benefits required of plans on the ACA insurance exchanges? To what extent should vision, hearing, dental, and behavioral healthcare be covered? How much long-term care should the program encompass? Should coverage of long-term care exclude institutions such as nursing homes, as Sanders proposes? Should there be any cost-sharing?

Other countries with national health insurance have faced the same challenges and have found their own solutions. Cost-sharing barely exists in Canada, but 12% of Canadians have private insurance that covers vision and dental care, prescription drugs, rehab services, home care, and private hospital rooms. In the United Kingdom, similarly, about 10% of residents buy private plans that primarily allow them to avoid long waits for elective surgery. In Germany, more than 90% of the population is in the statutory health insurance system (those with higher incomes can opt for expanded private coverage), but personal outlays on drugs, nursing homes, and other items accounted for 13% of health spending in 2014. The French have coinsurance of 20% for inpatient care, 30% for doctor visits, and 30% for dental visits. They also pay out of pocket for dental and vision services.[69]

Cost-sharing and some limitation on benefits could get us on the path to financing the extra costs of national health insurance if we don't favor large increases in taxes. High out-of-pocket costs or poor benefits, however, would limit access to healthcare.

Major Renovation Work

We don't have to wait for care delivery reform before implementing universal coverage. To control costs, though, our very inefficient, fragmented system needs major renovation work while we're in the process of covering everyone. In addition, we must find a way to reduce the costs of drugs and new technologies without stifling innovation (see Chapter 12). If we do all of this properly, we could have national health insurance within a decade, along with a care delivery system designed to control healthcare costs in a way that patients and providers could accept.

To understand how all of this might occur, let's turn first to the Affordable Care Act, which was the biggest healthcare reform in 50 years and which still affects our health-care system in myriad ways. The ACA has prompted many changes in both health insurance and healthcare delivery, so it's essential to see how it works and why it has fallen short of its promise. The next chapter lays all of this out.

CHAPTER 2

Obamacare: A Work in Progress

The Patient Protection and Affordable Care Act (ACA) is the most ambitious health-care reform legislation since the passage of Medicare and Medicaid in the 1960s. Although the law has serious flaws, the ACA has resulted in more than 20 million people gaining health insurance.

Obamacare, as it has become known, expanded Medicaid, created the ACA market-places for individual insurance, subsidized private coverage for poor and working-class people, allowed young adults to stay on their parents' insurance until age 26, prohibited insurance companies from excluding individuals with pre-existing health conditions, and required health plans for individuals and small firms to provide essential benefits.[1]

To create the conditions for long-term cost control, the ACA also included a number of provisions that sought to change how care was delivered to Medicare beneficiaries. The ACA's care delivery provisions were designed to set the healthcare industry on a course to get better results at lower cost. These arrangements are addressed later in this chapter.

Why Obamacare?

Barack Obama was not a strong supporter of healthcare reform when he was running for president in 2007.[2] So what brought Obama around after he was elected president? At the time, his fledgling administration was scrambling to deal with the fallout of the financial crash and the Great Recession. Looking beyond the immediate crisis, Obama and his advisers recognized that healthcare reform was essential to fixing the U.S. economy and reducing government debt in the long term.[3-4]

The reason was simple: healthcare was devouring federal and state budgets and consuming an ever-larger share of employers' revenues and workers' wages. Despite the most severe recession in 80 years, healthcare spending in the United States was estimated to have risen 5.7% to $2.5 trillion from 2008 to 2009. Even more alarming, the percentage of the GDP spent on healthcare had jumped to 17.3% from 16.2% in 2008—the largest one-year increase ever—and was projected to hit 19.3% in 2020.[5]

These financial facts were an important factor in Obama's decision to go all-in on health-care reform while Democrats controlled both houses of Congress. Explaining his decision to pursue the ACA in a 2016 speech to the National Governor's Association, he said,

"It was not just the compassion I felt for people personally being impacted—getting sick and losing their home, or not being able to get care for their kids, or having to go to the emergency room because of routine issues that should have been dealt with by a primary care physician. It also had to do with the fact that this system is hugely inefficient, and if we don't make it more efficient, then we're not going to solve our debt problem."[6]

HOW OBAMACARE WORKS

The ACA's expansion of individual insurance was based on three interrelated concepts:

1. Prohibiting insurance companies from excluding people with pre-existing health conditions;
2. Requiring all individuals not covered by employer-based plans or government programs to buy health insurance (the individual mandate); and
3. Providing government subsidies for the less affluent.

All three of these components had to be in place for the program to work properly, the law's architects reasoned. Without the protection for those with pre-existing conditions, many people would not be able to buy health insurance. Without government subsidies, lower-income people could not afford coverage. Without the individual mandate, some people would not purchase coverage at any price. Moreover, because some folks would apply for insurance only when they became sick, insurers forced to accept all comers would lose money as a result.

Medicaid was also expanded to cover everyone up to 138% of the federal poverty level, which greatly increased the pool of potential recipients in many states. The federal government pledged to cover 100% of the cost of this expansion until 2020, when its share would drop to 90%. However, in 2012, the Supreme Court ruled that states could not be forced to expand their Medicaid programs.[7] To date, 36 states and the District of Columbia have expanded Medicaid coverage, including 10 states with Republican governors.[8]

Insurance Exchanges

Obamacare created insurance "marketplaces," or exchanges, to help buyers choose between competing plans with standardized benefits. About 85% of those who purchase insurance in the marketplaces receive subsidies.[9] But these are sliding-scale tax credits that phase out when an individual's or family's income exceeds 400% of the federal poverty level. In 2019, that limit was $48,560 for an individual and $100,400 for a family of four.[10] In some sections of the country, this leaves out a significant portion of the middle class, which has been a concern ever since the ACA's inception.

The ACA set the penalties for individuals who did not buy insurance at $95 or 1% of income in 2014, $325 or 2% of income in 2015, and $695 or 2.5% of income in 2016. After that, the penalty was to increase with the cost of living.[11]

ACA critics said the penalties were insufficient to get young, healthy people to buy insurance; and in fact, an estimated 6 million individuals chose to pay a penalty rather than purchase coverage.[12] Yet in 2016, when the number of enrollees in exchange plans increased sharply, much of the rise was attributed to the increased penalty for not buying insurance. One commentator observed that for some low-income people, it was less expensive to buy a subsidized plan on an insurance exchange than to pay the fine.[13]

An employer mandate was also included in the ACA. Businesses with 50 or more employees were required to contribute a minimum amount to cover their workers' insurance premiums. If they failed to do this, they were subject to yearly fines of $2,000 per uncovered employee. Small firms affected by the law bridled at this requirement.[14]

The ACA's essential benefits provision guaranteed that coverage would be comprehensive enough to protect people financially when they got sick or gave birth. This was a big improvement over the low-cost, low-benefit individual plans that millions of people had. With government subsidies, many people could afford to switch from these bare-bones plans to comprehensive insurance. But other people were forced to drop inadequate plans—breaking Obama's campaign promise that "if you like your health plan, you can keep it."[15]

Another Obama promise that turned out to be dubious was, "if you like your doctor, you can keep your doctor."[16] To compete on the ACA exchanges and still make a profit, many insurers built narrow networks of hospitals, physicians, and other providers that were willing to accept relatively low payment rates. According to a 2016 study, 41% of exchange plans offered small or extra-small physician networks, compared to 25% of employer-based PPOs.[17] So in order to get federally subsidized insurance, some people had to switch doctors.

The ACA's original intent was for states to create their own insurance exchanges. The federal marketplace was designed as a backstop for states that lacked the resources to do this. But only a small minority of states had built their own exchanges by 2014, when the marketplaces were launched. The rest of the states enrolled individuals through the federal marketplace, known as healthcare.gov. Today, 12 states and the District of Columbia operate their own marketplaces; six other states have some involvement in exchange plans but rely on the federal IT platform. Healthcare.gov handles all marketplace functions for the other 32 states.[18]

THE PLOT TO KILL OBAMACARE

Soon after the passage of Obamacare, a poll found that 58% of Americans favored rescinding the legislation; only 38% opposed repeal. Fifty-two percent of those surveyed said the law was bad for the country and just 39% said it was good.[19]

Opposition to Obamacare helped fuel the rise of the Tea Party movement, and the energy in the anti-ACA coalition helped Republicans regain control of Congress in 2010. As soon as they were seated, Congress passed what would be the first of nearly 70 bills to repeal or modify Obamacare.[20] Although most of these bills couldn't pass the Senate, one bill that did pass, in January 2016, was vetoed by President Obama.[21]

After Donald Trump was elected president, another bill to repeal Obamacare failed in the Senate by one vote. But in their 2017 tax cut legislation, Republicans included a provision that zeroed out the ACA penalties for not purchasing insurance. This action did not undermine Obamacare as much as expected, but it did have serious legal consequences.

State Lawsuits

Soon after the ACA's passage, 26 Republican-controlled states filed a lawsuit against the federal government over the ACA's individual mandate. In 2012, that suit wound up in the U.S. Supreme Court. Leading a narrow majority of the court, Chief Justice John Roberts ruled that the requirement to buy health insurance was constitutional, because the penalty for not purchasing it was a tax, and Congress had the authority to levy taxes. As stated earlier, the decision also allowed states to decide whether to expand Medicaid.[22]

The second major lawsuit against the ACA was *King v. Burwell*. Brought by conservative activists, this suit alleged that the law permitted health insurance subsidies only in states that had created their own health insurance exchanges, not in those with federally administered marketplaces. The Supreme Court rejected this argument in 2015.[23]

In 2017, a federal judge in Texas struck down the entire ACA on the grounds that the individual mandate is unconstitutional and that the rest of the law cannot stand without it. In *Texas v. United States*, U.S. District Court Judge Reed O'Connor agreed with the plaintiffs' argument that when Congress removed the penalty for not buying insurance, it took away the justification for classifying the fine as a tax.[24] A federal appeals court agreed with O'Connor on this point, but sent the case back to him for further analysis of which other provisions of the ACA should be eliminated.[25] The ACA's legal defenders asked the Supreme Court to intervene. The High Court declined to do so immediately; but in March 2020, the court agreed to take up the appeal at a later date.[26-27]

While 20 Republican states brought *Texas v. United States*, a coalition of 17 Democratic-controlled states and the District of Columbia joined to oppose the suit in May 2018. (Four more states and the U.S. House of Representatives later intervened as well.) The Trump Justice Department, meanwhile, supports Judge O'Connor's ruling.[28] It is a hallmark of our divided politics that red and blue states are battling each other in this case while the federal government refuses to defend a law of the land.

Gutting Insurance Rules

Congress has also made it difficult to implement the ACA's insurance rules. In December 2014, for example, a spending bill amendment axed funding for "risk corridors" authorized by the ACA. Risk corridors were supposed to stabilize insurance premiums during the first few years of the exchange plans, when insurers were expected to have difficulty pricing the premiums in relation to insurance risk. Under the ACA, companies that set prices more than 3% below a set target would be reimbursed by the government, and those that overpriced premiums by the same margin would pay some of their profits to the government. The arrangement was slated to expire at the end of 2016.[29]

As a result of the amendment, the Department of Health and Human Services (HHS) had to inform the underpricing insurers that they would receive only a small fraction of the money owed to them. This saddled those health plans with huge losses.[30]

The next step in the GOP's plan to destroy Obamacare was to stop funding its cost-sharing reduction (CSR) subsidies. Under the ACA, health plans on the exchanges are supposed to reduce copayments and deductibles for people under a certain income level in order to make those plans affordable. The government promised to reimburse the insurers for their cost-sharing reductions. Without those payments, the health plans would have had to jack up their premiums by an average of 19%.[31]

Nevertheless, Congressional Republicans refused to fund the CSR subsidies, arguing that the ACA had not specifically appropriated money for that purpose. In October 2017, President Trump scrapped the subsidies. This was a big hit to insurers, which had expected $9 billion in CSR payments in the following year.[32] Naturally, they sued the government. So far, the insurers' suits have triumphed in the federal courts.[33]

Insurance Roller Coaster

When insurance companies entered the ACA marketplaces, they knew that their new plan members probably would have more health problems, on average, than people in employer-sponsored plans. That was, after all, the history of the individual market. But the insurers weren't prepared for the magnitude of the insurance risk they were about to take on. As a result, many companies initially underpriced their plans on the insurance exchanges.

United Healthcare, for example, discovered that the people who enrolled in its exchange plans were sicker than expected; consequently, it lost $650 million on the exchanges. In April 2016, United announced that it would exit most of the 34 states where it offered exchange plans.[34]

Aetna lost at least $300 million on its exchange business[35] and, in 2016, dropped out of the exchanges in most states.[36] Humana also considered exiting some marketplaces; however, most insurers stayed in the exchanges and their enrollment remained stable.[37]

The most successful insurers were those that had prior experience in the individual and Medicaid markets. The main expertise of United, Aetna, and other big national carriers was in administering plans for self-insured employers, so they weren't well prepared to operate their exchange plans. However, they also had Medicaid-managed care plans that profited mightily from the Medicaid expansion.[38]

Premium Explosion

In addition to insurer losses, Obamacare critics had another potent argument against the ACA: rising premium rates. In 2016, for example, average premiums on the ACA exchanges increased 8%. That was less than the 10% yearly rate increases in the individual market before Obamacare. Moreover, individuals who received ACA subsidies—85% of all exchange plan enrollees—saw an average premium hike of only 4%.[39] Yet presidential candidate Donald Trump and Congressional Republicans cited the rate increases—which were as high as 37% in some states—as proof that the exchanges were heading toward a cliff.

In the end, most of the plans that stayed on the exchanges did all right as they learned how to price their products. Anthem, for example, projected a net profit of 3%–5% on its ACA plans in 2016.[40] The concerted assault of the Trump Administration, however, would shake the foundations of Obamacare as the ACA faced its biggest survival challenge yet.

Repeal and Replace

Donald Trump's election in 2016 created a major new opportunity for the GOP lawmakers who controlled Congress: They could pass an ACA repeal-and-replace bill that would be signed by the new president. However, the Senate majority wasn't large enough to fully repeal the ACA, which would have required 60 votes. The best the Senate could do was to repeal the insurance-related portions of the law, which needed only a simple majority under the budget reconciliation rules.

The American Healthcare Act (AHCA), which the House passed on May 4, 2017, removed the ACA's individual and employer mandate penalties. It eliminated $900 billion in ACA taxes on the wealthy and on healthcare providers and insurers. It also cut Medicaid funding by an equivalent amount by phasing out the Medicaid expansion and giving states block grants or per capita amounts as the federal contribution to Medicaid. The bill provided tax credits to help consumers buy insurance, but these tax credits were much skimpier than the Obamacare subsidies.[41]

The Congressional Budget Office projected that the AHCA would save $337 billion over 10 years. However, the CBO said, 14 million people would lose their coverage by 2018 under the bill, and 24 million would lose it by 2026 because of the Medicaid cuts and the repeal of the individual mandate.[42]

Some AHCA provisions had to be jettisoned because they were ruled not germane to the budget process. In the end, a truncated version of the bill failed passage in the Senate, with the late Sen. John McCain providing the decisive vote against the measure.

This was the high-water mark of the campaign to kill Obamacare, but it wasn't the end of the movement. In December 2017, Congress passed the tax bill that effectively gutted the individual mandate. Meanwhile, the Trump Administration cut the annual enrollment period for exchange plans in half, slashed grants to the "navigators" who helped potential enrollees in ACA plans navigate the marketplaces, and cut back on advertising related to the insurance exchanges, which showed how much people could save on ACA plans.[43-45]

In July 2018, HHS released a rule that relaxed the restrictions on the sale of short-term health plans. These low-cost plans often are sold to people between jobs and don't have to include the benefits mandated by the ACA. Under ACA regulations, such plans could cover people for no longer than 90 days; the new rule gives them one-year terms and allows them to be renewed for up to 36 months.[46] In 2019, the number of people who bought these skimpy plans jumped from 100,000 to 600,000.[47]

THE BALANCE SHEET

Those who have benefited the most from Obamacare are low-wage workers, legal immigrants, and Hispanics.[48] Some are the working poor who make too much money to qualify for Medicaid but aren't covered by employer-based insurance. Many others have been able to qualify for Medicaid because of the program's expansion. Through April 2019, 13.1 million people had enrolled in Medicaid as a result of the ACA; 21 states that expanded Medicaid saw enrollment gains of 25% of more.[49]

Enrollment in the exchange plans has declined, however. In 2019, 11.4 million consumers enrolled in ACA health plans.[50] In contrast, 11.8 million enrolled in 2018, 12.2 million in 2017, and 12.7 million in 2016.[51]

Overall, the impact of the ACA insurance provisions has diminished in recent years. From 2017 to 2018, Census Bureau data shows the uninsured rate in the United States increased from 7.9% to 8.5%. This increase of 0.5 percentage points translated to nearly 1.9 million fewer people with insurance coverage.[52]

A report on the *Health Affairs Blog* attributed much of the increase in the uninsured to a decline in Medicaid enrollment. But overall, the report said, "Many of these trends have likely been impacted by the various policy changes or positions adopted by the Trump Administration."[53]

Inherent Flaws in ACA

There are other reasons 27.5 million people remain uninsured.[54] Some of them are "young invincibles" who gamble that they won't need healthcare. Many are undocumented immigrants who aren't eligible for ACA coverage. Others earn too much to qualify for government subsidies—a problem that has grown worse as premiums have increased. Unsubsidized ACA plans may cost middle-class Americans as much as 20% of their incomes.[55]

Even in heavily subsidized plans, out-of-pocket costs are too high for many poor people—the reason for the CSR subsidies that Trump eliminated. Moreover, the high deductibles and copayments of many ACA plans have decreased access for working-class and middle-class enrollees. More than half of the plans available on healthcare.gov in 2015, for example, had a deductible of $3,000 or more. In cities like Miami and Jackson, Miss., the median deductible was $5,000 or more.[56]

In some rural areas, it's even difficult to purchase an Obamacare plan because some insurers have cut back their participation in the exchanges or left them entirely. In 2019, 37% of counties had just one ACA insurer and 40% of them had only two. In 2018, 87% of ACA enrollees lived in metropolitan counties.[57]

Durable Program

Despite these problems, the insurance provisions of the law have proved durable. Even the disappearance of the individual mandate hasn't had as much impact to date as observers predicted, although young adults aged 19–34 are the age group most likely to be uninsured.[58] Most people who enrolled in exchange plans with the help of government subsidies have remained insured. Despite the elimination of risk corridors and CSR subsidies, insurers have found their footing in the exchanges. Marketplace premiums and insurer margins have stabilized, and new insurers are entering some of the exchanges.[59]

The ACA also has had a positive effect on the health of millions of Americans. People who previously couldn't obtain insurance because of pre-existing conditions can now buy it; as a result, many of them can get the care they need, and preventive services are covered under all health plans. Several studies have found a correlation between Medicaid coverage and improved health.[60]

In January 2019, Obamacare was more popular than ever. A whopping 51% of the adult population had a favorable opinion of the law, compared to 40% who had an unfavorable view, according to a Kaiser Family Foundation poll.[61] The improvement in the ACA's popularity since 2010 can be attributed to the major expansion in the number of people with insurance coverage as well as the ACA's new consumer protections.

The ACA's insurance reforms—including those that apply to the broader population—have had strongly positive effects overall; however, the uptick in the uninsured is a worrisome portent for the future. There also is virtually no chance that undocumented immigrants will be covered nationwide unless there is significant movement on immigration reform. While it's possible to build on the ACA to achieve universal coverage,[62] that's not likely to happen anytime soon.

CARE DELIVERY PROVISIONS

The ACA's care delivery provisions are likely to have a longer-term impact than those dealing with insurance, especially if the United States transitions to a single-payer system. Also, some of the care delivery provisions are particularly relevant to the physician-led reform model described later in this book.

Along with two other laws that addressed health information technology and physician payment reform, the ACA was designed to move the healthcare industry toward a value-based approach that would increase efficiency and improve patient outcomes. The ACA created provider incentives and penalties to raise quality in certain areas. It also authorized the Centers for Medicare and Medicaid Services (CMS) to conduct demonstration projects.

The Center for Medicare and Medicaid Innovation (CMMI), also established by the ACA, helps CMS implement these provisions and tests new models of payment and service delivery. In an unusual feature of the law, Congress gave the Secretary of Health and Human Services the authority to expand the scope and duration of a new model, including the option of testing it on a nationwide scale. CMMI has broad leeway in this regard, provided the program does not raise overall government spending and maintains or improves care quality.[63]

Among the programs that CMMI has tested are the Comprehensive Primary Care (CPC) Initiative and CPC+, the Bundled Payments for Care Improvement Initiative (BPCI), and the Independence at Home Demonstration. CMMI also has been instrumental in rolling out CMS's Quality Payment Program (QPP) for physicians and will play a key role in the new Primary Care First program.[64]

Value-based Care

The law's fundamental assumption is that if healthcare providers are paid for value rather than volume, healthcare will become more efficient and effective. "Value" is most often defined as delivering the highest-quality care at the lowest cost. In some cases, value is identified with the Triple Aim of the nonprofit Institute for Healthcare Improvement (IHI). Under the Triple Aim model, healthcare organizations strive to improve the patient experience of care, improve the health of the population, and reduce per capita costs.[65]

Under the insurance reimbursement system in effect when the ACA was passed—and largely still in place—most physicians were paid on a fee-for-service basis; that is, they were paid every time they provided a service to a patient. The more services they rendered, the more they were paid. They were paid only for face-to face encounters, which normally occurred in offices, hospitals, or other facilities. If they spoke on the phone with patients, visited them at home, or had a nurse call them or visit them, these services usually were not covered by insurance.

This payment system came into being many years ago, when patients sought care mainly for acute illnesses. But today, chronic diseases such as diabetes, asthma, COPD, and heart disease are the most common reasons for office visits,[66] and the management of these chronic conditions requires regular follow-up and monitoring. The fee-for-service system is not well-equipped to deal with chronic diseases, partly because it doesn't cover non-visit care. A volume-based payment system also invites physicians to overuse diagnostic and treatment services.

Hospital Incentives

Under Medicare's prospective payment system, hospitals are paid a prescribed amount for each "diagnosis-related group" (DRG) of services. If they perform additional services within a DRG, or if a patient's hospital stay is extended, they are not paid more for the DRG. For the most part, their revenues depend on how many patients are admitted to the hospital and the average severity level of the DRGs they assign to their patients. In essence, then, they also are paid for volume. The more they do for patients, and the more patients they treat, the higher their revenues.

Wherever healthcare is delivered, the fragmentation and poor coordination of care are responsible for much of the waste, the over- and under-utilization of services, and the less-than-optimal outcomes that characterize the U.S. healthcare system, according to a landmark Institute of Medicine report.[67] All of this is encouraged by an insurance system—including private health plans, Medicare, and Medicaid—that pays largely for volume rather than value.

The main alternative to fee for service is prepayment, which requires providers to take financial risk for the care they deliver. Providers are paid a prospective budget in the form of a capitation rate—a set monthly fee for each health plan member—or a global payment that covers all costs of care for a patient population. This is how group-model HMOs such as Kaiser Permanente operate. The insurance arm of the organization sets a budget for its physician groups and hospitals.

Prepaid group practices tend to have lower costs than fee-for-service healthcare organizations, while offering equal or better quality.[68] But as the United States discovered in the 1990s, when insurers launched HMOs across the country, most care is not delivered by organized systems that are prepared to manage care within a budget. Grafting prepayment onto a healthcare delivery system that was largely fee for service and unorganized proved to be a disaster.[69]

Payers learned their lesson. Today's value-based reimbursement models steer between the poles of unrestricted fee for service and pure prepayment. They combine incentives for cost containment with bonuses for improved quality and service.

Climbing the Ladder of Risk

The ACA's care delivery provisions attempt to move providers from pay for volume to pay for value in gradual steps. Essentially, this approach requires or incentivizes healthcare providers to take ascending levels of financial risk. At the bottom of the ladder is "Value-Based Purchasing," in which providers are financially rewarded or penalized for their performance on cost, quality, and patient experience measures. This "pay-for-performance" program is similar to those that many commercial insurers instituted in the 15 years prior to the ACA.

The next step up the risk ladder is "shared savings," in which provider groups try to reduce the total cost of care. If they're successful, and if they meet quality benchmarks, they can share in the savings. Under an upside-only shared savings arrangement, organizations may get bonuses for cutting costs, but they aren't liable for losses if they overspend their budget. In a two-sided arrangement, they must pay back some of the losses they incur to Medicare.

Some healthcare organizations take financial risk for overspending under one of the ACA's bundled-payment programs. Bundled payments require hospitals, physicians, and post-acute care providers to take financial responsibility for an episode of care such as a hospital stay plus 90 days of post-acute care.

Most of the ACA's care delivery provisions apply only to Medicare; however, this program accounts for about a fifth of U.S. health spending[70] and is hugely influential in the private sector. So, these aspects of the ACA are a lever designed to move the entire health system. In at least one ACA program, private insurers are already collaborating with CMS. Moreover, most insurers have value-based-care initiatives that complement those of the ACA.

HOSPITAL VALUE-BASED INCENTIVES

The ACA's value-based-payment provisions include initiatives to improve the safety and quality of hospital care. Alone among the ACA's care delivery initiatives, these programs have no upside for providers; they simply punish hospitals for poor performance.

The Hospital Readmissions Reduction Program, which was implemented in 2012, penalizes institutions that have an excessive number of readmissions. If a hospital's risk-adjusted, 30-day readmission rates for conditions such as heart attack, heart failure, and pneumonia exceed a benchmark, all of the hospital's Medicare payments are reduced slightly for a year.[71]

In fiscal year 2019, CMS imposed readmission penalties on 2,599 hospitals, or 82% of those participating in Medicare. Experts estimated that these fines cost hospitals a total of $566 million.[72]

Between January 2010 and January 2013, the average Medicare readmission rate fell from almost 19% to just over 17.5%.[73] While the readmission rate for the targeted conditions leveled off after that, it has been estimated that the lower rate resulted in 565,000 fewer Medicare patient readmissions between 2010 and 2015.[74]

The ACA also levies fines for high rates of hospital-acquired conditions (HACs) such as bed sores, falls, infections, and surgical complications. Since it went into effect on October 1, 2014, the HAC Reduction Program has penalized hospitals that rank in the worst-performing quartile of facilities. Medicare payments to these hospitals were lowered 1% in FY 2019.[75]

Like the readmissions reduction program, this initiative has been effective. The rate of hospital-acquired conditions among Medicare patients declined by 13% from 2014 to 2017, saving the providers $7.7 billion and averting 20,500 hospital deaths, according to the Agency for Healthcare Research and Quality (AHRQ). From 2010 through 2017, the average annual reduction in HACs was about 4.5%.[76]

Value-Based Purchasing

The ACA authorized two other major programs to rein in hospital costs: the hospital Value-Based Purchasing (VBP) program and the Bundled Payments for Care Improvement (BPCI) program.

The hospital VBP initiative, which began in 2012, is a pay-for-performance program in which CMS withholds a percentage of Medicare payments from hospitals—for FY 2019, this was 2%—and then redistributes the money to the hospitals based on their quality of care, patient experience, safety, and efficiency and cost-reduction.[77-78]

CMS launched the BPCI in 2013. Nearly 7,000 hospitals, physician groups, and post-acute care providers (nursing homes, home care agencies, and others) signed up for the BPCI, but most of them were just kicking the tires.[79] In 2015, when CMS began requiring BPCI participants to take financial risk for all program bundles, only 1,500 providers remained in the program.[80]

In 2016, CMS introduced a mandatory bundled-payment program, the Comprehensive Care for Joint Replacement Program (CJR). Approximately 800 hospitals across a large swathe of the country were required to participate in CJR, which covered all services for hip and knee replacements during hospitalization and for 90 days of post-discharge care.[81]

Under the Trump Administration, CMS cut in half the number of areas where bundled payments for joint replacement were mandatory. At the same time, it canceled the planned introduction of mandatory bundled payments for myocardial infarction, coronary artery bypass grafts, and surgical hip and femur fracture treatment.[82-83]

Early evidence from the CJR program was promising: Medicare payments for episodes of care decreased, and nearly 50% of hospitals achieved bonus payments by maintaining quality and reducing costs below a predefined benchmark. As of Feb. 1, 2018, 465 hospitals remained in the program,[84] which meant that most hospitals had dropped out in areas where CJR was no longer mandatory.

PHYSICIAN VALUE INCENTIVES

CMS's value-based incentives for physicians evolved from several sources that converged into the complicated regime now in effect. The ACA provisions in this area eventually merged with those of two other laws that were passed within the same decade. One of them, the HITECH Act, authorized a program that incentivized doctors to buy and implement electronic health records (EHRs).

The Quality Payment Program (QPP), which incentivizes physicians to provide value-based care, took effect in 2017. Authorized by the Medicare Access and CHIP Reauthorization Act (MACRA) of 2015, the QPP includes two tracks: one for pay for performance and the other for participation in what are called advanced alternative payment models (AAPMs).

The pay-for-performance track, known as the Merit-Based Incentive Payment System (MIPS), covers all eligible clinicians—including physicians, midlevel practitioners, and others—who have not chosen the AAPM track. MIPS bases rewards and penalties on clinicians' scores in four categories: quality, practice improvement, use of health IT, and cost and resource use.[85]

The negative or positive adjustments to clinician reimbursement started out at up to 4% of Medicare revenues in 2019; they were scheduled to rise to up to 9% in 2022, with additional bonuses for "exceptional performers."[86] But in practice, the bonuses and penalties have been small because most eligible clinicians have qualified for bonuses under CMS's very low thresholds. To keep the program revenue neutral, these payment increases must be funded from the penalties placed on the few doctors who score poorly. Hence there's not much money, although the program gives extra bonuses to "exceptional performers."[87]

AAPM Track

Physicians who derive a certain percentage of income from AAPMs are not subject to MIPS and are eligible to receive annual bonuses of 5% of their Medicare revenues for five years, starting in 2019. All of the AAPMs, unlike MIPS, require physicians to take some financial risk.

The AAPMs include the risk-based tracks of the Medicare Shared Savings Program (MSSP), the Comprehensive Primary Care Plus (CPC+) program, the joint replacement bundled-payment program, other bundled-payment models, and certain payment models for end-stage renal disease and cancer care.[88]

According to CMS Administrator Seema Verma, about 10% of QPP-eligible clinicians—including non-physician providers such as physician assistants and nurse practitioners—were recognized as qualifying AAPM participants in 2017.[89] In January 2020, she indicated that about 17% of eligible clinicians had made the cut in 2018.[90] While that's a sizable increase, it still represents a small fraction of QPP participants.

PRIMARY CARE SUPPORT

It has long been recognized that primary care is essential to curbing costs and improving population health. But, as Chapter 4 explains, the percentage of primary care physicians in the workforce is decreasing for several reasons.

The ACA architects included several provisions to buttress primary care and reverse its decline. First, Medicaid payment rates for primary care providers were raised to the level of Medicare rates from 2013 to 2014, after which they dropped back down. Second, the ACA provided a 10% bonus payment to primary care doctors for Medicare services from 2011 through 2015.[91]

CMS also launched two demonstration projects, the Comprehensive Primary Care (CPC) Initiative and its successor, CPC+, to help primary care physicians improve the health of their patient populations. Both projects emphasized care coordination, improved chronic-disease management, and greater access to primary care.

The CPC initiatives were derived from a private-sector concept called the patient-centered medical home (PCMH). Originally championed by primary care medical societies, the PCMH model is holistic primary care in which physician-led care teams coordinate and manage care. The National Committee on Quality Assurance (NCQA), a nonprofit quality improvement organization, has recognized more than 13,000 practices with 67,000 primary care providers as patient-centered medical homes. Encouraged by studies showing that PCMHs reduced costs, health insurance companies have given bonuses to many of these practices.[92]

The CPC program involved private payers, which helped CMS fund CPC in all seven of the targeted regions. These payers included commercial insurers as well as Medicare Advantage and Medicaid-managed care plans.[93]

Primary care practices received two forms of financial support for improving the care of their Medicare patients: a monthly, per-patient care management fee and the opportunity to share in any net savings to the Medicare program. Practices also received monthly fees from private-sector CPC payers.[94] Nearly two-thirds of the patients who were attributed to doctors in CPC sites belonged to private plans, but CMS funded 60% of the program's care management fees.[95]

CPC+, which began in 2017, continues on the same multi-payer track as the CPC, but on a larger scale and with more financial risk. The CPC+ is available in 18 regions rather than seven; includes 56 aligned payers, up from 40; and at latest report, included 2,851 primary care practices, several times as many as participated in the CPC.[96-97]

Track 1 of CPC+ is similar to the original CPC program, except that the performance-based payments are made prospectively. That allows practices to hire care managers and invest in other infrastructure upfront. Track 2 substantially raises the risk-adjusted care management fees, including higher fees for complex patients. The performance-based incentive is also higher than in track 1, and fee-for-service payments are reduced to balance that payment. In both tracks, performance incentives are retrospectively reconciled, and practices that exceed a benchmark must pay back the difference.[98]

Mixed Report Card

An independent study of the original CPC program delivered a mixed report card. While the participating practices achieved sizable gains in areas such as enhanced access to care and risk stratification of patients, they didn't cut costs or improve quality significantly, the study noted. Hospital admissions didn't drop, and the CPC practices didn't reduce Medicare hospital or outpatient spending enough to cover their care management fees. On the positive side, there was a slight decline in emergency department visits, and CPC practices provided more timely follow-up to patients after hospital and ED visits than comparison practices did.[99]

Whether the CPC+ program will achieve better results than its predecessor remains to be seen; however, health policy experts are optimistic about the program.

"I'm a fan of CPC+, track 2, which strikes a balance between fee for service and capitation," says Robert Berenson, MD, a senior fellow at the Urban Institute and a former CMS official. "You don't get windfall revenues if you're doing unnecessary services, but you're getting paid for your costs, and 40% of revenues come from the monthly capitation fee. That's the way to do it."

David Nash, MD, founding dean of the Jefferson College of Population Health, part of Thomas Jefferson University, also likes what he's seen of CPC+ in his health system's primary care practices. Thomas Bodenheimer, MD, professor emeritus of family community medicine at the University of California San Francisco, says CPC+ is "the best thing the government has pushed so far . . . They give you money to improve your practice, which is a good thing."

MEDICARE SHARED SAVINGS PROGRAM

The ACA's most ambitious attempt to promote value-based care was its creation of the Medicare Shared Savings Program (MSSP). The MSSP was designed to foster a new care delivery model known as the accountable care organization (ACO). ACOs are groups of healthcare providers that are accountable for the cost and quality of care for a defined population. Among the ACOs that participate in the MSSP are those created by practice networks, group practices, physician-hospital organizations, health systems and their employed doctors, and federally qualified health centers.[100]

The basic idea of the MSSP is that if ACOs meet quality goals and save Medicare money, they can share in those savings. ACOs that take no downside financial risk are eligible to receive 50% of the savings, and those that take risk receive a larger share.

A steadily increasing number of ACOs have enrolled in the MSSP since 2012; however, the program has not cut Medicare costs significantly. While some ACOs have profited handsomely from their MSSP participation, the majority have not.

Savings and Losses

The MSSP reported a net savings of $314 million in 2017 after paying off the ACOs. This was quite an achievement for the program, considering that it had lost money for the previous two years. On the other hand, the $780 million paid to providers went to just a third of the 472 ACOs in the MSSP. The other participating ACOs received nothing.[101]

In 2018, the net MSSP savings more than doubled to $739 million. This time, two-thirds of the ACOs produced gross savings of $1.7 billion.[102]

Meanwhile, the number of ACOs participating in the program steadily increased from 220 in 2012 to 548 in 2018. Between 2012 and July 2019, the number of assigned Medicare beneficiaries in the MSSP more than tripled, from 3.2 million to 10.9 million.[103-104]

In addition, the MSSP ACOs have raised quality across the board. ACOs that participated in the program in both 2015 and 2016 improved their average performance on 28 of the 31 MSSP quality measures; their performance declined slightly on the other three metrics.[105]

Resistance to Risk

In the first several years of the program, most ACOs joined the MSSP's track 1, which allowed them to share savings without taking any financial risk for spending in excess of a benchmark based on their historical costs.[106] ACOs could also select track 2 or 3, which provided ascending levels of risk and reward. If they spent more than their budget, they had to pay CMS a portion of the excess cost. Fewer than 10% of ACOs chose these risk tracks, so in 2016 CMS introduced track 1+, which allowed ACOs to take less risk.[107] In 2018, 10% of the MSSP ACOs were in track 1+ and 8% of them were in track 2 or 3.[108]

Because 82% of the ACOs still avoided downside risk, CMS made a further course correction. Starting July 1, 2019, MSSP participants were offered a basic track and an enhanced track. The basic MSSP track has five levels that start with upside-only shared savings and quickly ramp up to include some downside risk. The enhanced track is the same as track 3 of the old program. Eventually, all ACOs are expected to advance to the enhanced track.[109]

ACOs now must sign contracts with the MSSP for five years, instead of the three-year agreements they'd previously had. And instead of being able to avoid financial risk for six years, ACOs must start accepting it within two years of joining the program.

Observers expected that many ACOs would leave the MSSP because of the accelerated risk requirement; in July 2019, however, CMS reported that it had approved applications to the new enhanced-risk program for 206 ACOs. These included 41 ACOs new to the MSSP, 25 ACOs that reentered the program, and 140 ACOs that renewed their previous contracts. Including the ACOs in the middle of their contracts, the MSSP encompassed 518 ACOs in mid-2019, down less than 10% from the 561 ACOs in the program during 2018.[110] Meanwhile, the percentage of MSSP ACOs taking two-sided risk jumped from 19% to 29%—a significant change.[111]

By spring 2020, about 40% of the MSSP ACOs were in risk-bearing tracks. However, the emergence of the coronavirus pandemic changed the outlook of many ACOs. An April survey by the National Association of ACOs (NAACOS) found that 56% of MSSP ACOs at financial risk were likely to quit the program because of concerns that the COVID-19 crisis would worsen their 2020 performance. These ACOs had until May 31 to give notice to CMS if they didn't want to face the possibility of financial losses.[112]

In an April 13 *Health Affairs* post, experts on value-based care noted that at-risk ACOs might also see costs drop because of the postponement of elective surgeries and the drop in office visits during the pandemic. They acknowledged, however, that COVID-19 expenses were likely to outweigh these lower costs, leading to financial losses for many ACOs.[113]

ACA HITS AND MISSES

Experts offer mixed opinions on how much the ACA's care delivery provisions have moved the healthcare industry down the road toward value-based care. In the years immediately following the ACA's passage, many healthcare executives dismissed the value-based-care concept as a "flash in the pan," notes David Muhlestein, chief research officer for Leavitt Partners, a healthcare research and consulting firm. "But the ACA has fundamentally changed how people think about it and make strategic plans for the future. There are still major barriers to getting the models aligned with providers, which requires creating enough revenue to justify making the changes [in care delivery]. But the conversation has changed."

David Blumenthal, MD, president of the Commonwealth Fund and a former Obama Administration official, is disappointed that the Medicare Shared Savings Program hasn't done more to transform healthcare. "I don't think the MSSP has been as pow-erful as it could have been," he says. "It hasn't been a total failure, either. If you use value as the outcome, it has improved quality and generated some modest savings. So it's had some benefits."

Grace Terrell, MD, former CEO of the Cornerstone Medical Group in High Point, NC, and a board member of the American Medical Group Association (AMGA), supports the premise of the Comprehensive Primary Care program, but says it will be several more years before its impact on healthcare can be judged. Studies of patient-centered medical homes, she notes, show that practice transformation is slow and that it takes time for the downstream effect of those changes to become apparent.

By the Numbers

In January 2015, then Health and Human Services Secretary Sylvia Burwell announced lofty goals for the government's value-based payment program. By the end of 2016, she said, 85% of all payments in the traditional Medicare program would be tied to quality or value, and 90% would be value-based by the end of 2018.[114]

The government planned to tie 30% of Medicare payments to alternative payment models by 2017, according to Burwell, and hoped to reach the 50% mark by 2018.[115] In March 2016, HHS said it had reached the 30% goal a year ahead of schedule, mainly because of the MSSP.[116]

More recent data on the value-based-care movement comes from the Health Care Payment & Learning Action Network (LAN), a public-private partnership launched in 2015 by the Department of Health and Human Services. The LAN reported in October 2018 that public and private payers covering 226 million lives, or 77% of insured Americans, had tied 34% of their payments to value-based care. According to the organization, only 23% of total payments had been value-based in 2016.[117] A deeper analysis of the LAN data, however, shows that the vast majority of value-based payments—both in Medicare and in the larger healthcare system—were still limited to pay for performance, upside-only shared savings, and care management fees paid to patient-centered medical homes.[118]

More recently, the Catalyst for Payment Reform, a nonprofit firm funded by payers, found that 53% of commercial payments to hospitals and doctors in 2017 could be classified as value-oriented. However, the report said, 90% of value-oriented payments were built on fee for service and just 6% involved downside financial risk—about the same as in 2012.[119]

Without downside risk, most observers agree, providers will not significantly cut costs. Evidence to support this viewpoint can be found in MSSP data. In 2016, for example, ACOs in two-sided risk models accounted for only 10% of the ACOs in the MSSP, but generated almost 30% of the total savings. "The average ACO in a one-sided risk model saved $1.3 million against its benchmark," noted an article about this trend. "The average ACO in two-sided risk models saved $4.5 million—over three and a half times greater savings."[120]

Stuck on Fee for Service

What is the evidence that the healthcare industry is moving from fee for service to risk-based arrangements? Blumenthal replies, "As I listen to people in the healthcare sector talk about the future of payment, most accept the premise that value-based payment and risk sharing are going to grow in prevalence. But the evidence for risk sharing is not as strong as the evidence for pay for performance. So, I think it's an open question."

Muhlestein, who has studied ACOs and the evolution of risk, says there has been an increase in the number of providers who are taking downside risk, either through two-sided shared savings or capitated models. "But for the vast majority of providers, this is still a small minority of their total revenue. Even if you're fully capitated for 5% of your revenue, and the other 95% is fee for service, you're going to optimize [how you do business] around the fee-for-service component, not on that 5% capitation. And that's what we've seen: very few organizations have sufficient revenue through any level of risk that justifies making changes that cannibalize or in some other way hurt their fee-for-service revenue, which dictates their profitability."

Slow Walking to Value-Based Care

In Terrell's view, hospitals and healthcare systems across the country are "slow walking" toward value-based care. "Some hospitals are very good at fee-for-service medicine," she notes. "It's really hard to do these changes, and the slower it goes, the easier it feels to them."

She offers a startling example of how some hospitals have reacted to CMS's Value-Based Purchasing Program. A hospital chief medical officer privately told her that it was not financially worthwhile to reduce readmissions. "He said, 'We'll take the risk of the 30-day readmissions penalty [from Medicare], because we'll make so much from our continuous churn [of inpatient beds] that it's not worth bothering with.'"

Healthcare consultant Michael La Penna is not surprised by this story. Although such a sentiment would never be voiced in public or at a hospital board meeting, he says, hospitals' financial decisions tend to be based on how a particular course of action affects their throughput and occupancy rate. If they have to make a choice between hiring two new ER doctors to increase admissions or hiring nurses to manage high-risk patients at home, for example, they'll choose the ER physicians, he points out.

Hospitals are slow walking to value-based care, he says, because they need to fill beds, and the potential rewards from shared savings or risk contracts aren't enough to make up the difference if they reduce their admissions.

Muhlestein agrees that hospitals are taking their time in transforming their business model. "There's the view that the future belongs to these risk-based models, where you need to manage patients appropriately," he explains. "Then there's the present reality that fee for service dictates whether you keep the lights on. The health systems talk about better ways to manage high-cost, high-risk patients, but at the same time they continue to play the fee-for- service game they're good at."

Despite the pressure from some payers to assume risk, he adds, "It's just a reality that lowering average length of stay while improving your daily census and negotiating better contracts with payers is what moves the needle in the short-term, and that's where the focus is."

THE FINAL SCORE CARD

Overall, the Affordable Care Act has expanded coverage, improved the quality and safety of care, and made a start toward lowering costs. But the country's progress toward a value-based healthcare system is sluggish, to say the least. Fee for service still rules the roost.

CMS anticipates that the percentage of Americans who are insured will remain more or less stable at 90% over the next several years.[121] That tracks with the relative stability of ACA marketplace enrollment and the current size of the Medicaid expansion (assuming that the Supreme Court doesn't affirm the lower court decision to overturn the ACA). But it still leaves one in 10 people uninsured, and it doesn't address the festering issue of under-insurance. Moreover, this forecast was made before the COVID-19 pandemic led to mass layoffs and a rise in the uninsured.

Some experts believe the ACA has helped slow cost growth in the last several years.[122] That slowdown, however, isn't reflected in CMS's latest projections, which forecast that national health spending will increase by an average of 5.5% annually through 2028.[123]

In a recent evaluation of the ACA's first 10 years, David Blumenthal and Melinda Abrams pointed out that, from 2010-2017, per capita health care spending increased by an average of just 3.6% per year. This was low by historic standards and fairly close to the per capita growth in GDP for those years, they noted. Lower Medicare payments to hospitals and to Medicare Advantage plans—both authorized by the ACA—contributed to that outcome, they said.

They were skeptical, however, about claims that Obamacare provisions promoting value-based care have reduced costs. "Beyond its effect on Medicare prices, the role of the ACA in moderating health care costs remains to be definitely established," they concluded.[124]

In Muhlestein's view, the ACA has done little to control costs. "It has made a modest impact on quality and probably a small impact on cost. It's not going to solve our cost growth crisis in America."

Clearly, something else must be done to rescue our failing healthcare system. But the odds of this happening in the current environment are poor, whether we try to build on the ACA or move toward Medicare for All. A big part of the reason is the recent consolidation of the healthcare industry, which we turn to next.

CHAPTER 3

Industry Consolidation on Steroids

Since the 1970s, as U.S. antitrust enforcement has weakened, private economic activity has steadily become concentrated in fewer and fewer companies. From 1985 to 2017, the number of mergers completed annually rose from 2,308 to 15,361, Federal Trade Commission (FTC) data reveals. According to a non-FTC study, the concentration of ownership increased in 75% of U.S. industries from 1997 to 2012. This consolidation increased the market power of the remaining players. It also deterred market competition, increased labor monopsony, created barriers to entry by new firms, and was correlated with lower productivity growth.[1]

Until about 30 years ago, the healthcare industry appeared to be an exception to this trend. Standalone community hospitals, small physician practices, and locally owned home health agencies and nursing homes were the norm in healthcare. Medical practices, in particular, were viewed as a cottage industry of mom and pop operators.

Today, all that has changed. While independent private practices have not disappeared, their numbers are greatly diminished. Independent community hospitals are rare outside of underserved rural and inner-city areas. And many of the health systems that have risen on the ruins of the old cottage industry are multi-billion-dollar giants. Whether classified as for-profit or not-for-profit, these huge organizations have the same revenue-enhancing imperatives that other big corporations do.

The consolidation of the healthcare industry is not based solely on hospital mergers. In addition to engaging in horizontal integration, the healthcare systems have also gobbled up a steadily increasing percentage of physician practices, employing former practice owners and their associates. At the same time, most young doctors in their final year of residency plan to work for hospitals or physician groups rather than start their own practices.[2]

Health insurance companies also have consolidated in many markets. In 2016, United, Anthem, Cigna, Aetna, and Humana had 125 million members, representing 43% of the country's insured population and about 80% of the privately insured.[3-4] In 2018, the American Medical Association (AMA) reported that half of all states had insurance markets that were less competitive than they were the year before. In nearly three-quarters of the local areas studied, a few insurers controlled most of the market, and in 46% of the regions, one insurer had at least 50% of the market.[5]

The Bigness Imperative

As health insurers have grown, health systems have done likewise in order to maintain or improve their negotiating positions. That has proved to be an effective strategy in many cases. Even dominant health plans cannot do without the largest health systems in their areas, especially when they employ many of the local physicians. Therefore, while the plans may push back against the providers' demands—and now and then even threaten to walk away—they eventually capitulate and pass on the higher costs to employers and individuals.

Hospitals usually give other reasons for their mergers. For example, they often claim that the consolidation will lead to greater efficiency because of economies of scale. But that rarely happens, consultant Michael La Penna notes. "Hospitals may consolidate laundry services and supply purchasing, but they won't close a department in one hospital and concentrate those services at another. They won't close down one of the ERs."

A PwC study of 5,600 healthcare facilities and 525 healthcare systems found that large hospitals had a lower cost per patient encounter than small hospitals did. But PwC found that in health systems with multiple facilities, there was no relationship between size and cost. Hospitals within merged health systems didn't centralize functions or stop competing on procedures. The real purpose of mergers, PwC concluded, was to gain negotiating leverage with insurers.[6]

Some hospitals have asserted that they need to build larger systems to meet the challenge of value-based care. But, as explained in Chapter 2, this actually is the opposite of most hospitals' business models. "It's hard to find systems that are really moving in this direction," La Penna says. "Value exists, but only a few health systems have really plunged in."

There's also an argument that larger, more organized systems are better equipped to improve the quality of care and engage in population health management. But David Blumenthal of the Commonwealth Fund hasn't seen that happen very often. "I think it does happen in some cases. I wish there were better evidence of real quality gains," he says. Other experts have observed poorer patient outcomes when hospitals face less competition.[7] A recent study found that hospital mergers did not reduce readmissions or mortality rates, but were associated with a worse patient experience of care.[8]

In many mergers, large healthcare organizations acquire single hospitals or small hospital systems, La Penna observes. The smaller hospitals need capital and the large ones—which often include tertiary-care academic medical centers—are seeking patient referrals from the smaller institutions. He cites Northwell Health's acquisitions of hospitals on Long Island and New York City as an example.

Some mergers are designed as defensive moves against other large healthcare systems. In March 2019, for instance, Boston-based Beth Israel Deaconess Medical Center merged with Lahey Health to form a 10-hospital system with $6 billion in revenues. The systems maintained that they had to merge to counter Partners Healthcare, the largest healthcare organization in New England.[9]

Other mergers involve giants of similar size and scale. For example, Catholic Health Initiatives and Dignity Health completed their union in February 2019. The combined chains, which had roughly similar revenues, formed a new organization called CommonSpirit Health, which has 142 hospitals, 150,000 employees, and nearly $30 billion in revenues.[10]

Why do such large organizations merge? According to La Penna, it's primarily to raise capital. Not-for-profit healthcare systems can't sell stock so they have to borrow money. The bigger they are, the more they can borrow.

Mergers Proceed Apace

Other large health system mergers continue apace. In April 2018, for example, Chicago-based Advocate Health Care completed its union with Wisconsin's Aurora Health Care to create the 10th largest not-for-profit healthcare system in the country. The combined system has 27 hospitals and about $11 billion in annual revenues.[11] A month later, Atrium Health joined with Wake Forest Baptist Health (itself the fruit of an earlier merger) to form a system with 49 hospitals and combined revenues of $7.5 billion.[12]

According to a Kaufman Hall report, 90 hospital and health system deals were publicly announced in 2018. This was a decline from the 115 deals unveiled in 2017, but the average amount of the sellers' revenue hit a record high of $409 million.[13]

These well-publicized deals are just the tip of the iceberg. *The New York Times* reported in 2016 on a plethora of smaller deals, each involving just a handful of hospitals that, in some cases, dominated local markets. At the same time, some physician groups were also growing by acquisition, the *Times* reported. Altogether, at least 940 mergers of healthcare organizations occurred in 2015, compared to 480 in 2010.[14]

Where was the FTC to be found? Basically, nowhere. In 2014, a post on the FTC blog noted that the FTC challenged only two of 752 mergers, joint ventures, or other collaborations among healthcare providers on antitrust grounds. The following year, the FTC blocked a merger between Advocate Health Care and NorthShore University HealthSystem in Chicago and two smaller mergers.[15] But this flurry of activity was the exception, not the rule, for the FTC.

Extracting Higher Prices

A substantial body of research shows that health systems use their market power to raise prices. For example, a 2016 study found that hospital prices in California grew by an average of 76% per admission between 2004 and 2013. Prices at hospitals belonging to large, multi-hospital systems grew substantially more (113%) than prices paid to all other California hospitals (70%). By the end of the period, average prices per admission at hospitals in the largest systems exceeded prices at other hospitals by about $4,000, or 25%. After controlling for other factors, the authors concluded that the higher prices resulted from the greater market power of the biggest systems.[16]

Another study found that there were more than 1,400 hospital mergers in the United States from 1998 to 2015. In the end, nearly half of hospital markets were highly concentrated, dominated by one or two large health systems. Hospital admissions in these areas cost $2,000 more, on average, than admissions elsewhere, the authors noted.[17]

Another group of researchers showed how hospital costs drive the underlying growth in health costs. Focusing on the total cost of inpatient and outpatient care for four high-volume procedures, the study found that from 2007 to 2014, the amounts paid to hospitals by insurers and patients grew much faster than physician reimbursement. For inpatient care, facility payments rose by 42%, vs. 18% for physician payments. For care in hospital outpatient departments, facility payments jumped 25%, compared to a 6% growth in physician payments. Because hospital prices accounted for the majority of costs and increased faster than doctor prices, the study's authors concluded that the increase in the total price of care was driven by the growth in facility prices. Hospitals were able to get these prices, they said, because of their bargaining power.[18]

The RAND study mentioned in Chapter 1 found that commercial insurers paid hospitals an average of 241% of Medicare rates in 2017. This study encompassed 1,600 hospitals in 70 health systems—an average of nearly 23 hospitals per system. The private insurance payments to hospitals ranged from 150% to more than 400% of Medicare rates.

In discussing these results, the RAND researchers noted that some analysts interpret the high prices that hospitals demand from private payers as evidence that they need the money to cover the shortfalls from Medicare underpayments. "The other interpretation is that hospitals, especially 'must-have' hospitals, have used their negotiating leverage to extract unreasonable price concessions from health plans," the authors noted.[19]

David Muhlestein, chief research officer of Leavitt Partners, offers a franker assessment: "A dominant provider in the market can extract almost any price they want," he says.

Higher Insurance Premiums

As noted earlier, the insurance companies have also consolidated, and a few giants dominate many markets. In highly consolidated markets, this has led to increases in insurance rates.[20] A study of the Affordable Care Act marketplace in New York also found a correlation between fewer insurers and higher premiums.[21] Another study showed that adding one more health plan to a state insurance exchange reduced premiums by 4.5%.[22]

One might think that in a market with fewer insurers, they would have a greater ability to negotiate better rates with providers and would thus be able to lower premiums. But, even if health plans should be inclined to charge less than they can, the largest insurers have limited leverage with big health systems. Employers do not want to offer health plans with networks that omit major hospitals and physician groups; therefore, they accept the cost increases from their insurers or plan administrators and pass most of them on to their employees in the form of higher cost sharing.

Is There Hospital Competition?

If you've ever seen highway billboards claiming that one hospital has the best cardiac care or orthopedic care in the area—or is high up on the *U.S. News and World Report* rankings—you might have thought that that hospital was competing with other local facilities for patients. But those billboards are more likely public relations exercises than real signs of competition. Even where there is competition between hospitals, it rarely results in lower prices.

"Driven by a lack of competition, ever higher prices are being paid to hospitals, doctors and insurers without leading to better outcomes," declared health policy experts Martin Gaynor, Farzad Mostashari, and Paul Ginsburg in a 2017 *Forbes* article.[23]

Blumenthal agrees. "The evidence so far is that prices go up with more consolidation," he says. "The lack of competition increases the ability to charge high prices. But I don't think competition reduces prices in health care."

Competition among providers can lower prices in some cases, Muhlestein says, but this is the exception rather than the rule. Although a study he coauthored showed there was competition among health systems of comparable size in a few markets,[24] he cautions that these results are not generalizable across the country.

"What is meaningful competition?" he asks. "If you have 30 hospitals in an area, but their service areas hardly overlap, there isn't much competition."

In summary, the healthcare industry is going through the same transition to a high concentration of ownership that other industries have made. This process has allowed the merged healthcare systems to extract more and more money from employers and consumers. The fire of consolidation, however, hasn't just devoured hospitals and other healthcare facilities; it is now roaring through the ranks of independent physician practices, with unpredictable long-term consequences.

PHYSICIAN EMPLOYMENT

The American Medical Association (AMA) recently announced that, for the first time, more physicians were employed than were independent. While many of these doctors were employed by private practices, the AMA said, about 35% of physicians worked directly for a hospital or for a hospital-owned practice.[25]

This estimate was lower than that of other surveys. According to research conducted by the Physicians Advocacy Institute (PAI) and Avalere Health, a consulting firm, 44% of physicians were employed by hospitals in January 2018, compared to 25% in July 2012.[26] And that increase followed a doubling in the number of hospital-owned practices between 2004 and 2011, according to the Medical Group Management Association (MGMA).[27]

Many of the physicians employed by hospitals and health systems formerly were in private practice. They sold their practices to hospitals because of increasing overhead, dwindling reimbursement, and the rising administrative burdens of ownership, according to Jackson Healthcare, a physician recruiting firm. The Affordable Care Act also played a role in their decisions. Sixty-five percent of the doctors surveyed by Jackson had sold their practices since the ACA's passage in 2010, and many felt they didn't have the resources to comply with the ACA.[28] Other formerly independent physicians went to work for hospitals or larger groups because they couldn't afford to buy electronic health record (EHR) systems.

The many negative factors affecting primary care (see Chapter 4) also have impelled a growing number of primary care physicians to seek employment in recent years. In 2018, 47% of general internists, 57% of family physicians and 56% of pediatricians were employed.[29] There is evidence that this trend may be exacerbating the primary care shortage because employed doctors see fewer patients per day, on average, than do those in private practice.[30]

An increasing percentage of hospital-employed physicians are young doctors fresh out of residency training. A 2019 survey by Merritt Hawkins, another recruiting firm, found that 91% of final-year medical residents wanted to be employed and that only 1% wanted to start a private practice. Forty-five percent of the residents said they'd consider a job offer from a hospital—the highest percentage ever in Merritt Hawkins' ongoing survey.[31]

Why Hospitals Hire Docs

Hospitals say they acquire practices and build their physician groups to improve care coordination and lower costs, but some observers say it's mainly about patient referrals. According to a Stanford University study, a hospital's ownership of practices increases the odds that doctors will admit patients there instead of at another hospital. Because the hospitals that employ the referring physicians are not necessarily the best, hospital employment of doctors also boosts the chances that patients will go to higher-cost, lower-quality facilities.[32]

Hospitals and health systems benefit from employing doctors in other ways. Physicians in hospital groups order their tests from hospital labs and radiology centers. In addition, hospitals are able to bill Medicare for the ambulatory care provided by their doctors at a much higher rate than what Medicare pays to private practices for the same services. The hospitals have been allowed to do this because their employed physicians are considered to be part of hospital outpatient departments (HOPDs). HOPDs, which also include emergency departments and same-day surgery units, charge not only professional fees but also facility fees.[33]

Just how much of a difference this makes can be seen by comparing the Medicare-allowed fees for a medium-level office visit in the two types of care settings. In hospital-affiliated clinics that were considered part of HOPDs, the payment was $116 in 2018. In contrast, private practices received $81 for the same kind of visit.[34]

Pursuant to a regulation authorized by the Bipartisan Budget Act of 2015, the Centers for Medicare and Medicaid Services (CMS) began paying HOPDs and private practices the same for identical services in January 2019. But in September of that year, a federal district court ruled that CMS had overstepped its statutory bounds by implementing these "site-neutral" payments.[35] CMS had to repay the additional payments it had withheld from the hospitals, but has announced it will appeal the court decision.[36]

If the government is able to enforce site-neutral payments, it should reduce hospitals' incentive to acquire practices, says Farzad Mostashari, MD, a former national coordinator of health information technology and currently CEO of Aledade, a company that organizes and supports primary care-led ACOs.

Hospitals, however, have other incentives to employ physicians. Their most important motive, La Penna says, is to lock up physicians so that other hospitals can't control them. Even if there's little overlap between two hospitals' service areas, he says, they want to make sure that the other hospital doesn't employ some of their referring doctors.

"When I ask a hospital board, 'Would you be buying practices if St. John's wasn't buying practices,' they say 'No,'" he points out. "They're buying their own distribution chain, which they already have for free."

Higher Insurance Payments

Getting higher Medicare rates for their physicians is not the only way that hospitals have driven up costs by buying practices and recruiting doctors out of residency. When health systems employ physicians, they can use their market power to negotiate higher commercial payment rates for those doctors. A study of claims data from commercial insurers found substantial differences between the prices negotiated by employed groups and private practices across the country.[37] In two-thirds of the areas included in the study, physician prices increased as the result of practice purchases by hospitals.[38] Another study found that physician prices rise nearly 14% when a hospital acquires a physician group.[39]

The higher private insurance prices paid to many hospital-employed groups—like the higher Medicare payments to HOPDs—put additional pressure on independent practices. The physicians who own those practices must meet payroll and cover other costs, yet they're getting paid less than the much bigger hospital groups with which they're competing. Aside from the other reasons enumerated above, this factor has undoubtedly induced some private practice doctors to throw in the towel and go to work for a hospital.

Practice owners are also having an increasingly difficult time recruiting physicians to their groups. Because hospitals negotiate higher rates from commercial insurers, they can pay high starting salaries that private practices can't match.

Family physician David Boles, DO, says that when he interviews recent residency graduates, they want to start out at a salary "that's impossible to sustain under a production formula. If you start a family doc at $240,000 right out of residency—because that's the only way you can get one—the odds are that if that's a one-year contract, they're going to have to take a pay cut in the next year."

Practice Losses

Hospitals lose about $50,000–$100,000 per doctor per year on their employed practices, according to La Penna. MGMA, which represents independent groups, has estimated that hospitals and health systems lose nearly $196,000 per doctor annually.[40] Both estimates refer to losses on practice operations alone.

In an article posted on the website of the Healthcare Financial Management Association (HFMA), executives of consulting firm Kaufman Hall explained that hospitals often pay employed physicians more than they were making in private practice. This differential compensates them for signing restrictive covenants and for the value of practice assets.

These higher salaries, coupled with signing bonuses and rich benefit packages, often create losses for hospitals during the initial contract period. In addition, the consultants noted, the health system normally invests in upgrading the practice's EHR or converting it to the system EHR. And if the practice had its own lab, the charges formerly billed to that lab are now billed to the hospital, lowering practice revenues.[41]

What the consultants didn't say is that employed physicians don't usually work as hard as doctors who own their own practices. While productivity incentives are common, employed doctors are 12% less productive than practice owners, on average, according to a Physicians Foundation survey.[42]

In addition, hospitals are notoriously poor billing and collection managers for ambulatory care practices. Hospital billing offices are accustomed to handling large-ticket items such as procedures and don't usually have a process for chasing down small outpatient bills.

Downstream Revenues

Despite the losses that hospitals incur on practice operations, they derive large amounts of revenue from employed physicians who refer patients to them and order tests from their diagnostic facilities. To the extent that these doctors use the hospital that employs them more than they did in private practice, the hospital or health system can see a net gain in revenue, even if they have operating losses on their physician groups.

In 2016, the average net revenue that each employed doctor generated for his or her hospital was $1.56 million, up 7.7% from $1.45 million in 2013, physician search firm Merritt Hawkins found. In 2019, the same company conducted a survey showing that independent and employed physicians generated an average of $2.38 million each for their affiliated hospitals. These revenues included inpatient and outpatient income from admissions, tests, treatments, and procedures performed or ordered by doctors.

The Merritt Hawkins report also compares physician salaries to the revenues generated by doctors in each specialty. Family physicians, for example, earned $241,000, on average, and generated $2.1 million—nine times their salaries. General internists earned $261,000 and threw off $2.67 million, 10 times as much as they were paid. Orthopedic surgeons made $533,000 and created $3.29 million in revenue—six times their salaries.

"As these numbers indicate, physicians generate considerably more in 'downstream revenue' than they receive in the form of salaries or income guarantees," the report pointed out. "This is particularly true of primary care physicians. Though hospitals and other employers have been shown to lose money on physician salaries in some cases, they often recoup those losses from the downstream revenue physicians generate."[43]

Financial Value of Employment

As this report indicates, not all hospitals achieve financial gains by employing doctors. And, even if their practice losses are outweighed by downstream revenue, it's unclear how much of that revenue would have come to the hospital anyway if the doctors had been independent.

Independent physicians generate about the same amount of money for hospitals as employed doctors, La Penna says, but the hospitals want to make sure that no other institution can control those practices. "If nobody could buy practices, they'd have to do something else to get referrals," he says. "You'd probably end up with a stasis: the same ratio of referrals, just under a different relationship."

Travis Singleton, executive vice president of Merritt Hawkins, says that many hospitals do achieve net gains on their employed doctors. When hospitals suffer net losses on employed physicians after factoring in their referrals, he says, it's generally because the physicians are not productive and because some of them refer patients outside of the health system.

Employed physicians should refer at least 80% of their patients who need hospital services to the institution they work for, Singleton says. In some hospitals, however, there are physicians who refer only 20% of patients to their employer and send the rest elsewhere. When a hospital has that problem plus low productivity, he points out, it's bound to lose money on its physicians, even after the value of referrals and orders is factored in.

Health systems can't legally require their employed doctors to admit patients to their hospitals, Singleton observes. But the doctors know their contracts might not be renewed if they don't. The challenge for hospital management is riding herd on hundreds of physicians, many of whom came from private practices that haven't yet been amalgamated into the health system.

"There are areas of the country, especially in the Northeast, where systems struggle with that," he notes. "When this practice acquisition market started, it was the 200-man groups, the 50- man groups, the neurosurgeon groups you put under your wing. Today, there are hardly any of those left. Now we're talking about gobbling up 50 three-man groups, spread around the community. That's a whole different ball of wax, and it's a different thing to manage. And you do see serious leakage patterns where either physicians are not referring at the same pace as when you bought them, or not referring to your facilities at all."

What Young Doctors Want

Young doctors just out of residency have a different mindset than older physicians who have been in practice for many years. "They don't want to work hard and they want to make a lot of money," says David Zetter, a practice management consultant. "Most of them aren't entrepreneurial. They're not interested in dealing with the business side of medicine."

Singleton agrees, calling the current batch of residency graduates "worker bees" who have no yen to start a private practice. "Part of that is the desire to just practice medicine without administrative burdens, and there's also the uncertainty about the alternative," he says.

For many young doctors, he notes, working for a hospital is the only world they know. Even if they wanted to hang out a shingle, he says, they would have no idea how to build a practice. And most of them have so much student debt that it's hard for them to imagine borrowing more money to build the infrastructure that a private practice requires today.

However, Farzad Mostashari notes that, according to the Merritt Hawkins resident survey, 55% of third-year residents would accept a job offer from an organization other than a hospital. "That tells you something," he says. "It's all about whether we have alternatives for them."

Will the Pendulum Reverse Direction?

Mostashari says he has seen some physicians voluntarily leave hospital employment recently. "One of the reasons why these doctors bolted from the hospital is that they didn't like the hospital telling them they had to send their surgeries to the hospital's surgeon. They may not agree that that's the best surgeon for the patient. That's moral injury to a doctor when they feel like the duty they owe their employer is in conflict with the duty they owe their patient."

Hospitals lure physicians into employment by promising they'll have fewer administrative burdens and can just practice medicine, Mostashari notes. "Based on that, you'd imagine employed doctors would have lower rates of burnout. It turns out that it's exactly the opposite. The independent doctors have lower rates of burnout. It's because they have more control over their lives."

Zetter has helped physicians return to private practice after quitting hospital employment. "They have different reasons, but I hear complaints about no autonomy," he says. "Management communicates poorly, the support isn't there, and they're treated like second-rate citizens. They're also expected to practice in a certain way and refer in a certain manner. Their schedule is dictated, and they don't want to be seen as just pushing patients through."

Singleton, too, has detected a small groundswell of physicians leaving hospitals because employment didn't turn out to be what they expected. He also cites a Physicians Foundation study that asked independent and employed doctors whether employment was good for healthcare. About half of the hospital-employed physicians said "No."

Nevertheless, Singleton doubts that there will be a repeat of the mass exodus back to private practice that occurred around 2000 after the first big wave of hospital practice purchases. Even if hospitals and doctors wanted to part ways, he says, there's much more regulation and corporatization of medicine now than there was in the late 1990s. With the current emphasis on value-based care and the need to invest in EHRs, practices have to be larger than they used to be in order to survive in the current environment, he says. Moreover, physicians who have been out of the business world for 10–15 years may not be able to cope.

PHYSICIAN GROUPS

Whether a physician owns a small, struggling practice or is a final-year resident contemplating his or her future, the most viable alternative to hospital employment is to join a large independent medical group. Of the third-year residents surveyed by Merritt Hawkins in 2019, 20% said they'd prefer to work for a single-specialty group, and 16% said they'd like to be employed by a multispecialty group.[44]

In the 2018 Physicians Foundation survey, 31% of the respondents were practice owners, partners, or associates (usually on a partnership track); 19% were directly employed by a hospital; 17% were employed by a hospital-owned medical group; and 13% were employees of a physician-owned medical group. When asked what they planned to do in the next one to three years, fewer than 3% of the respondents said they intended to merge with another physician or group. Most of the doctors planned to continue what they were doing (54%), cut back on their hours (21%), or retire (17%).[45]

Comparing the results of these two surveys, it's evident that most of the new recruits for physician groups are young residency graduates. Most of the doctors who are still in private practice plan to stay put or retire.

Still, as the previously cited *New York Times* article on physician group mergers noted, there have been many mergers among small practices that created large groups. The article cited the DuPage Medical Group, which started as an eight-doctor practice in the Chicago suburbs in the 1960s. Numerous small mergers made DuPage into a big group. In the past five years, it has completed about 16 acquisitions and doubled in size to 500 doctors.[46]

Cornerstone Medical Group was a small practice when Grace Terrell, MD, founded it in High Point, N.C., in 1995. Over time, Cornerstone grew to include about 300 doctors. Now owned by the merged entity of Atrium Health and Wake Forest Baptist Health, the practice is part of a far larger physician group and is the nucleus of its accountable care organization.

Changes in Group Size

The average size of practices has grown significantly in the past few decades. According to the AMA, the percentage of physicians in solo practice dropped from 41% in 1983 to 18% in 2012.[47] The majority of physicians still work in relatively small practices, but the percentage of doctors in groups of 10 or fewer physicians fell to 56.5% in 2018 from 61.4% in 2012.[48]

Over time, the AMA reports, there has been a redistribution of physicians toward very large practices (50 or more doctors), with little change in the shares of physicians who practice in mid-sized practices (11–24 and 25–49 physicians). The percentage of physicians in practices with 50 or more physicians increased from 12.2% in 2012 to 14.7% in 2018.[49]

To put these numbers in perspective, just 9.5% of doctors practiced in groups of 20 or more in 2001. In that year, 82% of physicians worked in groups of one to nine practitioners.[50] So there has been a marked shift toward bigger groups, but far more physicians still work in small and medium-sized practices than in very large groups.

Lawrence Casalino, MD, chief of the division of health policy and economics at Weill Cornell Medicine in New York, says he's not seeing as many independent groups merging as he did in the early 2000s. "What we're seeing now is more hospitals acquiring physician groups or insurers like United/Optum acquiring groups," he says. "There are a lot fewer independent groups, especially big ones. Average group size, even among independents, is getting bigger, but there aren't many large-scale acquisitions. Some big groups are absorbing smaller ones, and some private equity firms are giving money to large medical groups to expand and bring in other practices."

Benefits and Drawbacks of Large Groups

Like proponents of hospital integration with physicians, reformers who favor the formation of large prepaid medical groups argue that they can efficiently provide high-quality care in a collegial professional environment.[51] But a 2003 survey by Casalino and his colleagues found that the most frequently cited benefit of large groups is that they can increase negotiating leverage with insurance companies. Bargaining clout was cited eight times as often as improving quality. The second most important benefit, according to respondents, was to achieve economies of scale.[52]

Today, Casalino says, the driving force behind physician group consolidation is still to negotiate better payment terms with insurers. That's much more important than the ability to get shared savings under value-based-care contracts, he argues. What concerns him is that even if large organizations provide poorer-quality care than small ones, they may squeeze out the smaller practices because they can obtain higher payments.

A 2014 paper, also coauthored by Casalino, looked at the question of whether large groups offer higher quality of care than do small practices. This study found that practices with one or two doctors had 33% fewer preventable hospital admissions than practices of 10–19 doctors; practices with 3–9 doctors had 27% fewer admissions. In addition, physician-owned practices had fewer preventable admissions than did hospital-owned practices.[53]

In our interview, Casalino noted that big organizations can afford to implement organized processes and hire additional staff to improve care. "The question is, if you get big, do you lose the personal touch or have dis-economies of scale?" he said. Also, he points out that hospital-owned groups and ACOs have less incentive than physician-led ACOs do to cut hospital utilization because filling beds generates more revenue for hospitals than shared savings.

OTHER EMPLOYMENT ALTERNATIVES

This survey of industry consolidation would be incomplete without mentioning insurers' acquisitions of physician groups, the return of private equity to practice ownership, and the growing involvement of pharmacy chains in care delivery.

The leading example of the first trend is Optum, a subsidiary of UnitedHealth Group. United began acquiring practices in 2008, and Optum currently is "affiliated" with about 47,000 physicians across the country.[54] These include 17,000 doctors who shifted to Optum when the company completed its purchase of the DaVita Medical Group in June 2019.[55] This made Optum the largest employer of physicians in the United States. In comparison, HCA Healthcare, a big for-profit hospital chain, employs about 37,000 doctors, and Kaiser Permanente has around 22,000 physicians.[56] The Veterans Health Administration (VA) system employs more than 11,000 physicians, not counting its many contract physicians and medical residents.[57]

A news report on Optum's plans notes that in some markets, UnitedHealth is directing plan members toward its acquired physician practices. For example, New West Physicians, a Denver-area group of 120 doctors that United bought in 2017, is included in a favored narrow-network plan. Members can see New West physicians for 20%–30% less in out-of-pocket expenses than if they saw doctors outside the network.[58]

In a more worrisome development, United Healthcare recently dropped hundreds of New Jersey doctors from its Medicaid-managed care network. Some of these physicians said the insurer was trying to shift patients to Riverside Medical Group, which is owned by Optum.[59]

Under the OptumCare brand, United also has purchased groups in Arizona, California, Connecticut, Florida, Indiana, Nevada, New York, Ohio, Texas, and Utah. In addition, OptumCare operates a chain of MedExpress urgent care centers and a national network of ambulatory surgical centers and surgical hospitals.[60]

Other health plans are building rather than buying primary care practices. For example, Blue Cross and Blue Shield of Texas plans to open 10 primary care medical centers in Dallas and Houston in 2020. These offices will provide not only primary care, but also urgent care, lab tests, and diagnostic imaging. The Texas Blues' partner in this venture, Sanitas USA, also operates medical clinics in conjunction with other insurers, including Florida Blue and Horizon Blue Cross and Blue Shield of New Jersey.[61] Partners in Primary Care, a subsidiary of Humana, operates senior-focused primary care centers in Texas, Kansas, Missouri, North Carolina, and South Carolina.[62]

Anthem, United's largest competitor, also has expanded its presence on the care delivery side. Its diversified business division includes CareMore, a 20-year-old company that provides intensive primary care and social services to Medicare, Medicaid, and dual beneficiaries. In June 2019, Anthem agreed to buy Beacon Health Options, the largest independently held behavioral health organization in the United States. The press release referenced "Anthem's strategy to diversify into health services . . . that personalize care for people with complex and chronic conditions."[63]

Venture Capital Strategies

Always on the prowl for investment opportunities, private equity rediscovered healthcare in the past decade. Worldwide, venture capital healthcare deals were worth $63.1 billion in 2018, their highest level since 2003. In the United States, there were 84 private equity (PE) transactions in various healthcare sectors, which were worth a total of $23.2 billion.

In many of these deals, PE firms acquired physician practices or companies that employed doctors. For example, PE firm KKR spent $9.9 billion to acquire physician staffing company Envision Healthcare. Summit Partners and Optum acquired a controlling stake in Sound Inpatient Physicians for $2.2 billion.[64]

Venture capital firms also have purchased practices in high-ticket specialties such as dermatology, ophthalmology, gastroenterology, urology, and allergy. The doctors in these practices may have been attracted by the large upfront payments they were offered. They also may have wanted to sell to relieve financial pressures and gain negotiating clout with health plans, according to one study.

However, the private equity buyouts may have some unfortunate consequences for both the quality and the cost of care, the study's coauthors suggest:

> Evidence comparing the quality of private equity firm–owned practices with physician-owned practices is limited . . . However, the need for private-equity firms to achieve high returns on investment (often at least 2.5×) on a fast time horizon (approximately 6 years on average) may conflict with the need for investments in quality and safety. Additionally, the need for generating returns may create pressure to increase utilization, direct referrals internally to capture revenue from additional services, and rely on care delivered by unsupervised allied clinicians.[65]

Pharmacy Initiatives

Pharmacy chains are also expanding their involvement in care delivery. CVS and Walgreens own the majority of the 2,200 retail clinics that use nurse practitioners to provide minor acute care. Walgreens has partnered with MedExpress urgent care centers adjacent to its pharmacies and is planning to open primary care clinics in the Houston area.[66] The pharmacy chain is also partnering with health systems to open retail clinics in several markets.[67]

Walmart recently opened a health center in suburban Atlanta—its second in Georgia—that goes far beyond its in-store convenience clinics. The health center, adjacent to a Walmart store, offers primary and urgent care, labs, x-rays, mental health care, and dental, optical, and hearing services. It charges 30%–50% less than physician and dental offices. The retailing giant is considering a rollout of similar health centers across the country.[68]

An even more ambitious program is emerging from CVS's $70 billion merger with Aetna, one of the country's biggest health insurers. In June 2019, CVS announced that it plans to launch 1,500 "Health Hubs" in its stores by the end of 2021. CVS said these in-store clinics will offer chronic-disease management, as well as the minor acute care featured in its 1,100 Minute Clinics, some of which may be expanded into Health Hubs. CVS reportedly will use Aetna's data on its members' health conditions to decide where to open the new clinics.[69]

CVS/Aetna's approach could improve access and the quality of care for some consumers. The availability of pharmacists onsite, for example, might improve medication compliance and patients' knowledge about their medications. But, as is explained more fully in Chapter 4, the expansion of pharmacy-owned retail clinics threatens the economic viability of independent primary care practices, which provide essential care to the majority of people. The corporate mandate to grow profits could thus "disrupt" a vital ecosystem.

REMEDIES FOR CONSOLIDATION

The rapidly increasing consolidation of the healthcare industry will continue to raise prices for consumers and employers, according to Paul Ginsburg, chair of the medicine and public policy department of the University of Southern California and a fellow of the Brookings Institution. In 2016 testimony to the California Senate Committee on Health, Ginsburg said that the government can play an effective role in addressing higher prices stemming from consolidation by pursuing policies that foster increased competition in healthcare markets.[70]

State insurance departments, for example, could prohibit contract provisions that prevent health plans from placing hospitals in "tiers" in which patients' out-of-pocket costs vary, depending on the cost and quality of the hospital they choose. States could also ban contracts that require insurers to include all of a health system's facilities, and they could prohibit "most favored nation" clauses that require providers not to accept lower rates from other insurers.

Since limited-network health plans can reduce premium costs, Ginsburg believes that states should remove barriers to these insurance models. Narrow networks, he notes, have lowered premiums by 15% compared to plans with broader networks. But employees feel trapped when their employers offer them such plans. Tiered networks have more appeal to consumers because they are allowed to see providers in higher-cost tiers. But hospitals often refuse to contract with insurers that don't place them in the preferred tier.

Policy Gaps

Federal antitrust policy hasn't addressed hospital acquisitions of physician practices, Ginsburg noted. "These acquisitions lead to higher prices to physicians because hospitals can negotiate higher prices for their employed physicians than the physicians were getting in small practices," he pointed out.

Hospital employment of doctors can also block physicians from referring patients to hospitals that offer greater value, Ginsburg observed, and it reduces the chances that doctors will form larger groups or networks that could participate in value-based contracts. One way for the government to increase the attractiveness of private practice, he said, is for Medicare to implement site-neutral payments for ambulatory care. However, as we've seen, a federal court has struck down CMS's site-neutral payment regulation.

Mostashari, who also favors site-neutral payments, suggests that the FTC strengthen its stance against anti-competitive behavior in the healthcare industry. One reason the FTC hasn't done more in this regard, he says, is that not-for-profit hospitals have been shielded from antitrust review. Congress could change that, freeing the FTC to oppose more mergers that are not in the public interest, he says.

Another area ripe for policy review, he adds, is barriers to market entry. "We have plenty of potential capital for startups that want to come in and do interesting things [in healthcare]. And there are policies that help new entrants and other policies that hurt them."

Encouraging new business models and technologies, Mostashari argues, could reduce the market dominance of big health systems. "As health care continues to move from the inpatient to the outpatient arena because of payment models, patient preference and new technology, the stranglehold of a hospital over time will be less important," he says.

Even if Mostashari's long-term prognosis is correct, however, consolidation of hospitals and physicians is continuing apace. And for the foreseeable future, it's likely that hospitals will continue to resist value-based care to the extent that it undermines their business model. Consequently, bolder steps must be taken to curtail the market power of hospitals. Chapter 8 explains how we can eliminate the ability of hospitals to block healthcare reform.

Now we turn our attention to the future of primary care, which holds the key to rebuilding our healthcare system and which is currently in a sorry state.

CHAPTER 4

Primary Care on the Ropes

Jeffrey Kagan, MD, a general internist in Newington, Conn., recalls an elderly patient who came to his office and complained about a burning sensation when he urinated. He also had a little back pain and fever. Kagan quickly determined that the person had a urinary tract infection. His heart rate was 95 and his blood pressure was 110/70, but the internist didn't think that was any cause for concern. The doctor prescribed an antibiotic and sent the patient home, instructing him to drink a lot of fluids. In a few days, the patient felt much better.

"If the same person had gone to the ER," Kagan says, "he would have been told, 'You have a urinary tract infection with sepsis. We know you have sepsis because your heart's a little fast and your blood pressure is a little low. You must be admitted to the hospital and get IV fluids and IV antibiotics.' I see this all the time."

If an older person visits the ER complaining of a bellyache in his or her side, "they get a CT scan and are told they have diverticulitis," notes Kagan. "They probably get admitted to the surgical service. They get put on IV antibiotics and are kept without food. Then the surgeon comes by and says, 'We're going to let things cool off for a few weeks and then you're going to come back and we're going to cut out your diverticulitis.'

"If they wander into my office with a pain in the side, I say, 'We're going to send you for a blood test and for a CT scan today. This afternoon, you'll come back to the office and we'll go over it. If you have diverticulitis, we're going to tell you to go on a clear liquid diet, and we're going to give you these two oral antibiotics, and we'll see you again in a week. Of course, if things get worse, you'll talk to us sooner. Then we'll see you again in a few weeks.' So this person avoids the hospital and, guess what, they don't have surgery."

Kagan will recommend surgery, he says, if the patient has three episodes of pain from the diverticulitis; but only about 25% of patients with diverticulitis need an operation. Generally, they can control the condition if they avoid eating seeds and stick to a high-fiber diet, he says.

Sometimes a patient just needs a little understanding from their primary care physician to avoid a bad outcome. Kenneth Kubitschek, MD, an internist in Asheville, N.C., recounts a story about an 86-year-old patient who, at his family's suggestion, self-referred himself to a neurologist for a persistent headache. This patient had a history of lung cancer, and it was possible that the cancer had metastasized to his brain. A CT scan showed that he indeed had a mass on his brain, and the neurologist referred him to a neurosurgeon.

After discussing the options, the surgeon recommended removing the mass, the man agreed, and he was scheduled for surgery.

But the patient was uneasy about his decision, so he went to see Kubitschek, who had been his primary care doctor for 30 years. Kubitschek asked him what he really wanted, and the patient said he'd prefer to stay at home and die there. It turned out that he'd consented to the procedure mainly because he wanted to please the surgeon. So Kubitschek sat down with the elderly man and his family for an hour, and they eventually decided to cancel the surgery, call in hospice treatment, and hire home health aides to help his family care for him. The doctor recalls that his patient was "very happy with that decision," and he died comfortably at home a couple of weeks later.

"Without primary care being involved, I think he would have gone down a different path," Kubitschek says. "Surgery probably would have been very damaging to a man of his age. Even if he'd survived it, he probably wouldn't have survived it well. And given that the cancer was metastatic . . . I just wanted to find out what he wanted, and sometimes that's what primary care's goal is."

What these stories show is that patients who receive good primary care from a trusted personal physician usually have better outcomes and cost the system less money than those who have no regular source of primary care. This is not news to most healthcare professionals; but unfortunately, many Americans don't have a primary care physician. They get their healthcare from walk-in clinics, ERs, and/or specialists.

What the Evidence Shows

Many other countries' healthcare systems outperform ours for one simple reason: They place a much greater emphasis on primary care, which occupies the central place in their systems. "The evidence is that where you have more primary care physicians, where you coordinate care, and where you pay to keep people healthy, you get better outcomes at lower cost," says David Nash, MD, founding dean of the College of Population Health, part of Thomas Jefferson University in Philadelphia.

The evidence that Nash mentions includes studies by Barbara Starfield and her colleagues at Johns Hopkins University. In a 2005 *Health Affairs* paper, they showed that a higher ratio of primary care physicians to the population is associated with a lower mortality rate from all causes and from heart disease and cancer; in contrast, having more specialists in a particular area does not decrease the overall mortality rate or deaths from cancer and heart disease.[1]

Another study of Medicare data found that states where a higher percentage of physicians were PCPs had higher quality care and lower cost per beneficiary. This factor alone accounted for nearly half of the variation in Medicare spending from one state to another.[2] A separate study found that in the areas of the country that had the most primary care providers, the average Medicare cost per beneficiary was a third lower than in areas with the least PCPs.[3]

One reason for this is that primary care doctors provide comprehensive, continuous care, including preventive and routine chronic care. Chronic illnesses drive 90% of health costs, and some studies show that intensive primary care can reduce ER visits and hospital admissions and improve the health of chronically ill people.[4]

In addition, primary care physicians strive to understand the whole patient, both physically and mentally. Besides having an in-depth knowledge of each patient's health factors, "I know what's going on in their lives," Kagan says. "I know who's getting divorced and who's lost their job and who has some stress in their life."

This comprehensiveness is an essential feature of primary care. "We don't miss an opportunity to fix the things that down the road are going to be significantly greater problems for you," says Russell Kohl, MD, an official of the American Academy of Family Physicians (AAFP). "That's the challenge we have around a specialty-driven approach, where patients say, 'let me see a bone doctor for my bone problem or a heart doctor for my heart problem, or a kidney doctor for my kidney problem,' and not see those three things are integrally connected with each other. It's that comprehensive approach that makes sense for you long term."

A "Sick" System

Not all primary care physicians provide this level of holistic care. But in general, primary care is oriented to keeping people healthy as well as treating them when they're sick. And primary care is "upstream" of the more costly, specialized care that may be required when people get really ill.

Overall, Nash notes, the U.S. healthcare system is designed to treat sickness, not to maintain health. "If we had a focus on going upstream and shutting off the faucet rather than mopping up the floor, primary care would have a central role," he says. "But the system is focused all downstream, which reduces the prestige of primary care physicians and the range of skills that they need. If the system were focused upstream, they'd be paramount."

The difference in how primary care physicians are regarded in the United States and in other nations is reflected in the amount of resources devoted to them. In this country, one study finds, only 7% of the total cost of care goes to primary care (other studies estimate it at 5%). In contrast, around 20% of healthcare spending in other advanced countries is allocated to primary care.[5] The ratio of specialists to primary care doctors in the United States is about 2:1. In other countries, the ratio is about 50/50.[6]

Since these other nations rely much more heavily on primary care than we do, their systems are organized differently from ours. So, if we want to achieve results similar to theirs, we should restructure our system to emphasize primary care. However, the indicators for U.S. primary care are moving in the opposite direction.

CURRENT STATE OF PRIMARY CARE

First, we have a worsening shortage of primary care. In 2010, there were 246,000 primary care physicians in the United States, of whom 208,800 were practicing full time.[7] No comparable figures are available for 2020; however, from 2005 to 2015, one study found, the number of jobs for primary care doctors grew by 8%, while the number of jobs for specialists grew six times faster. At the same time, the share of the physician workforce devoted to primary care decreased from 44% to 37%, while the number of primary care doctors per capita remained flat.[8]

A portion of the demand for primary care is being met by non-physician clinicians such as nurse practitioners (NPs) and physician assistant (PAs). When these clinicians were included in the total, the study noted, the supply of generalist providers grew 17% between 2005 and 2015.[9] However, this was still much less than the growth in the specialist workforce, and midlevel practitioners cannot do as much as primary care doctors can, as will be discussed below.

"Worst Shortage in 20 Years"

A wide range of experts agree that there is a primary care shortage. Nash sees this shortfall as the main reason the business of retail clinics and urgent care centers is booming. Travis Singleton, the executive president of physician search firm Merritt Hawkins, describes the current situation as "the worst primary care shortage we've had in 20 years."

And things are expected to get even worse. Only 20% of young doctors are going into primary care,[10] and the percentage of PCPs in the physician workforce has fallen to 32%.[11] By 2030, forecasts the Association of American Medical Colleges (AAMC), there will be a shortfall of between 14,800 and 49,300 primary care doctors. The AAMC also predicts a shortage in non-primary care specialties of between 33,800 and 72,700 physicians.[12]

To some extent, Nash notes, the shortages may reflect the maldistribution of U.S. physicians, who are concentrated in major urban centers. The PCP-to-population ratio in rural areas is only 39.8 per 100,000 people, compared to 53.3 in urban areas, according to the CMS.[13]

Consultant David Zetter points out, however, there would still be a primary care shortage even if PCPs were better distributed. "Take Houston," he says. "It's classified as a physician shortage area, although it's a very large metro area. A lot of primary care doctors are booked up there, and they're not taking new patients."

Midlevel Practitioners

The numbers of NPs and PAs have grown rapidly in recent years, along with opportunities in primary care and other specialties. Currently, more than 270,000 NPs are licensed in the United States, compared to 106,703 in 2010. Nearly three-quarters of today's NPs deliver primary care, up from 52% in 2010; there are now about 200,000 NPs in primary care—nearly four times as many as there were a decade ago.

During the same period, the number of PAs has increased from 70,383 to over 131,000. Of these clinicians, however, just 24% deliver primary care.[14-16]

Studies have shown that NPs can manage 80%–90% of the care provided by PCPs with comparable patient outcomes. Moreover, training an NP takes only half the time required to train a primary care doctor, and NPs earn less than half of what PCPs make, on average.[17]

Thomas Bodenheimer, MD, professor emeritus of family and community medicine at the University of California San Francisco and a leading expert on primary care, says that NPs and PAs can do most of what a primary care doctor does. "I think they're indistinguishable. They can handle acute and chronic care and behavioral problems. NPs and PAs are dealing with all that stuff, and a lot of them are doing a very good job."

But David Boles, DO, who works closely with NPs, says they're not the same as doctors. For one thing, he notes, a midlevel practitioner is much more likely than an experienced physician to refer a patient to a specialist. "For example, when you have a diabetic patient, you have to document that you're looking at their kidneys. Virtually all of the midlevels think that means a nephrology consult."

Nash takes an intermediate position on this issue. Non-physician clinicians are fine for handling routine visits, he says, but a complex patient requires more expertise. "If a patient has multiple chronic conditions, the doctor ought to be much more intimately involved," he says. "But thankfully, in primary care, most people are well most of the time. So that's perfect for the NP or the PA."

Alternative Care Settings

Millions of consumers receive primary care in alternative care settings such as retail clinics, urgent care centers, and standalone ERs. These facilities mainly treat minor acute problems, although some retail clinics are starting to morph into full-service operations. Telehealth services also deliver primary care on an episodic basis.

In recent years, these alternative care settings have mushroomed across the country. From 2016 to 2017, for example, the use of retail clinics increased 7%; use of urgent care centers rose 14%; and the number of insurance claims submitted for telehealth services jumped 53%. From 2008 to 2017, urgent care center usage increased by 14 times and that of retail clinics, nearly seven times from a very small base. Telehealth utilization increased by a factor of 12 from 2012 to 2017.[18]

Meanwhile, the number of alternative care facilities also has grown rapidly. There are now about 2,200 retail clinics, of which half are operated by CVS or Walgreens.[19] The number of urgent care clinics jumped from 6,100 in 2013 to 8,774 in November 2018, according to the Urgent Care Association.[20] And in 2017, there were between 550 and 600 standalone ERs.[21]

Hospitals and health systems have become major players in the urgent care business. Ownership of urgent care clinics (UCCs) helps hospitals recapture some of the business that independent UCCs have diverted from their emergency departments (also true of standalone EDs). In addition, hospital-owned or identified UCCs provide a branding opportunity that can help pull patients into the parent health system for more complex needs. In 2014, hospitals owned 37% of UCCs. More recently, they have partnered with independent UCC operators to tap their expertise in retail care.[22-23]

Comparable primary care services are reimbursed at about the same rates in physician offices and retail clinics, which are staffed mainly by nurse practitioners, but urgent care centers and standalone ERs receive higher payments. What is more concerning to primary care physicians like David Boles is that these alternative venues are taking many of the easy cases that are the most profitable because they require the least time.

"It's the icing that they [alternative care settings] are taking," Boles says. "If I see 25 patients in a day, it will be 25 complicated patients. During the flu season, we used to be covered up in flu patients. I used to see those people between the harder patients, and they're not there now."

Another problem with the episodic care provided in alternative sites—including the one-off consultations with telehealth doctors—is that it's not connected to the patients' ongoing healthcare. About half of the 40 million consumers who visit retail clinics don't have a regular primary care physician, notes Nash. And for those who do, it's unlikely that the notes from their encounter with an urgent care physician or a telehealth doctor will be transmitted to their PCP. So, U.S. healthcare, which was already fragmented, is becoming even more chaotic.

"There's nothing wrong with the urgent care or the retail clinics, as long as there's a primary care physician that the patient has a relationship with," Bodenheimer comments. "And if a person goes to a retail clinic or urgent care clinic, the data from the encounter should come back to the doctor. But generally, they're quite separate."

As we've seen, more competition from alternative care settings is on the horizon as CVS and Walgreens gear up to provide full-spectrum primary care in their pharmacies. And Humana is taking telehealth in a radically new direction by offering a low-cost health plan that emphasizes virtual care in partnership with telehealth service Doctor on Demand.[24]

The prevalent explanation for the explosion of alternative care settings is that, because primary care providers are in short supply, patients' access to them has been reduced. There *is* a primary care shortage, as discussed earlier, and some doctors don't want to expand their hours to see more patients. But the majority of family physicians have walk-in hours or offer same-day access to their practices,[25] and many offer extended hours. So it's not just a lack of access that's driving many people into retail and urgent care clinics. Consumers are also looking for convenience, and millennials, in particular, may not see the need to have a personal physician, Bodenheimer notes.

Self-referral to Specialists

Back in the 1990s, during the first wave of managed care, primary care doctors were designated as HMO "gatekeepers" who controlled access to specialists. Patient dissatisfaction over not being able to see whichever physician they wanted to see contributed to the collapse of the managed care trend. To mollify their employer customers, insurance companies offered wider physician networks and allowed their members to self-refer to specialists.

Today, many people, especially in the Northeast, go directly to specialists for a wide variety of complaints. At the same time, primary care physicians have become prone to refer their more complex patients to specialists, even if they could handle some of these cases themselves.

Robert Berenson of the Urban Institute recalls that when he needed surgery for spinal stenosis, all his primary care physician did was clear him for surgery. "He compared my new EKG to the old EKG and said it's abnormal, but it's always been abnormal. He's very well trained, but he's made it clear he doesn't want to get involved in the more challenging diagnoses. Chronic back pain? Not his problem. He's happy to refer me."

Not all physicians welcome this turn of events. As recently as 10 years ago, Boles says, if a patient had a minor laceration, he'd take care of it in the office. Now he refers the patient to a specialist. There also are orthopedic practices with nurse practitioners who do primary care orthopedics, he notes. That takes away the strains and sprains that his practice used to handle.

The economics of primary care largely explain why generalist physicians refer out so frequently. "It's related to the rat-race factor: you have to see a certain number of patients each day to survive," says Boles. "It takes the physician less time to fire off a consult [with a specialist]."

Over time, this deference to specialists has resulted in primary care doctors losing skills and confidence in their ability to provide complex care. For one thing, PCPs no longer follow their patients in the hospital; hospitalists and specialists do that now. Even services that family physicians were trained to provide, such as sewing up minor cuts and setting simple fractures, seem more daunting when they haven't done them in a long time.

"When I trained in primary care, you were trained to feel like you should be able to handle a lot of stuff, and only refer patients when you couldn't," says Lawrence Casalino, MD, of Weill Cornell Medicine. "The main reason that PCPs refer out today is the pressure to see a lot of patients each day. And then gradually it becomes a habit and they lose confidence."

Decline in Primary Care Visits

One of the most telling indicators of where primary care is headed is this statistic: Office visits to primary care physicians declined 18% from 2012 to 2016 for adults under 65 years old with employer-sponsored health insurance. Office visits to NPs and PAs in primary care practices increased 129% during the same period. Balancing the decrease in PCP visits against the rise in visits to midlevel practitioners, however, office-based primary care encounters dropped by 160 per 1,000 people, or nearly 11%. Specialty office visits, in contrast, did not decline.[26]

Some of the drop in primary care office visits undoubtedly stems from the concurrent growth in the use of alternative care settings. Nash suggests it may also have something to do with the out-of-pocket costs that patients face with higher copayments and deductibles. With 40% of Americans only one paycheck away from poverty, he says, it's not surprising that doctor visits are down. Many patients only go to the doctor when they're really sick, he says, and that physician may well be a specialist.

Casalino agrees. "I wouldn't be surprised if more people are going straight to specialists, now that they don't have to go through [primary care] gatekeepers. It could be there's less access to PCPs. Urgent care centers are probably a factor, too."

Young Doctors Avoid Primary Care

Relatively few young physicians born in the United States are seeking careers in primary care. Of the 32,194 first-year residency positions offered in 2019, nearly half were in primary care fields. But about three-quarters of doctors who train in internal medicine will go on to subspecialize in fields such as endocrinology, allergy, and critical care. So roughly 30% of the 2019 residency slots were offered to doctors who planned to become PCPs. Most of these jobs were filled, but U.S.-born doctors matched to only 41% of the internal medicine positions, 39% of the family medicine positions, and 60% of the pediatric positions. The rest went to foreign-born physicians.[27]

The biggest reason for the reluctance of U.S. doctors to go into primary care is the disparity between the earnings of PCPs and specialists.[28] According to Medscape's 2019 survey of physician compensation, primary care physicians earn $237,000 a year, on average, compared to $341,000 for specialists. Some primary care doctors, such as pediatricians, make far less than the average; some specialists, such as orthopedic surgeons, earn far more.[29]

Medical school debt also plays a role in young doctors' avoidance of primary care. Nearly half of U.S. medical school graduates leave residency owing more than $200,000; therefore, the prospect of taking a primary care job at a comparatively low salary is not attractive to many new physicians.[30]

The Rule of the RUC

Why do specialists—and particularly surgeons—earn so much more than primary care physicians? In a nutshell, it's because surgical procedures and specialized knowledge are much more highly remunerated than primary care. And who decides the relative amounts that should be paid for different kinds of work? Specialists.

Here's how it works: The Medicare physician fee schedule is based on a nearly 30-year-old system known as the Resource-Based Relative Value Scale (RBRVS). This system weights the value of every medical service according to the amount of work required, the associated practice expense, and malpractice costs. Every five years, the RBRVS is updated by the American Medical Association's Relative Value Scale Update Committee (RUC), which is composed mainly of specialists. CMS generally accepts the RUC's recommendations and uses them in determining the Medicare fee schedule. Private insurers also follow the RUC's weighting system, but many health plans pay specialists even more compared to primary care doctors.

The gap between specialist and primary care incomes has widened further because of the increasing volume of many specialist procedures. The number of colonoscopies, minor surgeries, and imaging tests paid for by Medicare, for instance, has risen at a much faster rate than the number of evaluation and management (E&M) services performed by primary care doctors. Multiplying the higher reimbursement for procedures times the increased number of those services largely explains why specialists earn so much more than do generalists.[31]

There are other reasons primary care is unattractive to young doctors and why so many older PCPs burn out and leave the field or retire. "The work is unbelievably difficult," Bodenheimer points out. "There are other specialties where the work is difficult. But a PCP, NP, or PA has to deal with a thousand different diagnoses, and a lot of people don't have diagnoses. Whereas if you're a urologist, you're dealing with about three things. Even a cardiologist is dealing with maybe 10 things. So primary care is really hard. Burnout is high among some specialties, but it's massive in primary care."

Death by EHR

On top of the inherent difficulty of the work, primary care physicians now have to deal with EHRs. Many doctors find these systems hard to use, and EHR documentation often spills over after hours, reducing their family time. In addition, there is a growing sense of frustration that computer data entry is coming between doctors and their patients.

A time-motion study of 57 doctors, 23 of whom were in primary care, throws this malaise into stark relief. During a typical office day, the physicians spent 27% of their work hours on direct clinical face time with patients and 49% of their time on EHR and desk work. During patient exams, doctors were tapping on their computers 37% of the time. Twenty-one of the physicians reported they did one to two hours of after-hours work each night, mostly on their EHRs.[32]

The researchers observed that in 2016, 54% of U.S. physicians experienced some sign of burnout, up from 46% in 2011–2014. This is not proof that EHRs were to blame, but the period of increasing burnout coincided with the major growth in physicians' use of these systems.

Jeffrey Pearson, DO, a family physician in Carlsbad, Calif., left his solo practice to join a large group in 2012, mainly because of the expense of buying an EHR. He left the group recently to restart his private practice, largely because he was burned out from using the EHR. Between these work situations, he took off four months and says he spent two hours a day for half of that time just catching up on his electronic charts.

Partly because of the amount of time devoted to entering data in EHRs, physicians have less time to interact with patients than they used to. This and the "checkbox mentality" fostered by the relentless quality measurement to which physicians are now subjected have harmed the doctor-patient relationship, suggests Timothy J. Hoff in his book *Next in Line: Lowered Care Expectations in the Age of Retail and Value-Based Health*.[33] Thus, technologically driven efforts to standardize care and improve quality have undermined one of the foundational elements of good healthcare.

Other factors in physician burnout include too many "bureaucratic tasks" related to compliance with government and insurance requirements; spending too many hours at work; insufficient income; feelings of depersonalization and emotional exhaustion; and poor work-life balance.[34]

Farzad Mostashari, the former national coordinator of health IT and the CEO of Aledade, cites a study showing that physician burnout is less prevalent in independent practices than in employed practices. That result may be counterintuitive, considering that hospitals promise to take administration burdens off doctors, he says. "But the independent doctors have lower rates of burnout because they have more control over their lives and more clinical autonomy."

DIRECT PRIMARY CARE

Numerous initiatives to save independent primary care have been launched over the years, with varying degrees of success. These initiatives and trends fall roughly into three categories: prepayment for primary care outside of insurance, practice reengineering, and value-based contracting through ACOs and larger primary care groups. The rest of this chapter explores these efforts to resuscitate primary care.

Prepayment for primary care is usually associated with a capitation payment—that is, a set amount per member per month—from an insurance company. In contrast, the kind of prepayment discussed here comes from patients, usually in addition to a patient's insurance.

Such arrangements are further subdivided into "concierge" arrangements and "direct" primary care. A concierge practice usually accepts private insurance and government programs. In addition, it offers enhanced services and enhanced access to a primary care physician for annual or monthly fees. Because these fees are fairly high, the concierge approach is designed for affluent people. As a result, the approach is inherently limited. Also, while this strategy can increase physician incomes, practices must still cope with insurance requirements.

A direct primary care (DPC) practice, in contrast, doesn't accept insurance or participate in Medicare or Medicaid. The practice derives all of its income from monthly membership fees. In return for these fees, which are generally lower than those of concierge practices, patients receive extended visits, clinical, lab and consultative services, care coordination, and comprehensive care management. Most DPC practices advise patients to purchase high-deductible insurance to cover any non-primary care services they may need.[35]

Growing Trend

There are around 800 DPC practices in the United States, and the number is growing.[36] Many primary care physicians find the idea of not having to deal with insurance companies appealing. It's a leap to give up all insurance payments, but there seems to be a market for direct primary care, especially among people who are uninsured or have high-deductible plans.

DPC practices usually charge less than $100 a month.[37] Rob Lamberts, MD, a Georgia primary care doctor who is board-certified in internal medicine and pediatrics, charges just $50 a month. That keeps his practice affordable for most patients, including those on Medicaid, he says.

Lamberts launched his solo DPC practice after leaving a group practice in 2012. In that practice, he handled between 2,000 and 3,000 patients, and his office visits were usually very brief. In his current practice, he has only about 800 patients and can spend up to half an hour with any patient who needs it.

The majority of Lamberts' interactions with patients occur via text messaging or email. He has three times as many of these virtual visits as in-person visits. Lamberts averages eight to 10 face-to-face encounters with patients daily; on his busiest day, he might see 15 patients.

Despite this, he says he is earning as much as he was before. Moreover, he doesn't have to deal with all of the administrative and billing-related tasks that take much of a physician's time and effort in traditional practices. And he doesn't have to pay someone to file insurance claims and follow up on them.

The DPC financial numbers are compelling. At $50 per month, or $600 per year, 800 patients generate nearly $500,000. As a rule of thumb, primary care physicians earn about half of their gross, and Lamberts has less overhead than most primary care doctors do. Therefore, his income must be equal to or above the average for a primary care physician.

Just as important, he enjoys his work and feels much better about the care he provides than he used to. Many doctors see 30–40 patients a day, he says, "and they go home feeling abused and dirty and like they haven't given good care, and I don't have that problem in my practice."

Low Overhead

Jeff Pearson, the California family physician, launched a cash-only primary care practice in 2018 after being in a large group for several years. While he doesn't charge patients a monthly fee, he charges less than other practices in his area for the same services. He can do that, he says, because his overhead is very low.

Pearson sees only 10 people a day, on average, compared to 20–25 people in his previous practice. He spends 20 minutes to half an hour with each of his patients, rather than the seven minutes he gave each of them, on average, when he was with the group practice. Although he doesn't accept insurance, he says, his patients may pay him less out of pocket than they'd pay a traditional practice if they have high-deductible insurance or no insurance.

Lamberts and Pearson like their cash-only practices because they don't have to cope with insurance rules, have low overhead, and can spend more time with patients. This approach also benefits their patients, who receive better care in some ways than they would in a practice that accepts insurance. But as some observers point out, the cash-only approach has one glaring flaw: if a significant fraction of practices adopted it, it would reduce patients' access to care.

"If these physicians really cut their panel size dramatically, you say, 'What if all primary care doctors did that?'" Bodenheimer notes. "The capacity for primary care practices to meet demand would be much less than it is now—and it's already too low."

In Lamberts' view, however, "access is in the eye of the beholder. If your access is to a doctor who sees 30 patients a day, and you get five minutes of their time and you wait two hours, that's true. We can't give all those people a sliver of our time like they do. But my patients have far more access to me."

PRACTICE REENGINEERING

The most widespread initiative to improve and strengthen primary care is the patient-centered medical home (PCMH) movement. Originally propounded and piloted by the AAFP, the PCMH concept was endorsed in 2007 by medical societies representing family physicians, internists, and pediatricians. Since then, the PCMH movement has grown rapidly, partly because many private insurers pay bonuses to practices that have been officially recognized as PCMHs. A 2017 AAFP/Humana survey found that nearly half of family physicians worked in such practices.[38]

While practices don't have to be recognized PCMHs to participate in CMS' Comprehensive Primary Care Plus (CPC+) program (see Chapter 2), CPC+ requires roughly the same capabilities that PCMH recognition does. In addition, the PCMH goal of delivering higher quality care at lower cost aligns with the incentives of CMS's Merit-Based Incentive Payment System (MIPS), in which the majority of primary care physicians are required to participate.[39]

In a 2010 article, Nash provided this definition of a PCMH:

> The patient-centered medical home (PCMH) is essentially delivery of holistic primary care based on ongoing, stable relationships between patients and their personal physicians. It is characterized by physician-directed integrated care teams, coordinated care, improved quality through the use of disease registries and health information technology, and enhanced access to care.[40]

The 2007 statement by the primary care medical societies says that a PCMH requires:

- A personal physician who is the first contact for his or her patients and who provides continuous and comprehensive care;
- A physician-led care team that takes collective responsibility for care;
- A "whole person" orientation, meaning that the personal physician will provide for all of a patient's health needs and arrange referrals to other health professionals as needed;
- Care coordination across all care settings, facilitated by information technology and health information exchange;
- An emphasis on delivering high-quality, safe care in partnership with patients and their families;
- Enhanced access to care through open scheduling, expanded hours, and improved communication among physicians, staff, and patients via secure email and other modes; and
- Additional reimbursement to reflect the value of the PCMH's activities and the costs of setting up the necessary infrastructure.[41]

The National Committee for Quality Assurance (NCQA), one of the entities that certifies medical homes, has broken down these requirements into more specific categories and criteria, but the fundamental idea remains the same: rebuild primary care from the ground up based on the principle that the patient, rather than the physician, should be at the center of healthcare. Secondarily, primary care is posited as being at the center of the healthcare system. From this viewpoint, patients are best served if they allow their PCP to guide them through the system. In addition, the PCMH is viewed as a cost-saving innovation that can succeed only if it receives additional resources from payers, including an upfront investment in infrastructure.

Grueling Process of Change

The process of transforming a primary care practice into a patient-centered medical home is grueling, expensive, and time-consuming. In an evaluation of the practices in the AAFP's first PCMH pilot, researchers noted that "transformation to a PCMH requires a continuous, unrelenting process of change. It represents a fundamental reimagination and redesign of practice, replacing old patterns and processes with new ones."[42]

One obstacle participating practices faced was that their EHR systems were not up to the task. A number of the features required for improving care coordination and managing population health were missing from the EHRs, requiring the addition of new software. Physicians also had to move from a doctor-centered workflow to one in which they delegated more to office staff. Moreover, they had to learn how to consult patients about their goals rather than simply follow practice guidelines or the care processes they were used to. Change fatigue was also a real challenge for most of the practices.

The NCQA, which claims that 24% of primary care doctors practice in a PCMH it certified, has systematized the measurement of a practice's progress toward becoming a medical home.[43] However, Bodenheimer wonders how many practices recognized as medical homes have truly transformed themselves and how many have just checked the required boxes.

"What I've found is that a lot of people want to get PCMH recognition for marketing purposes," he says. "So they fill out the checkboxes and send all these documents in, but their practices don't change at all. Other practices get their recognition, and they realize that that's just step number one. What they now have to do is make the changes. But I don't think just getting the [PCMH] recognition is associated with better care, necessarily."

Positive Results

Several health plans have documented positive results from PCMHs. The PCMH program of Blue Cross Blue Shield of Michigan, for instance, includes about 4,500 primary care doctors in 1,600 practices. According to the company, these PCMHs were instrumental in reducing adult ER visits by 15% and in cutting preventable adult hospitalizations by 21%.[44]

The Patient-Centered Primary Care Collaborative (PCPCC) and the Robert Graham Center, both nonprofit research organizations focused on primary care, assessed 45 peer-reviewed papers on PCMHs. The majority of the 13 studies that looked at cost found that the PCMH was associated with a lower total cost of care. The association was stronger for mature PCMHs and for those that cared for patients with more complex conditions.

However, the review paper noted, "Few peer-reviewed studies that showed cost savings commented on the cost of transformation or whether they took this into consideration in their analysis."

The results were also mixed for quality improvement, with fewer than half of the studies reporting the PCMH had a positive impact. In his earlier-cited book, Hoff cites research showing that the achievement of PCMH recognition "does not always guarantee better patient care, patient experiences or doctor-patient relationships."[45]

Besides the challenges of practice transformation noted above, and the reluctance of some PCMHs to do the hard work required, the biggest barrier to achieving the potential of the PCMH is the relative powerlessness of primary care practices. In the early years of the movement, it was hoped that specialists, hospitals, and other providers—known collectively as "the medical neighborhood"—would cooperate with PCMHs to improve care and lower costs. But on the whole, these hopes have not panned out.

A report from the PCPCC and the Robert Graham Center cited this issue in explaining the somewhat disappointing results of PCMHs in many studies.

> Where results were mixed, some observers noted expected returns on overall cost and quality from PCMH transformation were unrealistic, given the isolation of these interventions to primary care and the lack of buy-in from a broader medical neighborhood of providers in other health care settings, such as specialists and hospital-based providers.[46]

Team-based Care

Despite the barriers that PCMHs have encountered, the practice reengineering trend has continued, with an increased emphasis on how to duplicate what high-performing practices have achieved. In a 2014 paper, Bodenheimer and his colleagues described the 10 building blocks of such groups after studying 23 of them. The building blocks included a wide variety of characteristics, ranging from engaged leadership, data-driven improvement, and population health management to continuity of care, prompt access to care, and comprehensive care coordination. But at the heart of their success formula was the use of care teams.

The need for care teams is based on the fact that primary care providers are expected to deliver all recommended care for large and growing patient panels. "Clinicians without teams caring for a panel of 2,500 patients would spend 17.4 hours per day providing recommended acute, chronic and preventive care," the building blocks study said. By sharing the care with well-trained non-clinicians in a care team, the coauthors noted, practices can add capacity and reduce the burden on clinicians.[47]

In a recent article, Bodenheimer described how these teams work. Advanced primary care teams, he wrote, include a core team or "teamlet" and an extended team. The core team, to which individual patients are attached, consists of a physician or a midlevel practitioner and one or more medical assistants. The extended team, which may include registered nurses, pharmacists, social workers, and behavioral health providers, supports several teamlets. These health professionals always work together, and patients on the care team's panel receive all of their care from the core and extended teams.

According to Bodenheimer, the medical assistants in the core teams can be trained to "independently identify and close care gaps" such as overdue cancer screenings, immunizations, and routine diabetes services. RNs and pharmacists can be empowered to "independently care for patients with uncomplicated diabetes or hypertension, including titrating medication doses within standing orders."

Bodenheimer cited several studies showing that team-based care of this type can have a major impact on the cost and quality of care. In one study, chronically ill patients in 18 Boston-area primary care practices that used team-based care had an 18% reduction in hospitalizations and a 36% reduction in ambulatory care-sensitive ED visits, compared to control practices. Among healthier patients, however, there was an increase in outpatient visits and hospitalizations.

At Intermountain Healthcare, which has a long history of team-building, diabetic patients treated in practices that used team care, compared with patients in practices that didn't, had higher rates of diabetes control, lower lipoprotein cholesterol levels, and fewer hospital admissions and ED visits.

"The survival of primary care depends on sharing the care," Bodenheimer's article concluded. "Primary care panels are too large and cannot be reduced because of the clinician shortage."[48]

Better Care for More People

In an interview, Bodenheimer said he believed that primary care physicians could provide excellent care to 2,000 patients each "if they had dramatic changes in their teams. I firmly believe that nurses and pharmacists could take care of 90% of people with diabetes and hypertension without a doctor spending one second with those patients. They'd need standing orders and protocols, but they could do it."

The big problem is insurance reimbursement, he added. Most PCPs are paid fee for service for encounters with patients. Any services provided by staff members are incidental to the doctor's work and aren't separately paid for. Risk-based arrangements could eliminate this issue, but the payment system is still predominantly fee for service, he noted.

Another challenge is the high cost of the ancillary team members. "Care teams are a good idea," Casalino says. "But the jury is still out on whether you can increase revenue enough to pay for all those extra people."

In an unpublished study submitted to Mayo Clinic Proceedings, Bodenheimer found that, at the Bellin Clinic in Green Bay, Wisc., the addition of a second medical assistant to each doctor's team more than paid for itself because clinicians were able to see more patients as a result. He hypothesized that an extended team of RNs, pharmacists, and physical therapists could increase practice capacity by up to 200%.[49] That would increase revenues, but it's not clear whether it would cover the cost of the additional team members. What is clear, Bodenheimer told me, is that only larger groups or ACOs have the resources needed to implement this approach.

PHYSICIAN-LED ACOS

As noted earlier, ACOs led by physicians have a much better track record on cutting costs and improving quality than those dominated by hospitals. Because their incentive is to rein in utilization of specialists, hospitals, and expensive tests, physician-led ACOs tend to focus intensively on population health management and care coordination/care management. There is some evidence that primary care-only ACOs function best, perhaps because they are furthest upstream and can address chronic conditions while they are still manageable.

According to Mostashari, physician-led ACOs are the way forward for primary care physicians. In the fee-for-service world, he notes, "primary care docs are the lowest on the totem pole. They're paid less, and they become susceptible to being scooped up, whether it's by a larger group or a hospital. But in a value-based world, whether they participate in an ACO, a patient-centered medical home or CPC+, they can benefit from some real [health] outcomes, like lower hospitalization rates. A PCP that's taking Medicare Advantage risk in Florida or California can make urologist money, as much as $400,000–$500,000 a year. So that to me is the way forward for primary care. It's the unique edge that they have in value-based care."

Mostashari's own company, Aledade, which helps primary care practices form ACOs, is an exemplar of this trend. In 2018, Aledade's ACOs in the MSSP saved Medicare more than $69 million, according to a company news release. All of the Aledade ACOs—which now number 38 MSSP ACOs and 42 non-MSSP ACOs and average about 100 doctors each—improved the quality of care and the health of their patients.[50]

Of course, that's Aledade's story. But several experts interviewed for this chapter praised what the company has done, and Aledade recently partnered with the California Medical Association to recruit physicians for new ACOs in California.[51] The company currently has 25 commercial contracts and recently announced national deals with United and Aetna, Mostashari says.

Besides contracting on behalf of its client ACOs, Aledade also provides services and coaching to help them succeed in their risk contracts. For example, the firm sets up interfaces between practice EHRs and hospitals to facilitate data exchange, obtains claims data from payers, and installs a population health tool that rides on top of the 90 different EHRs used by its ACOs. This tool pulls relevant clinical data out of the EHRs and combines it with claims data to facilitate quality reporting to the MSSP and private payers, Mostashari explains.

Aledade splits the shared savings payments it receives from the MSSP with its doctors. Physicians that take upside-only risk get 50%, and those that take two-sided risk receive 60%. All of Aledade's expenses and profits come out of its share of the savings.

ACO Medical Director's View

To find out how this works at the level of the frontline doctor, I interviewed Jennifer Brull, MD, a family physician who is part of a small practice in Plainville, Kans., and is also a regional medical director for Aledade. When I first encountered Brull in 2014 as a reporter for *Medical Economics*, she was working hard with her colleagues to improve the quality of care in the practice.[52] Later, the practice won recognition as a patient-centered medical home.

Brull's group joined the Aledade ACO in Kansas in January 2016, and she soon become its medical director. At that time, the Kansas ACO included 12 practices. Now, as regional medical director, she manages four ACOs that include 35 practices, of which 19 are in Kansas. Nearly all of them are primary care-only groups.

Brull's original ACO did not take downside risk initially, because its practices had had no experience in risk management and were geographically separated. The Kansas ACO entered the MSSP in 2016. The next year, it added a contract with Blue Cross and Blue Shield of Kansas, and in 2019, it started working with Medicare Advantage and Medicaid plans.

The ACO practices did not qualify for MSSP bonuses in 2016 or 2017. However, they did reduce their costs and, when Brull was interviewed, they expected to receive shared savings for 2018. The ACO also achieved MSSP quality scores in the 98th percentile—the highest for any Aledade ACO.

The Blues contract gave the ACO quality bonuses from the get-go. The largest group in the ACO received a check for $500,000 in the first year, and Brull's practice took home $100,000. In 2019, the ACO initiated a two-sided risk contract with Blue Cross

Blue Shield. That will give the ACO the potential to earn bonuses for reducing the total cost of care.

Care Management Tools

The ACO benefits in several ways from the Aledade app integrated with its members' EHRs, Brull says. First, a statewide health information exchange sends admission-discharge-transfer (ADT) alerts for hospitals and EDs to Aledade, which populates the data in the app's dashboard. This is important information that helps the ACO manage care more effectively. The tool also extracts clinical data for quality reporting and analysis, and combines it with claims data to populate the dashboard for each practice. This not only saves a lot of time on manual chart review to report quality data, but also keeps physicians informed on their performance.

In some regions, Brull notes, Aledade hires care managers that work with multiple practices. In contrast, all of the practices in her ACO hired their own care managers. "Early on, we discovered that practices with care managers were doing much better than those that didn't," she says. "So we required it as practices joined the ACO." Her own practice, she adds, employs two care managers—an RN and a social worker—whom she regards as essential.

When her group first joined the ACO, it participated only in the MSSP. "About 25% of my patients were on Medicare, so 25% of them were in value-based care," she notes. "We've since added commercial and Medicare Advantage contracts, and right now about 80% of my patients are under value-based care. That's really good, because you want to do these things for all your patients, and you can do them and their insurance pays for it."

Overall, Brull feels that the ACO is helping her practice remain independent. "I don't know whether Aledade is the ACO partner that will do this, but I do think if an independent practice can successfully make the transition from fee-for-service-based care to value-based care, that's how they're going to stay alive. So joining an ACO like this is one of the solutions."

CONCLUSION

U.S. primary care is in poor shape, but there are opportunities for it to climb out of its slump. In fact, as value-based reimbursement grows and fee for service declines, primary care physicians are bound to become more important in healthcare than they are today. Primary care doctors are ideally positioned to work with patients to maintain their health and to detect and treat chronic conditions early; by providing intensive care management, their practices can also help sicker patients control their diseases so that they don't end up in the hospital or the ER or being handed off from one specialist to another. What this all adds up to is better outcomes for patients and lower costs for those who pay the bills.

The plight of primary care, however, will not be resolved under our current system. A large portion of primary care doctors work for hospitals, which, as we've seen, are less than thrilled about the idea of value-based care. Physicians need to be liberated from hospital employment so they can form independent groups capable of taking financial risk. When that happens, and when primary care controls the healthcare system, primary care doctors working as part of care teams will be able to show what they can do to reduce the total cost of care.

Nevertheless, we're a long way from that promised land. Hospitals are still intent on filling beds, and 70% of physician practice revenue, on average, remains tied to fee for service,[53] which encourages the provision of wasteful services. The next chapter examines where all the waste in American healthcare comes from and how we can cut it down to size.

CHAPTER 5

Waste Not, Want Not

Vertebroplasty is a surgical procedure designed to alleviate severe, disabling back pain caused by a compression fracture in a vertebra. Unfortunately for patients with this condition, there is no solid evidence that vertebroplasty is effective.

In 2009, a pair of randomized controlled trials of vertebroplasty were published in the *New England Journal of Medicine*.[1-2] These studies found that one month and six months after the procedure was done, there were no significant differences in the amount of pain reported by patients in the study and control groups. A similar study published in 2018 in the *BMJ* reported the same results through a year of follow-up.[3] A 2018 review paper by the international Cochrane Collaborative stated, "High-quality evidence shows that vertebroplasty does not provide more clinically important benefits than placebo."[4]

Despite these findings, surgeons frequently perform vertebroplasties—as well as a related procedure, kyphoplasty—"because they are highly profitable," says Grace Terrell, MD, the former CEO of the Cornerstone Health Care Group. Claire Neely, MD, president and CEO of the Institute for Clinical Systems Improvement (ICSI) in Bloomington, Minn., which has created a clinical practice guideline for low back pain, agrees that vertebroplasties are overused.

This is just one example of the systemic waste that drives up health costs without improving patient outcomes. The Institute of Medicine (IOM), in its landmark book *Crossing the Quality Chasm*, said:

> A highly fragmented delivery system that largely lacks even rudimentary clinical information capabilities results in poorly designed care processes characterized by unnecessary duplication of services and long waiting times and delays. And there is substantial evidence documenting overuse of many services—services for which the potential risk of harm outweighs the potential benefits.[5]

Since 2001, when the IOM published this book, clinical information has been largely digitized, and health information exchange has improved. But healthcare waste is still widespread. In fact, it has been estimated that 30% or more of U.S. healthcare spending is unnecessary.

In 2010, an IOM panel calculated that the annual excess cost from systemic waste was approximately 30% of total health costs, or $765 billion in that year. Nearly half of that total represented unnecessary services ($210 billion) and inefficiently delivered services

($130 billion). The rest included $190 billion in excess administrative costs, $105 billion in excessively high prices, $55 billion in missed opportunities for disease prevention, and $75 billion in fraud.[6]

In a 2012 paper, Donald M. Berwick, MD, who had just stepped down as acting CMS administrator, and Andrew D. Hackbarth, a RAND Corp. researcher, estimated that healthcare waste, including unnecessary treatments, overpriced drugs and procedures, and the underuse of preventive care, represented 34% of U.S. health spending. The coauthors stated:

> In just six categories of waste—overtreatment, failures of care coordination, failures in execution of care processes, administrative complexity, pricing failures, and fraud and abuse—the sum of the lowest available estimates exceeds 20% of total health care expenditures. The actual total may be far greater.[7]

Administrative Waste

Administrative complexity was the largest single category of waste in these researchers' analysis. In 2011, they found, it wasted between $107 billion and $389 billion. Under their definition, these unnecessary costs stemmed from the "inefficient or misguided" rules of government, private payers, accreditation agencies, and others. One example is the lack of standardization in billing forms, which forces physicians and staff members to do extra work unrelated to patient care.

The Institute of Medicine in 2010 estimated that about 14% of healthcare spending was generated by billing and insurance-related activities.[8] Today, the Center for American Progress estimates, the United States spends nearly $500 billion a year on billing and insurance processing—far more than any other country as a percentage of our national health expenditures.[9]

As explained in Chapter 1, there's a debate over how much Medicare for All would cut these administrative costs. It would be a substantial drop, but there are other ways to reduce administrative spending besides going to a single-payer system.

For example, former Obama Administration official Ezekiel Emanuel, MD, pointed out in a *New York Times* op-ed that an independent commission "could create a clearinghouse for processing all medical bills with uniform standardized electronic formats for all insurers." This approach has been very successful in Germany and Japan, he said.[10]

In an interview, Berwick told me that administrative complexity encompasses not only a failure of cooperation among payers, but also "silly rules, unnecessary restrictions, and reporting requirements that have no value." With "good solid leadership and a rational payment system," he added, administrative costs could be greatly reduced without instituting Medicare for All.

If the United States did move to a single-payer system, he said, he hopes it would result in a switch from fee-for-service payments to global budgeting and "population-based payments." If that happened, he added, insurance- and billing-related waste would be largely eliminated.

Meanwhile, the processes of care delivery would continue to drive up costs, as noted earlier. Much of this spending growth stems from overuse, misuse and underuse of services, safety issues, poor care coordination, and a lack of adherence to best practices.

Overtreatment Is Widespread

The full extent of overtreatment in U.S. healthcare is unclear; however, landmark research by Elliott Fisher, MD, the father of the ACO, and his colleagues at Dartmouth Medical School showed that nearly a third of Medicare spending pays for services that don't improve health. Medicare costs in the most expensive areas of the United States, the researchers found, were about 60% higher than those in the least expensive areas,[11] but the extra spending didn't improve patient outcomes. Patients hospitalized in the low-cost areas for hip fracture, colorectal cancer, and acute myocardial infarction had outcomes that were just as good as those of similarly ill patients in the high-cost regions.[12]

While rates of major surgery didn't vary greatly across the country, one of the Dartmouth studies found, patients had more tests and more minor procedures in the high-cost areas. The paper concluded that regional differences in Medicare spending "are due almost entirely to use of discretionary services that are sensitive to the local supply of physicians and hospital resources: more frequent physician visits, greater use of specialists, and greater use of the hospital and intensive care units as sites of care."[13]

Some of these services are provided despite clear evidence that they don't help and may even harm patients. One study of geographical variations in healthcare found "significant levels of inappropriate use: 17% of cases for coronary angiography, 32% for carotid endarterectomy, and 17% for upper gastrointestinal tract endoscopy."[14]

The McAllen Syndrome

In a famous *New Yorker* article published in 2009, Atul Gawande, MD, explored the overutilization of healthcare in McAllen, Tex. Although McAllen was one of the poorest cities in the country, it was the second most expensive market in the country for Medicare. The relatively poor health of McAllen area residents wasn't to blame; El Paso, Tex., had similar health statistics, yet half as much was spent on Medicare patients in El Paso as in as McAllen. Doctors also received similar training in both cities.[15]

One surgeon interviewed by Gawande attributed the high costs in McAllen to overutilization of procedures. For example, surgeons operated right away on gallstones rather than waiting to see if the pain went away. Patients with chest pain were immediately catheterized. So the difference in costs between McAllen and other areas of the country appeared to be at least partly linked to differences in practice patterns.

Similar relationships between practice patterns and costs have been observed in other parts of the United States. One study found that those patterns were principally responsible for the difference in Medicare costs per beneficiary between Miami ($13,596) and Minneapolis ($7,998).[16]

In a follow-up *New Yorker* article in 2015, Gawande reported that between 2009 and 2012, McAllen's health costs had dropped by almost $3,000 per Medicare recipient. Inpatient visits had decreased by 10%, and home health spending by 40%. In total, these changes saved Medicare half a billion dollars, Gawande said.[17]

The national focus on McAllen as a result of his first article had something to do with this, he wrote. Federal prosecutors had cracked down on fraud in the market, and a local hospital had launched a campaign to reduce unnecessary care. But the major reason for the change, Gawande said, was local primary care physicians who changed their practice patterns to garner bonuses from Medicare Advantage plans. One top-performing doctor, for example, built a team around his patients, including cardiologists and surgeons. He selected specialists who didn't order no-value care and persuaded his patients to shift to them.

Another factor driving up costs in McAllen was home healthcare. The area had hundreds of home health agencies, some of them owned by physicians. One local primary care-led ACO, the Rio Grande Valley Health Alliance (RGVHA), used data analysis to determine that some non-ACO physicians were ordering home care at a rate far above the national average and that many of these orders failed to meet Medicare requirements. By persuading these physicians to provide better care coordination, RGVHA cut its home care costs by 41% over two years, said Victoria Farias, the ACO's program administrator, in a *Group Practice Journal* article.[18]

Underuse of Services

Besides overtreatment, underuse of recommended services also generates waste when a lack of appropriate preventive and/or chronic-disease care leads to preventable ED visits and hospital admissions. Patients also may be harmed because of underuse. For example, cancer diagnoses may be delayed when patients aren't screened in a timely manner. Similarly, patients with diabetes who don't receive timely care and don't manage their condition may become severely ill and may have limbs amputated in extreme cases.

It's difficult to measure underuse because it consists of potentially beneficial services not provided to patients.[19] But an often-cited study by Elizabeth McGlynn and her RAND colleagues found that U.S. adults received only 55% of recommended acute, preventive, and chronic care services. Adherence to these care processes ranged from

52% for screening tests to 59% for follow-up care. There were wider variations in adherence among different health conditions.[20]

Overall, the researchers found underuse to be a greater problem than overuse. For example, patients with hypertension received 65% of recommended care. High blood pressure is linked to increased risk for heart disease, stroke, and death, and poor blood pressure control contributes to over 68,000 preventable deaths annually, the paper noted. Although the study didn't look at financial costs, the underuse of recommended care for hypertension undoubtedly drives a lot of avoidable ER visits and hospital admissions.

Safety Issues

Medical errors—estimated to cause upwards of 98,000 deaths per year in hospitals alone[21]—also account for a significant amount of waste in the system. To prevent these errors, a hospital must develop a "safety culture" as part of its quality improvement efforts, says Kedar Mate, MD, chief innovation and information officer at the Boston-based Institute for Healthcare Improvement (IHI).

"In a safety culture, the causal pathway to increasing value is through the avoidance of defects," Mate says. He draws an analogy to the continuous quality improvement process used by Japanese auto manufacturers to improve their cars and to prevent errors and slowdowns on the assembly line. "If you prevent defects, you avoid rework, which is where the true cost to the system lies," Mate notes. "Safety culture helps avoid the rework that is a source of waste and a source of bad outcomes for the individual patient."

Besides increasing complications, readmissions and other kinds of rework, the lack of a safety culture also leads to inefficient processes and a lack of reliability, Mate says. One example is poor planning of the patient flow in a hospital. "Failing to achieve hospital-wide patient flow—the right care, in the right place, at the right time—puts patients at risk for suboptimal care and potential harm," states an IHI white paper.[22]

IHI has found that when cost data are supplied to nurse supervisors and physician leaders in a hospital, they tend to tackle the sources of financial waste, Mate observes. "In many cases, we're seeing 20%–30% reductions in the cost basis of service delivery in these units," he says. "That's a combination of changing consumables [drugs and supplies], improving locums tenens utilization, and improving patient flow and throughput."

Hospitals are concerned about this kind of waste because it directly affects their bottom line in Medicare diagnosis-related groups (DRGs), which limit the amount Medicare pays for each case. When it comes to low-value care, however, many hospitals have a different attitude. For example, Mate says, healthcare resources are often wasted on inappropriate hospital admissions.

"I'm an inpatient physician and I've seen plenty of people admitted to the hospital who could have easily been managed in an outpatient environment, and were thereby exposed to the harms and risks of being hospitalized. And this becomes even more of a factor as patients age. We tend to hospitalize folks who have relatively minor ailments that can be treated in an outpatient setting."

Poor Care Coordination

Chronic diseases generate most healthcare spending. Hence there is a need for healthcare providers to build an infrastructure that can provide the full complement of services required by people with chronic conditions such as heart disease, diabetes, and asthma, the Institute of Medicine noted in *Crossing the Quality Chasm*. Yet this is the exception rather than the rule, the IOM pointed out:

> Physician groups, hospitals, and other health care organizations operate as silos, often providing care without the benefit of complete information about the patient's condition, medical history, services provided in other settings, or medications prescribed by other clinicians.[23]

Twenty years later, not much has changed. And it isn't just health information exchange that's inadequate; there's also a lack of coordination and teamwork across care settings. Hospitalist physicians and ambulatory care physicians don't usually have close working relationships, and ambulatory care doctors often don't receive discharge summaries before the patient makes a follow-up visit.[24] Primary care doctors count themselves lucky when they receive a report from a specialist they referred a patient to, and specialists frequently don't understand why patients were referred to them.[25] Ambulatory care coordinators are rarely employed except in practices that take financial risk, belong to ACOs, or qualify as patient-centered medical homes.

In Berwick and Hackbarth's paper on eliminating healthcare waste, failures of care coordination were estimated to cost between $25 billion and $45 billion in 2011—a relatively small sum compared to other major sources of waste. Yet inadequate care coordination, the authors noted, can lead to complications, hospital readmissions, and a decline in patients' abilities to function on their own.[26]

A bigger driver of waste, according to Berwick and Hackbarth, are failures of care delivery related to "poor execution of known best care processes, including, for example, patient safety systems and preventive care practices that have been shown to be effective. The results are patient injuries and worse clinical outcomes."[27]

GUIDELINES AND MEASURES

To promote the use of best care processes, specialty societies have created thousands of clinical practice guidelines. Healthcare systems and regional quality improvement organizations often tweak these guidelines for local use and/or develop their own guidelines for certain conditions, tests, and treatments. Currently, there is no up-to-date national database of guidelines. The Trump Administration defunded the National Guidelines Clearinghouse, which had been maintained by the Agency for Healthcare Research and Quality (AHRQ).

At one time, practice guidelines were based largely on expert opinion. Today, they're much more likely to be based on the best available evidence from clinical trials. The Institute of Medicine defines practice guidelines as "statements that include recommendations, intended to optimize patient care, that are informed by a systematic review of evidence and an assessment of the benefits and harms of alternative care options."[28]

This sounds reassuring, but in fact there are still large areas of ignorance and many gray areas in medicine. Solid, high-grade evidence justifies less than 50% and perhaps as little as 15% of what doctors do.[29] This is partly because there is no money to fund certain kinds of randomized clinical trials—the gold standard of medical evidence. In addition, there may be ethical issues involved in performing sham vs. real surgery. Also, as former ICSI Executive Director Gordon Mosser, MD, told me years ago, there are any number of decisions that doctors make for which there is no protocol, such as how to respond when a patient says they have an odd pain in the right side of their chest.

Even where there is good evidence, expert opinions still play a role in guidelines. "It is difficult to produce clinical practice guidelines that are completely evidence-based," Earl Steinberg, MD, and Bryan Luce, MD, stated in a 2005 *Health Affairs* article.[30]

Guidelines are still often based partly on expert opinion and community consensus, notes Ken Cohen, MD, chief medical officer of Denver-based New West Physicians and senior medical director of OptumCare, a division of the group's corporate parent. Wherever possible, he notes, New West selects guidelines based on large randomized controlled trials and large meta-analyses of studies. Specialists convened by New West then examine the evidence and make whatever changes they feel are necessary to each guideline. Even after that, he says, physicians can follow a guideline for only about 85% of their relevant patients; the other 15% require clinical judgment outside of the algorithm.

Barriers to Guideline Adherence

Even if a systematic literature review or a large, well-conducted clinical trial shows that a particular technique or drug is superior for treating a certain condition, the majority of physicians may not adopt it for many years. Among the reasons for this are inadequate dissemination of the data, poor educational methods, and a resistance to change. In some cases, physicians don't believe that their patients will accept certain treatments. This might explain why they were so slow to embrace antibiotic treatments for ulcers and why many doctors are still reluctant to prescribe diuretics as the first-line treatment for hypertension.

Physicians have good reasons for disbelieving the results of some clinical trials, based on the affiliations of the researchers with drug companies and other interested parties. Also, the subjects of clinical trials may not resemble the patient sitting in front of a doctor in an exam room. For example, researchers often exclude certain patients from a study because they have a comorbid condition in addition to the condition being studied. Yet the patient in the exam room may have one or more comorbidities.

Many clinical trials exclude people over 65. Consequently, the physician has no way of knowing whether the study's results apply to a Medicare patient. The same problem applies to children: pediatricians can't assume that because a particular medication worked in adults, it will help their patients. Women and minorities have long been underrepresented in clinical trials, Grace Terrell notes.

It's also hard for physicians to keep up with the literature. With more than 150,000 new studies being published each month,[31] doctors can only skim the surface of new knowledge. Online services that search the medical literature and boil down the most pertinent research—including UpToDate, DynaMed, the Cochrane Collaborative, and specialty-based "journal clubs"—help fill this gap. But high subscription costs deter many physicians from using these services.

Still, there are good evidence-based guidelines that cover many of the conditions that doctors diagnose and treat day in and day out. Why don't clinicians consistently follow these guidelines to reduce the amount of inappropriate and useless care they deliver?

One reason is that the guidelines are extremely long and detailed. Doctors aren't going to browse through a 30-page or a 100-page guideline to figure out how best to manage a patient who has a condition they have been treating for years. Moreover, they may not want to apply what they regard as "cookie cutter" guidelines to individual patients.

Malpractice concerns also affect how doctors approach guidelines. An old country doctor, asked why he didn't use a well-established rule to determine whether a patient had an ankle fracture without X-raying it, responded, "It's the patient's ankle, but it's my ass. I would rather X-ray 100 sprained ankles than go through the hassle of defending a single missed fracture in a malpractice suit."[32]

Crunching Down Guidelines

The Institute for Clinical Systems Integration (ICSI) has developed practice guidelines with input from Minnesota health organizations since the 1990s. In its formative period, ICSI was putting out one or two new evidence-based guidelines each year, creating a total of 56 protocols over a 12-year period. The ICSI guidelines were all derived from those issued by national specialty societies, but local physician input on portions of these protocols encouraged their adoption.[33]

Today, largely because of improvements in guideline development, ICSI takes ownership of only eight guidelines, says ICSI CEO Claire Neely, MD. Some of the other guidelines it has published summarize parts of existing protocols such as the massive stroke guideline released by the American College of Cardiology and the American Heart Association. "We consolidated that for the initial treatment—the first 48 hours after a stroke—to make it more usable," Neely says.

Even when ICSI crunches down guidelines to make them usable at the point of care, they can be several pages long. To make them more digestible, all ICSI guidelines have an algorithmic first page to help doctors think through how they build processes, develop workflows, or run through a diagnosis, Neely says.

ICSI has had a considerable impact in Minnesotan medicine, she notes. "In other parts of the country, I still hear about how do you get doctors to use guidelines and whether cookie cutter guidelines don't limit how people practice medicine. No one asks those questions in Minnesota anymore. People understand the value of a group of experts, clinical and operational, getting together to look at the evidence and deciding what makes sense to do. Not everybody likes every guideline, but it's accepted that this is an aid to practice."

Over the years, Neely adds, ICSI has moved from developing guidelines to exploring complex areas of medicine where the evidence is unclear, including opioid addiction, mental health problems, and patients with multiple comorbidities. In addition, ICSI focuses on the implementation of existing guidelines and on optimizing practice.

"Writing a guideline doesn't change anything," she declares. "Building a system that supports people in making those changes, educating folks, creating reminders and things like that is more where our work is."

Performance Measures

Many guidelines have been boiled down into quality measures that have real-world implications for physicians and hospitals. Specialty societies, CMS, and other parties are the stewards of these metrics. The National Quality Forum (NQF), a nonprofit organization, convenes multi-stakeholder committees that recommend submitted measures for endorsement. CMS has been using selected NQF-endorsed measures in its quality programs since 2011. Today, about 300 of these metrics are used in more than 20 federal public reporting and pay-for-performance programs, as well as private-sector quality initiatives. These metrics are related to clinically reported outcomes, patient-reported outcomes, intermediate outcomes, processes, efficiency, and cost/resource use.[34]

One might expect that these measures—especially when they're imbedded in EHRs—would spur greater adherence to best practices. But there is little evidence of that. Studies of insurer pay-for-performance programs failed to demonstrate that they moved the needle on quality.[35-36] Similarly, the average quality scores of ACOs in the Medicare Shared Savings Program (MSSP) were 95% in 2016, about the same as in 2012/2013.[37] This fact suggests that many clinicians were simply "checking off the boxes" to meet MSSP requirements for getting a portion of shared savings.

That's exactly the problem in today's value-based-care programs, says David Nash, MD, dean of the College of Population Health at Thomas Jefferson University. "Even though we're on the road to redemption with value-based care, the measures to get us there are blunt instruments—mostly process measures. It becomes a check-the-box mentality: did you order the mammogram, did you get the cholesterol checked, rather than a set of measures such as whether we're preventing hospitalization and self-reported measures of health."

Patient outcomes are notoriously hard to measure, Cohen notes. "[Intermediate] quality outcomes are easy to measure at a primary care level: what's the hypertension control of your population, the diabetes control, cancer screening rates. When you get to specialists, it becomes incredibly difficult to measure outcomes. The only way to do it is through what are called PROMs: patient-reported outcomes measures. How is the patient actually doing a year or two after a back operation? The vast majority of providers in this country are not measuring that."

Aside from the fact that there is no financial incentive for providers to measure long-term outcomes, many physicians are skeptical about the validity of patient reports. Moreover, if patient-reported data is to be used to measure outcomes, it must be integrated with electronic health records, probably through patient portals connected to EHRs. While this is feasible,[38] it isn't clear how patient-reported data could form the basis for outcomes measures.

In any case, physicians are already overwhelmed by a proliferation of quality measures from myriad private and public payers. As Nash quips, he's not sure how well he'd score on all of these metrics after having been in practice for 30 years. "There's no way to effectively keep up with the checklists."

Other physicians agree. In addition to having to pay attention to a variety of tasks that are not germane to the reason for a patient's visit, they must also document everything they did in the EHR—a very time-consuming chore. This is one reason around half of physicians say that EHRs reduce their efficiency.

In the current environment, physicians tend to view the emphasis on quality improvement as an onerous assignment that does not actually improve quality but does reduce their time with patients. "Physicians want to provide our patients with the best care possible, but today there are confusing, misaligned and burdensome regulatory programs that take away critical time physicians could be spending to provide high-quality care for their patients," commented Robert M. Wah, MD, then president of the American Medical Association, in 2014.[39]

CHOOSING WISELY

Quality measures aside, some physician leaders are concerned about how much unnecessary and inappropriate care is being provided to patients. In 2012, the American Board of Internal Medicine (ABIM) Foundation teamed with *Consumer Reports* to create a mechanism to inform doctors and patients about treatments and tests that specialty societies view as low-value. The Choosing Wisely campaign, which grew out of a proposal made by Howard Brody, MD, in the *New England Journal of Medicine*, now encompasses more than 80 specialty societies that have made more than 550 recommendations regarding unnecessary services. Choosing Wisely also has made available 110 patient handouts to inform discussions between doctors and patients. Nineteen other countries have started similar campaigns.[40-41]

The Choosing Wisely recommendations cover a broad range of situations. For example, one patient handout notes that some physicians place blood clot filters in patients who don't have leg clots but are at high risk for getting them. But filters don't prevent clots—only blood thinners can do that, the handout notes. Also, the filters present a number of health risks.

Another patient resource discusses bladder catheters that are placed in patients in hospitals and nursing homes when they have problems with bladder control. The handout notes that antibiotics should not be given to these patients unless they develop urinary tract infections. Indiscriminate use of antibiotics can lead to complications and more pathogen resistance.

Choosing Wisely also recommends against whole-body scans to screen for cancer, noting that these scans rarely find cancer in asymptomatic people and that many of these tumors would never cause a problem if left alone. Whole-body scans create health risks and can cost from $500 to $1,000 each, not counting follow-up tests, a handout observes.[42]

Impact of Choosing Wisely

Frontline physicians recognize the problem of low-value care. In a 2017 survey, the ABIM Foundation found that three of four U.S. physicians said the frequency with which doctors order unnecessary medical tests and procedures is a serious problem for the health system. Sixty-nine percent of respondents said the average physician orders unnecessary tests and procedures at least once a week.[43]

Yet studies suggest that there has not been a significant drop in the use of low-value or unnecessary care since the Choosing Wisely campaign began. For example, a 2017 study found there had been only a 4% decrease in low-value back imaging two and a half years after the program was launched.[44] Another study showed that of seven services that Choosing Wisely had recommended against, only two had showed a modest decrease in usage.[45]

Other research based on data from a large commercial insurer found that the growth in spending on five low-value services decreased an average of 1.7% annually from 2014 to 2016. However, the drop was less than expected. Among the low-value services in the study were vitamin D screening tests; PSA tests in men over 75 years old; unnecessary testing and lab work prior to low-risk surgery; imaging for uncomplicated low back pain within the first six weeks after onset; and the use of brand-name medications when generics are available.[46]

The ABIM survey showed that while doctors were aware of the problem, they were not necessarily disposed to change their own practice patterns. Just 59% of the doctors exposed to the Choosing Wisely campaign said they were likely to have reduced the number of times they ordered a test or a procedure after learning it was unnecessary.[47]

Seventy-five percent of the primary care physicians aware of Choosing Wisely agreed with the statement that the campaign had empowered them to reduce the use of unnecessary tests and procedures. When that figure is compared to the 59% of all doctors aware of the campaign who decreased the use of low-value care, it can be deduced that specialists are less likely than primary care doctors to heed these recommendations.

Why Doctors Don't Follow Advice

Richard J. Baron, MD, president and CEO of the ABIM Foundation, agrees that this is the case. "Specialists are often more narrowly focused on doing their procedures well," he says. Moreover, he adds, "A lot of specialists believe that if a primary care doctor refers a patient to them, it's because the doctor expects them to do the procedure. Specialists worry that if they don't do the procedure, the referring doctor won't send them more patients, because they'll feel like they're being criticized."

Financial incentives also play a role in many a specialist's decision to go ahead with a test or a procedure, Baron says. "And often it takes longer to explain why the procedure isn't needed than to go ahead and schedule it. That's clearly part of it."

This is also true in primary care, "where it's easier to order the test than to have a long conversation with a patient about why the test isn't necessary," he adds. "From a business viewpoint, you're burning your resources in having the conversation about why it's necessary, and you're not deriving any financial benefit from the fact that it didn't get done."

Baron, a general internist, recalls a case in which he spent 45 minutes convincing a patient that he didn't need a procedure recommended by another physician. Baron ultimately was successful, saving the healthcare system about $10,000. "But if we want to construct a healthcare system where a bunch of doctors will spend 45 minutes losing money to save somebody else $10,000, that's not going to be a winning strategy or a scalable strategy," he points out.

The odds of being sued for malpractice are also on the minds of practicing physicians every day. For that reason, the American College of Emergency Physicians (ACEP) originally declined to participate in Choosing Wisely, Baron says. "They were concerned if they didn't do an MRI for a headache, and the patient had a brain hemorrhage, they'd get sued." But ACEP eventually came on board.

Because the Choosing Wisely recommendations are evidence-based and come from specialty societies, Baron adds, they can be a defense in a malpractice suit. Also, if physicians discuss these recommendations with patients upfront, the risk of being sued declines, he says.

Patient Demands

While some doctors are concerned about not ordering tests or medications that patients expect, Baron downplays that issue as a factor in poor compliance with the Choosing Wisely recommendations. For example, he notes, many patients with upper respiratory infections expect to receive an antibiotic prescription, even if it they don't need one. "But some doctors extend that assumption to other patients who don't have that wish at all," and prescribe antibiotics to everyone with that condition.

Nevertheless, he notes, some patients distrust the motives of insurance companies, ACOs, and providers that take financial risk. When a doctor tells them something is unnecessary, he says, "Patients ask, 'are you doing that because an insurance company or administrator wants you to—somebody who doesn't care about me but does care about the bottom line?'"

Choosing Wisely provides a strong argument against that viewpoint, he notes, since the recommendations come from specialty societies. Still, when a doctor says that something isn't necessary, some patients are surprised and suspicious.

Recommendations not Made

One study of the campaign's impact notes that the specialty societies tended to omit services that physicians frequently performed and to target services that were performed infrequently.[48] For example, vertebroplasty is not the subject of a Choosing Wisely recommendation.

Cohen lists some other low-value procedures that have been left out of the database, including carotid endarterectomy in asymptomatic carotid artery stenosis, the aggressive treatment of low-risk prostate cancer, the overuse of lumbar spinal fusion, and the overuse of arthroscopy for osteoarthritis of the knee. In his view, Choosing Wisely is moving in the right direction but hasn't gone far enough.

Berwick agrees. "Choosing Wisely is a very good step in the right direction. I agree with the observation that a lot of the tests and procedures that were involved in Choosing Wisely don't represent the mainstream activities of these professions. It's a good first step, but should be bolder."

Baron doesn't deny that some societies have pulled their punches in making recommendations; but he says that some of them *have* addressed services that generate a lot of income for their members. The society of radiation oncologists, for instance, has recommended against proton beam therapy in most cases, he notes.

"The value of Choosing Wisely was that it got a lot of people into the value-based conversation, and it engaged a lot of professional societies in that conversation," he concludes. "It gave consumer organizations credible information to convey to patients about how to think about low-value care. And it created some tangible tools for people to use when they wanted to put these conversations forward."

NEW WEST PHYSICIANS

Since the inception of managed care at Kaiser Permanente and other group- and staff-model HMOs, scores of medical groups have figured out how to provide high-quality, efficient healthcare and eliminate much low-value care. But these groups are largely limited to certain states, including Arizona, California, Colorado, Florida, Massachusetts, Minnesota, Nevada, and Texas. By far the largest concentration of such groups is in California, where Kaiser has led the way.

While some primary care groups have risen to this challenge, multispecialty groups have more commonly undertaken it. These groups are usually larger than primary care practices and have greater resources to create the infrastructure required for managed care. Nevertheless, a primary care-driven national model will be required to fully wring the waste out of our system, because primary care physicians are in the best position to limit unnecessary referrals and coordinate care across care settings.

Hence, the rest of this chapter will highlight the long-running success of one primary care practice in eliminating waste and improving the quality of care. This is the previously mentioned New West Physicians (NWP), which is now infusing its proven principles into the other groups owned by OptumCare. Based in Denver, NWP now includes 130 physicians. Most of them are family physicians and general internists, along with a few hospitalists, a cardiologist, a gastroenterologist, a psychiatrist, an endocrinologist, and a neurologist.

Founded in 1994, in the midst of the first managed care wave, NWP started taking financial risk from Medicare plans in 1997, later graduating to commercial risk. At first, Cohen recounts, the group limited itself to full professional risk, which encompasses care delivered outside the hospital. Soon the group broadened its financial responsibility to 50/50 gain sharing on the hospital side. NWP now splits 70% of the insurance premium with United Healthcare—which is under the same corporate umbrella as OptumCare but is only one of the insurers it contracts with—and plans to increase that to 85% in 2020.

It would be an understatement to say this is a lot of risk for a primary care group to take. Initially, NWP hedged its bets by purchasing "stop-loss" insurance, which took over when the losses on a case hit a particular level. Because the group always had a surplus after paying for services, Cohen notes, it began to bank a certain amount per patient per month until it built up enough reserves to cancel its stop-loss policy in 2003.

Cutting out Waste

Under NWP's risk contracts, the group's leaders recognized from the outset that care delivery was a cost center, not a profit center. Consequently, they decided not to own ancillary facilities such as imaging centers or laboratories. This vision also impelled the group to "critically select" its network of specialists, hospitals, and ancillary providers based solely on their quality and efficiency, Cohen explained in a 2015 article.[49]

"Our primary care-centricity has allowed us to work closely with our narrow specialty network to eliminate much of the wasted care in our healthcare system," he wrote.

In selecting this network, the group first made sure that all the specialists it was considering provided high-quality care. However, that was just the price of admission. "Inherent in our model was the recognition that high-quality care afforded only small improvements in efficiency," Cohen wrote. "We recognized that cost of care was not linked to quality of care and that excessive care was both costly and dangerous to patients."

In a recent interview, Cohen explained that NWP's method was to plot cost vs. quality for a group of specialists on a graph. "Within that graph, there's a subset of providers who are practicing at the optimal intersection of quality and efficiency, and those are the providers we selectively sought out."

If a chosen specialist still provided a significant amount of low-value care, he added, a group medical director would meet regularly with the doctor. "By repeatedly feeding information back to our specialists and by orienting referrals to the specialists who are doing the best job, over time you quickly gain alignment on optimal care."

What's In It for the Specialist

If a specialist were doing just fine under fee for service and NWP asked him to limit some of his most profitable tests and procedures, why would he be interested?

"The reason is this: Think of a situation where it takes, say, 10,000 patients to fill an orthopedic surgeon's practice with the surgeon performing procedures at the current rate," Cohen said. "Imagine what would happen if a primary care group funneled all of its referrals to that orthopedic surgeon. With the primary care physicians doing most of the legwork, the orthopedist could take care of a population of 20,000 patients. There will be the same number of procedures in that population of 20,000 as there were in the population of 10,000 people, but now all of the procedures are indicated [i.e., appropriate]."

Under this model, the primary care physicians work up patients further before referring them, start more often with conservative therapy, and ensure that the patients are properly vetted as surgical candidates. "By the time the orthopedic surgeon sees these patients, there's a much lower likelihood that they will be subject to low-value care, because the PCPs have done a good job of working with those patients prior to referral," Cohen noted.

One challenge that the group has had all along is how to deal with patients who prefer to see specialists outside its network. If there are qualified specialists in network, Cohen said, the patient will be referred to one of them; if they still want to see someone else, that doctor will refer them to a non-network specialist.

Bench to Bedside

We earlier looked at how NWP selected and modified clinical practice guidelines. In addition, it developed a Bench to Bedside program—the basis for OptumCare's Optimal Care model—that was designed to accelerate the incorporation of important new evidence-based-medicine studies into practice. In his article, Cohen noted that this transition can take five to 10 years for many doctors. NWP and OptumCare have fast-tracked that to just 12 weeks.

In a more recent piece, Cohen said that Optimal Care starts with cultural transformation—no small matter. The OptumCare groups focus on educating clinicians about the value of evidence-based medicine and the need to eliminate low-value care. Experts deliver CME-accredited lectures in each specialty area.[50]

In addition, the OptumCare Forum for Evidence-Based Medicine distills recent high-quality studies into easily deployed recommendations. Infographics serve as point of care reminders on low-value care metrics. EHR tools show specialists their outcomes and quality scores and their total cost of care for specific procedures and diagnoses. They also identify the most efficient site of service for any test or procedure.

Both primary care physicians and specialists also receive reports on quality and utilization in which they're compared to themselves, to others in their specialty, and to national benchmarks. The doctors regularly meet to share and analyze this data.

How It Works in Practice

Most people have back pain at some point in their lives. But how that back pain is treated can make a big difference, not only to the patients, but to overall health costs. The cost of imaging for lower back pain alone rose 44% from 2014 to 2016, and there's every reason to believe it has continued to grow.[51]

In one of OptumCare's publications on evidence-based medicine, Michael Daubs, MD, an orthopedic surgeon with Southwest Medical Associates, explains that after initial conservative treatment of back pain, a primary care doctor may order an imaging test. A CT or an MRI image may show evidence of spine degeneration. But that's common in middle-aged people and is not by itself an indication for spine surgery, he said. A Cochrane Collaboration review of six studies, he adds, found that irregular CT or MRI images couldn't be correlated with incidence or severity of back pain. So, doctors should stop ordering imaging studies in patients with lower back pain unless they have features that suggest a serious underlying condition, he concluded.[52]

In another OptumCare piece for physicians, Cohen noted that in spine care, there's an overreliance on MRIs and procedures such as steroid injections and vertebroplasties. Too many drugs are prescribed, including opioids and antidepressants. And there's too much surgery, particularly lumbar fusion procedures. The evidence for spinal surgery is strongest where a patient has acute lumbar disc herniation or spinal stenosis that did not improve with conservative therapy, he said.[53]

In our interview, Cohen noted that OptumCare PCPs are urged to refer patients who don't respond to physical therapy or other conservative treatments to a physiatrist. This non-procedural specialist not only guides their rehab but can also help patients decide whether they should have surgery—a decision that some primary care physicians may not feel qualified to make with the patient. "So there's a lower likelihood of referral, and when a patient is referred, it's more likely they're a good candidate for surgery."

Patient Engagement

Selective contracting and working closely with doctors to root out waste aren't the only tools in NWP's toolbox. Over the years, the group has also carefully chosen the most efficient, high-quality hospitals and ancillary providers. It has zeroed in on keeping people out of the hospital and the ER. It has done population health management with a focus on high-risk patients. And it has contracted with health plans that reward the group for improving outcomes and keeping costs down.

NWP and OptumCare are also increasingly trying to engage patients in their own care. This is not only about teaching them how to manage their chronic conditions. In some cases, patients are also being encouraged to participate in making key decisions about their care.

"Shared decision making should apply to any significant procedure, whether it's a heart catheterization, heart surgery or abdominal surgery," Cohen said. "It should be applied in virtually all clinical situations. But it isn't actively utilized for several reasons: first, it's not rewarded in a fee-for-service model. Second, it's time-consuming to do, and practitioners often won't take the time to do it. And third, there aren't good [software] platforms out there to do shared decision making."

One exception, he says, is an app called Lumbar Fusion Calculator. Available online, the tool prompts the doctor to ask the patient a number of questions in the exam room. "It takes about five minutes to complete, and at the end of it, it shows patients what the statistical likelihood is that they'll be improved one year after surgery. That's an incredibly powerful tool, and it's not always what they hear from the surgeon."

THE WAY FORWARD

As Berwick and Hackbarth noted in their 2012 *Health Affairs* article, it makes a whole lot more sense to cut waste than to limit access to necessary services or slash provider payments to the bone. In their telling, a significant reduction in waste would allow us to bend the cost curve without hurting healthcare quality or access.

Berwick shared with me that he doesn't know how much unnecessary care physicians or hospitals could safely eliminate. "Some of it is marbled into the daily activities of healthcare organizations," he said. "There would have to be systemic changes to get it done. But it's a matter of will. With enough will, a lot of it could be eliminated. And when you're talking about $1 trillion [worth of waste], even if you get 10% of it, that's a tremendous amount that could be applied to other activities."

Risk-based contracts, whether shared savings or capitation, can incentivize physicians to reduce waste. From the viewpoint of long-suffering primary care physicians, value-based-care agreements that let them share in the savings they generate are a godsend. Family physicians David Boles and Jen Brull, whom we met earlier, can attest to that. Of course, not all primary care doctors are willing to take financial risk or change their practice patterns. But if maintaining their current income depends on it, most physicians will embrace change.

Specialists, too, can benefit by embracing the new paradigm. If they're mainly being paid fee for service, they'll have to forgo a lot of lucrative tests and procedures. But as Cohen explained, they can still keep their incomes up by delivering more-appropriate procedures and tests to a larger patient population.

In this scenario, it might seem that fewer specialists would be needed. But the Association of American Medical Colleges predicts we're going to have an increasing shortage of specialists as the population ages and develops more chronic diseases. If that's true, there will continue to be plenty of work for specialists. And as primary care doctors rise to the top of the food chain, with the chance to reap higher earnings, more and more young doctors will become primary care physicians rather than specialists.

Where Hospitals Stand

Hospitals might also be motivated to cooperate with physician groups in reducing waste if those practices were paying them out of a global budget. But provider groups must be very large and experienced with managed care before they're ready to take on inpatient risk. Also, there are limits to what hospitals can do to cut waste when services are ordered by physicians. That's why New West Physicians hires hospitalists, who ride herd on specialists in the hospital.

Berwick points out that hospital consolidation has led to a big increase in the cost of healthcare. But that trend could be reversed, he suggests, if hospitals were paid differently than they are today. "A shift to population-based payment should make hospitals more interested in keeping people home and well or recovering smoothly," he says.

Some hospitals have moved in the direction of taking financial risk, such as bundled payments or ACO shared savings, but not enough to swing the needle on health costs. When will hospitals see the light and adopt a philosophy more congenial to at-risk physician groups?

"Here's Berwick's test for successful health policy: do hospitals want to be empty?" says the emeritus president of IHI and the former acting administrator of CMS. "We will know when things have gone in the correct direction when hospitals are trying to help people stay well rather than keeping beds filled. But that's habit, and it's hard to change."

CHAPTER 6

Population Health Management

Rio Grande Valley Health Alliance (RGVHA), the small primary care ACO we encountered in Chapter 5, saved $9.8 million in 2018 in the Medicare Shared Savings Program (MSSP). The ACO was in a two-sided risk track of the MSSP, meaning it could receive up to 75% of what it saved Medicare. Since its quality rating was 93 out of a possible 100, its gainsharing percentage was reduced to 70%. At that ratio, the McAllen, Tex., ACO garnered $6.8 million in earnings. Even after accounting for the ACO's expenses, its 21 primary care physicians made out very well on their participation in RGVHA.

They had done well in the MSSP for several years. The ACO had achieved much of its success by reducing certain kinds of waste, such as the overordering of home care by area physicians. In addition, notes Bo Bobbitt, a North Carolina attorney who helped start RGVHA, the ACO had the advantage of starting with a very high MSSP benchmark because of the unusually high Medicare costs in the area. This benchmark—in effect, an annual budget for the total cost of care—made it relatively easy to achieve savings, at least initially.

But the not-so-secret-sauce of RGVHA—and the reason it's still cutting Medicare costs after six years of operation—is the ACO's commitment to population health management (PHM). With strong physician support, RGVHA has invested in the requisite PHM infrastructure, including health IT. It also has hired five nurse care managers who provide telephone support to the 15% of the ACO's patients who are at risk of becoming sicker. RGVHA also has field nurses who look after the sickest 5% of patients, making home visits as necessary.

Meanwhile, the ACO uses PHM software to stratify its 6,100 MSSP patients by health risk and to compile lists of patients with gaps in preventive care and chronic-disease care. The physicians try to make sure these patients get the recommended care when they come into the office, and their practices reach out to patients who are overdue for the necessary services. All of this has not only bolstered the ACO's quality scores in the MSSP but has also improved patient outcomes. From 2015 to 2016, for example, the ACO reduced unplanned hospital admission rates for its patients with diabetes and congestive heart failure.[1]

National Opportunity for Physicians

If a group as small as RGVHA could accomplish this, it's theoretically possible for other small and medium-sized ACOs to do the same thing, says Victoria Farias, the ACO's administrator. The success of Aledade's primary care ACOs (see Chapter 4) lends credence to this hypothesis.

However, such efforts face a number of obstacles. First, the doctors must be fully engaged and must be willing to take a certain amount of downside risk. If they're poorly managed or don't implement the PHM model well, they could lose money on risk contracts. But at least in a shared savings model where the payer retains ultimate risk, there's a limit to how much they can lose. Under the latest CMS regulations, for example, ACOs like RGVHA that are in the enhanced track of the MSSP can earn a maximum of 75% of their savings up to 20% of their benchmark; if they come in over budget, they have to pay back 40%-75% of the difference between the benchmark and actual costs up to 15% of the benchmark.[2]

Second, ACOs and groups may find it difficult to obtain risk contracts from health plans. "That's probably true in most of the country," says David Nash, MD, founding dean of the College of Population Health at Thomas Jefferson University. "The payers are very reluctant to participate in sophisticated, complex reimbursement schemes because most stuff is still fee for service and that's easier to administer."

Even where insurers are willing to delegate risk to providers, only some of them will supply claims data, which is critical in population health management. Nash believes this is mainly because the insurers don't want to reveal what they're paying particular providers in a market.

Still, as the RGVHA example shows, there are major opportunities for risk-bearing physician organizations to increase revenues by learning how to manage population health. If they can hold down costs and improve outcomes, they can benefit both now and in the future as public and private payers offload more risk to ACOs and other provider organizations. This chapter explains how physician groups and ACOs are leveraging population health management to manage risk under value-based contracts.

PLANNED CARE

Risk contracting turns fee for service on its head. Instead of rewarding providers for volume, it rewards them for value—which, as previously discussed, is high-quality care provided efficiently. To succeed financially under risk agreements, healthcare organizations must do population health management, which fundamentally changes how care is delivered. In place of fragmented episodes of care, for example, PHM focuses on planned care that may encompass multiple care settings. And, unlike fee for service, which pays only for the care delivered by a particular physician or institution to an individual patient, PHM also seeks to improve the health of a defined population within a predetermined budget.

While aspects of PHM have been around for a long time, the concept became popular after Donald Berwick, MD, and his colleagues at the Institute for Healthcare Improvement (IHI) articulated the Triple Aim referred to in Chapter 2:

- Improve the experience of care.
- Improve the health of populations.
- Reduce the per capita cost of care.[3]

In the IHI model, the aim is to raise the quality of care and improve care coordination across all care settings, including acute care, ambulatory care, and post-acute care. Secondly, care is seen as ongoing and longitudinal, not confined to single episodes. And as the second aim makes clear, healthcare organizations must improve not just individual, but also population health.

Group-model HMOs such as Kaiser Permanente and large integrated delivery systems like Intermountain Healthcare and the Geisinger Clinic have long deployed major components of population health management. Today, an increasing number of ACOs and risk-bearing physician groups use PHM to manage risk. The main tenets of this approach include:

- An organized system of care.
- Care teams that include physicians and allied health professionals.
- Coordination across care settings.
- Easy access to primary care.
- Centralized resource planning.
- Continuous care provided both during and between office visits.
- Patient self-management education.
- Focus on health behavior and lifestyle changes.
- Interoperable electronic health records.
- Electronic registries that track patients by disease state.
- Focus on social determinants of health.[4]

A Little Background

The large organizations that originally implemented PHM represented a small portion of the U.S. healthcare system. But, starting in the late 1990s, health plans sought to deploy some aspects of PHM more widely through an approach known as "disease management." Using nurse care managers who telephonically interacted with very sick patients, the plans tried to ensure that the patients received recommended care and that their care was being properly coordinated. The impact of these care managers was limited, however, because they usually were not connected with the patients' physicians.

Some group-model HMOs also pursued disease management using what was known as the Chronic Care Model. Pioneered at Group Health Cooperative in Washington State, this model attempted to integrate care for patients with chronic diseases across care settings and over time. This approach required the resources of large groups or health systems; it could not readily be implemented by smaller groups and independent practice associations.

Patient-centered medical homes (PCMHs) were the next major effort to coordinate care and to ensure that patients received ongoing, appropriate care for their chronic conditions. Some healthcare organizations have adopted the PCMH model as preparation for more extensive forays into value-based care. But, as noted in Chapter 4, many primary care practices are medical homes in name only because real practice transformation requires too much work and cultural change. In addition, the efforts of PCMHs to improve care coordination have not gained much cooperation from specialists and hospitals.

Nevertheless, PCMHs did pave the way for ACOs, and there is some evidence that the two models reinforce one another. A review paper on the topic noted that the characteristics that lead to the success of ACOs are also central to the success of advanced primary care models such as the PCMH. Moreover, studies show that ACOs led by advanced primary care teams experience positive results in cost, quality, and utilization. ACOs with PCMHs are more likely to generate savings and also demonstrate higher quality than ACOs that lack these crucial building blocks, the paper said.[5]

Whatever mechanism is used to organize care, there's general agreement that population health management is required to manage financial risk. Conversely, says Karen Handmaker, former vice president of population health strategies for IBM Watson Health, the amount of risk assumed by a healthcare organization usually determines how interested it is in PHM.

Is PHM Poised to Go Mainstream?

As noted in Chapter 2, more than half of commercial payments to healthcare providers are now tied to some kind of value-based model. Yet the percentage of payments that involve two-sided risk is still in the single digits.[6] If Handmaker is right, the low prevalence of financial risk means that not many organizations have fully implemented population health management.

Nevertheless, Paul Grundy, MD, founding president of the Patient-Centered Primary Care Collaborative (PCPCC) and the former chief medical officer of IBM's healthcare and life sciences team, believes population health management is now poised to go mainstream in the United States. He cites three reasons.

First, he says, the biggest barrier to PHM is physician culture, which is still attuned to fee for service. But in his view, progress is being made by some medical schools, which are training young doctors in population health management.

Second, the percentage of provider reimbursement that is value-based is rising fast. "Everybody is figuring out how to step up to that, and if they don't, they won't survive," he says.

Finally, he says, many health plans and government payers are demanding that healthcare providers start to take financial risk.

That pressure is real; but, so far, most providers have not responded to it. The healthcare system and physician incentives will have to be substantially restructured before they will.

PHM INFRASTRUCTURE

Population health management depends on the availability of timely, comprehensive information on patients. The digitization of health records over the past decade has provided a key element of the requisite infrastructure. But electronic health records are still far from interoperable (see Chapter 10), and providers often don't have access to vital information about the care that their patients received elsewhere.

Providers must also have access to insurance claims data to form a full picture of a patient's health and the care they've received. But, as previously mentioned, many health plans are reluctant to share that data with providers; even if they do provide it, the data can be three to six months old by the time a physician sees it. By then, it's usually too late for the doctor to do anything with the information.

Specialized software is also required to analyze claims and clinical data so that it can be useful in population health management. The ability to aggregate disparate kinds of data and map them to a standard format is especially important in ACOs where practices use multiple types of EHRs—which is to say, most ACOs based on physician networks.

Among the common types of data analysis for PHM are:

- Risk stratification, which classifies individuals by their level of health risk.
- Care gap identification, which shows which patients have not received recommended preventive and/or chronic care services.
- Provider measurement, which shows how well individual providers perform in delivering evidence-based care and managing the utilization of healthcare resources.
- Utilization of services, broken down to primary care and specialist physicians, hospitals, and post-acute care providers.
- Reports on out-of-network care.

Many ACOs and groups also have implemented software that, in conjunction with or as part of the EHR, is used to automate the routine aspects of PHM. One example is patient outreach software that automatically calls patients when they're overdue for preventive or chronic care services and that can even make appointments for them. Automation software also can be used to electronically send tailored educational materials and alerts to healthy patients and people who are in the early stages of a chronic-disease such as hypertension or diabetes.

A PHM infrastructure also includes health IT experts, care managers, disease educators and coaches, nutritionists, pharmacists, and other ancillary providers. The number of these care team members varies with the size, resources, and philosophy of a healthcare organization. But the use of care teams itself is a core principle of population health management.[7]

Reducing Hospital Admissions

Besides physicians and other providers, the most important members of the care team are nurse care managers. These nurses typically call high-risk patients to make sure they're following their care plans and are not getting sicker. This is different from the health plan disease management approach, because these care managers are calling in the name of the patient's doctor. Many care managers are imbedded in medical offices, where they meet with patients and teach them how to care for themselves. Care managers also facilitate transitions of care for patients who recently have been discharged from the hospital. They may even visit certain patients at home.

Care managers try to ensure that their patients don't make avoidable visits to the ER and aren't admitted or readmitted to the hospital unnecessarily. Because these are the most expensive care venues, keeping people out of the hospital can significantly decrease the total cost of care. This is one way in which population health management contributes to the financial health of risk-bearing organizations.

HIGH RISK VS. WHOLE POPULATION

A healthcare organization that invests in PHM infrastructure needs to see a return on that investment. The organization can get this return fastest by focusing on high-risk patients who have conditions that are already bad and likely to get worse. Often known as "super-utilizers" or "frequent flyers," these patients may see several different specialists for multiple chronic conditions. An ACO can reduce spending quickly by coordinating their care and keeping them out of the hospital, by handling their discharges appropriately, and by dealing with their mental and behavioral issues, Bobbitt points out.

Supporting this viewpoint is the fact that the sickest 5% of patients account for about 50% of health costs.[8] Only 30% of the high-risk patients, however, were in that category a year earlier[9]; and by the time an organization knows they're high risk, there is a limit to what it can do for them. So ACOs and risk-bearing groups also have to manage the next group of patients in the risk hierarchy. Known as "rising-risk" patients, these people form another 15% of the population. High-risk and rising-risk patients generate about 80% of health spending.[10]

The patients in these two categories are the central focus of RGVHA's population health management efforts. But the ACO also tries to ensure that its physicians fill as many care gaps as possible for all their patients. In addition, the practices contact people who are overdue for recommended services.

"It's really hard to manage patients under care coordination if they already have a malignancy," Farias says. "We know there's not a lot of impact we can make, unfortunately. So, we want to target a step down from that and we want the physician offices to help us with the patients in the lower-risk categories."

Grundy maintains that "the only approach that makes sense is to have a 360-degree view of your entire population and manage their health." Early medical home pilots that focused on managing only high-risk patients failed, he recalls. "They failed because you don't know who's going to be the sickest few tomorrow if you don't have the information about your entire population," he says. "You have to understand the 80% of people who are not at risk and send them some preventive care reminders on their cellphones."

Based on interviews with several organizations that are managing population health, it appears that most of them have adopted some type of whole-population approach. For example, Prevea Health, a 300-doctor multispecialty group in Green Bay, Wisconsin, targets its entire population in order to intervene with patients who might get sick or sicker if they don't control their chronic diseases.

"At the end of the day, if you don't manage what you can't see, the emerging problem is your next problem, your next high-risk patient," says Ashok Rai, MD, CEO of Prevea. "It's all about risk mitigation, and risk doesn't start at your sickest patients. It starts at that middle population, who have the potential for risk."

Heritage Provider Network (HPN), a physician-led managed care organization, takes full risk from health plans for nearly 700,000 people in California; it also has operations in New York, Arizona, and Missouri. Mark Wagar, president of Heritage Medical Systems, an affiliate of HPN, says the organization focuses on all segments of its population but assigns a higher priority to its sickest patients.

"We do focus on all of them," he says, "but the highest risk ones are most at risk, and you have to engage them at a different level of intensity. Then you have cohorts of people who are at other levels of risk. They might have a chronic condition and are somewhat stable; they could benefit from changes in their lifestyle or surrounding them with some additional care management. And there are people who, as you move down the risk scale, don't believe they're at that much risk. So how you approach them is not the same as someone in a high-risk category, who is very aware they're sick and needs help."

STRATEGIES FOR HIGH-RISK PATIENTS

Cornerstone Health Care, a North Carolina multispecialty group, developed viable strategies for dealing with high-risk patients and documented the first year of its experience in a published study.[11]

Cornerstone's approach was to redesign the underlying care models for five of its highest-risk populations: patients with late-stage congestive heart failure (CHF), cancer patients, Medicare-Medicaid dual eligibles, people with five or more chronic conditions, and complex patients with multiple late-stage chronic conditions.

A wide range of interventions were designed to improve care for these population segments. For example, a special heart function clinic was designed for CHF patients. Instead of focusing only on preventing the readmission of previously hospitalized patients, as many health systems do, "Cornerstone sought to proactively identify patients at high risk of hospitalization and keep them out of hospital by focusing on reducing exacerbations, improving quality of life, and providing palliative care," the paper said. The clinic was staffed by cardiologists, and a pharmacist and a psychologist were also imbedded in the site.

Another program provided comprehensive, coordinated care for very complex patients with multiple chronic conditions, including the 3% of Cornerstone's patients at highest risk. These patients were directed to a standalone facility that had easy access for the frail and elderly. "A care team consisting of an internist, a nurse practitioner, a clinical pharmacist, a nurse patient navigator, and a social worker collaborated closely with other caregivers, specialists, home health agencies, and palliative care agencies. The program focused on improving patient quality of life, functionality, and self-care ability, while reducing cost and unnecessary health care utilization," the paper noted.

The results of Cornerstone's initiative after just one year were eye-opening. Overall costs for the patients studied dropped by 12.7% compared to the year before enrollment. The four fully implemented programs delivered cost savings of 10%–16%. Hospitalizations dropped by 30% across all these programs.

DATA-DRIVEN APPROACH

As mentioned earlier, data is the fuel of population health management. EHR data is rich in clinical detail, but it doesn't show what happened to patients outside of an ACO or a practice. Claims data from a patient's insurer, whether the insurance is commercial, Medicare or Medicaid, provides a much broader view of the patient's medical history.

Medicare claims data is available to any ACO that participates in the MSSP. Claims data from commercial insurers is another matter. Only ACOs and groups that take full risk have access to claims data while it is still clinically actionable. Other organizations use older claims data from Medicare and private payers to measure their own performance and that of their providers.

One such organization is the Austin Regional Clinic (ARC) in Austin, Texas. A physician-owned group with 340 physicians, 60% of whom are primary care doctors, the practice includes an ACO that has shared savings contracts with the state of Texas, as well as several commercial insurers. A broader ACO that encompasses ARC, some smaller groups, and a local hospital participates in the Medicare Shared Savings Program.

All of ARC's commercial contracts require the payers to provide claims data, says Anas Daghestani, MD, the group's CEO and the director of its population health department. "It's still a challenge, because there's a claims lag of 90 days and you also have the time for the health plan to curate the data, aggregate them, and run an attribution model on them," he notes. "It's usually a 6- to 9-month delay. Claims data is very helpful in managing quality and getting a more comprehensive picture. It's less helpful in managing financial risk. That's why I think the current ACO model is not sustainable long term without evolution. Because I don't see taking risk when I don't know about something happening outside of ARC until nine months later."

On the positive side, Daghestani adds that some commercial plans, including Humana and Wellcare, alert ARC beforehand about major patient events, such as planned surgeries. "As soon as an authorization request hits their system, it's coming to us. It's not as good as paid claims, but it's more of a live feed. We want to know when there's a request for a heart surgery, whether it's authorized or not, so we can know what's happening."

RGVHA has a shared savings contract with Blue Cross Blue Shield of Texas through a larger ACO. The claims data provided by the Blues is very limited, Farias says, "because they don't want to reveal the negotiated prices with different hospitals."

In North Carolina, Bobbitt notes, Blue Cross and Blue Shield is offering value-based contracts to some ACOs. But "it's pulling eye teeth to get data," even though this information is vital to ACOs that are taking financial risk. His explanation for this is "institutional rigidity."

Mark Wager of Heritage Provider Network, similarly, points out that health plans have a hard time changing how they deal with providers. Where HPN is globally capitated, as in California, it has instant access to claims data. "But it's a slower process in newer markets where payers aren't ready for that."

In those markets, he notes, "Some plans may just want to show you the claims data at the six- month point when you're reconciling payments, but that's too late for the high-risk patients. And it delays intervention for those at moderate risk and people who are healthy but have heuristics for future risk. So why wait? The management organization needs to be able to give the providers that information right away."

Software Tools

Electronic health records (EHRs) were designed to maximize billing, not for population health management. Thus, it's not surprising that most organizations rely on third-party software that focuses on specific aspects of PHM. RGVHA, for instance, uses an application that aggregates the clinical data from its members' eight different EHRs and combines it with claims information. This software delivers monthly reports that the ACO shares with its doctors. These reports inform doctors about their patients' care gaps and the outside services they have received. RGVHA care coordinators also have access to the analyzed data and use it to reconcile the medications that have been prescribed to patients by various providers.

PHM also requires the use of electronic registries that show each patient's health conditions, the services they have received, when the services were provided and by whom, the patient's recent lab values, when they were last seen, and when they're due for preventive and/or chronic-disease care. Registries can be used to compile lists of subpopulations that need particular kinds of care, such as annual mammograms for women in a particular age group or HbA1c tests for diabetic patients at prescribed time intervals.

Applying analytics to registries can reveal care gaps at both the individual and population levels. Patient-focused analytics can be used to alert providers and care teams so they can fill patients' care gaps. Using population-based analytics, a management team can evaluate how the organization is doing in comparison with past performance or benchmarks based on data from similar organizations. Registries can also be combined with outreach tools to alert patients when they need to come in for health maintenance. And they can generate work lists for care teams, such as making sure that every diabetic patient who visits an office has a foot exam.[12]

EHRs Still Not Up to Snuff

The leading EHR systems include registries and other population health management tools. These have been steadily improving, says Karen Handmaker. Moreover, Epic, the EHR that dominates the market, has become more interoperable so that it can ingest key data from other EHRs, she notes. Nevertheless, EHR-based PHM tools still can't combine claims and clinical data, and EHR registries are regarded by some observers as inferior to those of third-party developers.

Nathan McCarthy, a consultant with ECG Management Consultants, says that PHM tools from EHR vendors like Epic, Cerner, and eClinicalWorks are indeed getting better. "But I tell our provider clients that they can't solely rely on their EHR vendors, especially in population health. They're going to need some of these other tools out there. The third-party companies that are vendor-agnostic are able to bring in more comprehensive data for your population and pull it in a better and more meaningful way than your EHR vendor can."

Ashok Rai of Prevea is more bullish about Epic's Healthy Planet PHM suite. "We left some of the products we had in the past because they weren't doing anything that we couldn't do ourselves now that Epic has become more robust," he says. But Prevea is still using an outside application for patient outreach, he adds.

Daghestani, whose group also uses Epic, says ARC employs Healthy Planet mainly as a population registry. "You can assign a nurse or case manager a list of patients, and they can use some of the documentation and tasking [in the software]. To use it as a robust tool for care gaps or risk stratification, however, you have to bring in external data. You have to bring in claims data, otherwise you're doing risk stratification and management of care gaps based only on what's in the EHR."

Currently, he adds, ARC is building an Epic data warehouse known as Caboodle. While this will cost a lot of money, he says, it's necessary to bring together all the disparate kinds of data needed for PHM. When the data warehouse is completed, he says, it will allow a seamless transition of data from outside to inside the group and vice versa.

THE MEDICAL NEIGHBORHOOD

To manage population health effectively, ACOs and other risk-bearing groups must gain the cooperation of specialists, hospitals, and post-acute care facilities. On one level, the biggest barrier to enlisting other providers in this collaboration is to persuade them to act against their own short-term financial interest in a fee-for-service world. On another level, large multispecialty groups must change the mindset of their own physicians.

With only 21 primary care physicians, the Rio Grande Valley Health Alliance has had to cope with the suspicion and opposition of other providers in its own medical neighborhood. For example, when RGVHA discovered that home health spending in the area was four times the national average and that some specialists were referring patients inappropriately to home care, the ACO sent a letter to all the physicians caring for its patients stating that RGVHA wanted to coordinate the patients' care with the specialists.

"Some doctors got really upset and had attorneys call us," Farias recalls. But after the ACO put the physicians on notice and warned some of them that they were violating CMS rules, there was a big drop in home care referrals.

Local hospitals also didn't like what RGVHA was doing because they believed the ACO was trying to prevent patients from being hospitalized, Farias says. "But when we met with the hospitals, we told them, 'We're not trying to keep patients from going to the hospital. Patients will always have to go to the hospital. We're trying to prevent unnecessary readmissions and ER visits and have a better coordination of care between hospitals and PCPs, many of whom no longer round in the hospital.'"

Because the hospitals didn't want Medicare to penalize them for excessive readmissions, she notes, they supported that part of RGVHA's mission. But it's still difficult for the ACO to get timely hospital data after seven years of trying, she says. To coordinate care for their patients, the ACO needs admission-discharge-transfer (ADT) data feeds, but the hospitals refuse to provide this information, saying that it goes to the ACO's doctors individually. "That's great, but sometimes our doctors' staffs don't check it, and we need it at the ACO level so we can manage our patients," Farias points out. Just this year, she said, the hospitals finally gave the ACO access to their EHR systems, allowing it to get notifications of admissions and discharges.

One value of this information is that before a patient is discharged, the ACO is alerted and has input into the decision on where the patient will go. In one case, Farias notes, a hospitalist was going to send a patient to inpatient rehab. Her outpatient doctor in the ACO recommended that she be sent to a skilled nursing facility (SNF) instead, and the change was made.

Inpatient rehab is now being overutilized in the McAllen area as much as home health care was previously, Farias says. "We're about four-five times the national average for inpatient rehab right now, which is unacceptable." RGVHA has talked to every hospital and hospital case manager about this, she says, and "we're starting to see a decrease. But we want to make sure. That's our new goal."

Daghestani says the hospitals in the Austin area cooperate with the group on population health management to some extent; however, it's still difficult to get ADT alerts from the hospitals. The facilities require that patients have a primary care physician at ARC—which the hospitals don't always capture—before they'll release the data. "So we give them an active roster [of ACO patients] twice a year, and they compare it to their inpatient census and send us daily reports of ER visits and inpatient census," he says.

Whether or not hospitals cooperate, ACOs and groups can usually place their own hospitalist physicians or care managers at facilities to which they refer patients. This has shaped up as a standard strategy for ACOs. While hospitalists employed by or contracted to a facility are supposed to manage inpatient care, their incentive is to do what the hospital, not the ACO, wants. So, to ensure that patients receive appropriate care, many ACOs employ their own hospitalists or specialized nurses. For example, ARC has inpatient care managers who round on patients, in some cases along with a hospitalist or a specialist.

Vetting Specialists

As discussed in Chapter 5, it's imperative for groups at financial risk to choose the right specialists to whom to refer patients. At-risk ACOs and groups would prefer to use specialists who provide high-quality care efficiently. But it's not easy to identify those doctors without full access to claims data, Bobbitt notes.

Austin Regional Clinic, while a large group, is 60% primary care. Therefore, ARC and its ACO must find the right outside specialists to refer to. "This is one of our Achilles heels, and I suspect that's true not only for us, but for 80% of the doctors in this country," Daghestani says. "We don't have enough insight to determine who's high quality and reasonable cost. For the most part, referrals are based on gut instinct and word of mouth."

Another problem is that some high-value specialists practice at expensive hospitals or outpatient facilities. "They might be the best one to do this heart surgery, but they do it at the most expensive place in town," Daghestani says.

ARC doesn't have access to meaningful data on specialists from Medicare or private payers, he observes. "Health plans offer star ratings, but that's superficial. It's based on HEDIS [quality ratings from the National Committee on Quality Assurance] and doesn't factor in costs. Health plans say they're not allowed to share stratification [of specialists] based on cost. And we need that data if we're going to manage risk."

Even if ARC had the average spending for each specialist in a particular specialty so he could compare their costs, he notes, "I don't know what their downstream charges are. Does this specialist who has below-average costs send all patients who need kidney operations to their neighbor? The data is fragmented and requires a lot of massaging."

Full Risk Has Benefits

ACOs that take full risk for the cost of care, like those of the Heritage Provider Network, are in a better position to assess the performance of specialists because they have immediate access to claims data. When the organization risk-stratifies patients, Wagar says, "we also profile and stratify the providers we need to refer to. We use that data to identify the higher performers and try to help the lower-performing specialists and facilities to improve."

Primary care physicians are incentivized to refer to high-value specialists, and HPN decides which physicians—both generalists and specialists—it wants to include in its network. "The PCPs and the specialists that do that the best, their performance shows forth and they're typically the most popular with patients," he says. "And those are the people you want in your practices and in your IPA [independent practice association] networks."

Keeping It All in the Family

Prevea Health, in contrast, refers mostly within its group, which includes a large chunk of the specialists in its area of Wisconsin. Therefore, the group focuses on helping its own specialists improve their performance.

Prevea has the data it needs to do that because, while independent, it co-owns a health plan with six hospitals. That health plan covers about 40,000 people, some of them hospital employees, and represents 14% of Prevea's commercial business.

"Because we have the health plan data, we can look at the specialists' cost of care and their utilization management, and we educate them," Ashok Rai says.

Co-owning a health plan also gives Prevea the data it needs for population health management. "We're not dependent on someone to give us that, we get it live," Rai notes. "This allows us to give providers and care managers timely, actionable data. We know about ED utilization. We know to contact somebody who's on that third ED visit in three weeks, so we can intervene not three months later, but that week."

The hospitals that co-own the health plan—and therefore have a stake in lower costs—are extremely cooperative, Rai says. Since the hospitals are on the same EHR as the group is, he adds, Prevea gets ADT alerts immediately and can easily exchange data with the hospitals.

MANAGING POST-ACUTE CARE

As RGVHA discovered, post-acute care (PAC) spending on nursing homes, rehab facilities, and home health care is one of the key drivers of health costs. It also is the area that has the greatest variations in spending. These variations are often unrelated to patient outcomes.

One study, for example, compared age-adjusted PAC costs of Medicare patients and commercially insured patients around age 65 who'd been discharged from a group of Michigan hospitals. PAC spending was between 68% and 230% greater among fee-for-service Medicare beneficiaries than among similar commercially insured people, yet there was no difference in their readmission rates.[13]

"These findings suggest that post-acute care utilization is highly sensitive to payer influence, and there may be an opportunity for additional savings in Medicare without sacrificing quality," the authors concluded.

Until a few years ago, hospitals didn't care how much SNFs and home care agencies pumped up their own Medicare revenues. Then CMS launched the Bundled Payments for Care Improvement (BPCI) program and the Comprehensive Care for Joint Replacement Program (CJR), as explained in Chapter 2. The Trump Administration reduced the number of hospitals for which CJR was mandatory and canceled CMS' planned expansion of bundling to additional procedures. But by then, many hospitals were already beginning to expand and integrate their PAC networks to control costs during the 30 days after discharge.[14]

While bundled payments affect only a minority of hospitals, the ACA provision that penalizes hospitals for excessive readmissions impacts all hospitals and helps drive their interest in post-acute care. Hospitals that aren't at risk for the cost of care but are concerned about readmissions are more likely to discharge their patients to SNFs than to home health care, despite the higher cost of nursing homes.[15]

Medicare patients discharged to home health care had a 5.6% higher 30-day readmission rate than those sent to a SNF, one study found. But home care saved Medicare $4,514, on average, during the 60 days after discharge.[16]

Since 2009, there has been a steady decline in Medicare SNF days per 1,000 beneficiaries, a study by Avalere Health reveals. But that isn't because hospitals are trying to save Medicare money. Avalere attributes the drop-off to the decline in inpatient admissions, as well as to the rise in "observation stays" that hospitals use to game the readmission penalties.[17]

What does all of this mean for risk-bearing ACOs and physician groups? First, post-acute care spending must be controlled in order to reduce the total cost of care. Second, the choice of a PAC setting and the ability of physicians and PAC providers to communicate with each other can be critical to patient outcomes.

Post-Acute Care Interventions

Well aware of these facts, Prevea has started its own nursing home service. "We have offices in all the nursing homes that meet our quality standards, and they get our patients," Rai says. In addition, a cadre of Prevea physicians, whom Rai calls "SNFists," round on their patients in these facilities daily.

Rai, who does this work himself, explains, "We're embedded inside the nursing homes that we've chosen to work with. We do admissions and take care of issues with patients. We monitor their rehab and medications. We have the Epic EHR in there to look at the records in the hospital and tie it into the nursing home records, and patients are managed significantly better."

While the SNFists have access to Epic when they round in the nursing homes, the SNFs themselves have a different kind of EHR. Most PAC providers, in fact, use information systems that are incompatible with those of hospitals and ambulatory care providers. But Rai says the SNFs can use Epic's Care Everywhere application to pull his notes out of Epic.

As for home care, he says, the hospitals that co-own Prevea's health plan "handle that pretty effectively with the home nurses. Our hospitals own their own home care companies, so we're in the home more than most groups."

Other at-risk groups aren't as far down the road as Prevea is on post-acute care. Austin Regional Clinic, for example, is just getting ready to manage home visits with the help of an outside post-acute care company, Daghestani says. It has trained some staff and created some connectivity between EHRs.

Handmaker sees opportunities for nursing homes and other PAC providers to start offering care management services that extend the reach of ACOs. Those that do so, she says, could "act as the feet and the eyes on the ground to support the ACOs."

While Handmaker agrees that the incentives of PAC providers are not usually aligned with those of at-risk organizations, she notes that SNFs have the resources needed to improve the quality of care. "It's not that different from home health, except you have a bunch of people living in the same place," she says. "So, you could deploy care teams. A partnership could emerge between a nursing home provider and an at-risk provider to have onsite support for all their patients who are in that facility."

PHYSICIAN CULTURE

Bobbitt, who has helped start several ACOs besides RGVHA, says much of an ACO's success is determined by its physician culture. Because most practicing doctors haven't been trained in anything other than clinical care, he says, "physicians are really unprepared in the new environment, and it's a big lift to think in terms of population health management. It's hard for the doctors to get off the volume train, even if they have had time to reflect and have some sort of understanding of the value-based world."

The key to an ACO's success, Bobbitt says, is having a physician champion who can communicate the need for change to his or her colleagues. Farias agrees. At RGVHA, she notes, Luis Delgado, Jr., MD, the ACO's cofounder, has been a driving force in getting the other physicians engaged. "Doctors work very hard, and they like peer-to-peer communication," she points out. "If an administrator tries to tell a doctor what they need to do, it's hard to do that."

Another obstacle to many physicians' engagement in PHM is that, if only a small portion of their revenue is at risk, they're less inclined to support major changes in how they work.

"If you're a provider and 70% of your business is commercial and 30% is Medicare, and some of those patients are in Medicare Advantage plans that still pay fee for service, and you've got an upside-only shared savings ACO, you're not going to have a big infrastructure just for that ACO," Handmaker observes. "When you build this infrastructure, you want it to be for all of your population. Nobody likes to practice one way for some patients, and another way for others."

In California, Wagar notes, HPN supplies the PHM infrastructure for all its practices and contributes the majority of their revenues. That incentivizes the doctors to deliver high-quality care as efficiently as possible and "to have conversations about the majority of their patients concerning utilization, care management and patient outreach." But in other markets, he says, HPN has to "get several payers to wake up" and offer risk contracts so that physician practices can manage population health for more than 10%–15% of their patients.

"You have to get past the chicken-and-egg stage and get more than one payer working with you in a market," he notes. "Unless it's a Kaiser, where they only deal with their own patients, no single payer can fill up a physician's practice. So, you need a multi-payer provider network, and that's what we're trying to do."

Culture Trumps Incentives

Of the organizations interviewed for this chapter, Prevea Health has taken the most unusual path to physician engagement. More than half of Prevea's business comes from fee-for-service contracts, and the group pays its doctors based mostly on their production. Yet Prevea expects its physicians to treat all patients the same, whether they're under fee-for-service or risk-based arrangements. The group also applies population health management to its entire patient panel, Rai says.

Asked whether this creates a psychological problem for doctors who are paid on the basis of how much they produce, Rai replies, "They should know that, whether a patient is a risk patient or a fee-for-service patient, they should be practicing good medicine every time. I'm frustrated when I hear people saying they're preparing for population health. I think, 'So you finally decided to practice good medicine?'"

This emphasis on practicing the right way and following evidence-based protocols is stronger than financial incentives, in Rai's view. "I'd rather fix the culture than pay for something that's broken. We have some financial incentives [for improvement], but it's a very small amount. The majority of it is just to bring attention to the fact that we had a discussion on it."

Getting Specialists Aboard

In Chapter 5, we looked at how New West Physicians persuaded its chosen specialists to forgo unnecessary tests and procedures that were lucrative for them. The solution was to refer all the group's patients to those specialists, who made up for the loss of revenue by having a larger patient population.

For ACOs and groups that refer to a lot of outside specialists, Bobbitt agrees, this is the way to go. "I work with a large ACO that has 300 PCPs, and they plan to send all their referrals to high-value specialists. And those specialists can double their referrals," he says.

What has amazed him, he adds, is "how hard the doctors not in the ACO have worked to get referrals. Before, it was about sucking up to PCPs in ways that don't violate [the] Stark [anti-self-referral law] or the Anti-Kickback Act. Now it's about getting on the same page with the ACO on clinical pathways and best practices and ACO continuum-of-care initiatives. That's how they get referrals legally, and they'll stand on their head to do that, and don't even ask for any of the shared savings."

Of course, this approach won't work in groups that refer most patients to their own specialists. Those organizations have to rely on discussions between their medical directors and their specialists to ensure that those doctors cooperate with PHM initiatives.

Heritage Provider Network does some of each. By showing specialists data on their performance, the organization tries to persuade them to improve. At the same time, Wagar says, it has created a network of high-value specialists outside of HPN, and it gives its primary care doctors data on those physicians to aid them in referral decisions.

Beyond population health management, Wagar stresses, ACOs and groups must make sure to select the most cost-effective care settings in order to manage financial risk. For example, he says, "Some important cancer drugs can be very expensive, but many of the infusion companies and other companies that offer those in a high-quality way can charge different amounts. Some infusion centers charge $7,000–$9,000 per infusion, while hospitals in the same market charge $47,000. So, providers have a responsibility to identify the most cost-effective sites."

There's always more waste to eliminate, Farias notes. Since Medicare ended competitive bidding for durable medical equipment, for instance, there has been an upsurge in orders for equipment that patients don't need, she says. "I don't know how they get our patients' names, but doctors from all over are ordering $2,000 or $3,000 braces for them, and the patient doesn't need it. It's just in a box in their living room. It's such a waste of dollars."

OVERCOMING BARRIERS

There's an adage that "you have to spend money to make money," and this is as true for at-risk ACOs and groups as for any other business. For example, Daghestani estimates that ARC has netted $30 million over six years in ACO shared savings. But he says the group has probably spent that much money on infrastructure, including the data warehouse and PHM software tools. "Each one of these pieces has an implementation fee, a software fee, and a per-user fee, plus the time to build it," he says. "It doesn't come out of the box ready to use. Each one of those is a half million-dollar investment."

Moreover, to serve the 220,000 patients covered under its value-based contracts, ARC has built a PHM department that now includes 70 people. Of those people, about 40 are care managers, and the rest include health IT staff who manage the PHM software and the data warehouse and analyze the data.

Epic's Caboodle warehouse costs too much for a smaller group or ACO, even one with 100 doctors, Daghestani says. "That's what's driving a lot of the consolidation [in the industry]. Smaller groups would have to stretch their financials just to buy an EHR, and if you buy a cheaper EHR, it doesn't come with this tool."

Yet small ACOs like RGVHA are managing population health and taking risk successfully. They have far smaller populations and fewer providers than ARC does, and they can't afford all the bells and whistles of a full-blown PHM infrastructure. But with the help of lower-cost third-party software, engaged physicians and a little innovation, they get by just fine.

Some smaller ACOs and groups, such as those affiliated with Aledade and OptumCare, are using the infrastructure of a larger organization. The same is true of Heritage Provider Network, an umbrella organization for a host of large and small practices. An increasing number of management companies for primary care groups, such as Oak Street, One Medical, and Iora, are being funded by private equity. However, David Nash doesn't think the latter route is a long-term solution, since venture capitalists are mainly interested in taking such companies public as soon as possible.

Nash is of two minds about the ability of smaller ACOs to compete with large organizations on population health management. On one hand, he says, smaller groups and ACOs have fewer resources to invest in PHM, which partly explains the consolidation in the industry. On the other hand, he thinks many groups could "do a good job" of managing risk and that some already are. "Could an agile multispecialty group, unencumbered by the expensive capital of hospitals, make a go of it? Sure."

Marketplace Barriers

It has already been noted that many health plans don't offer risk contracts and that even those that do may not share much, if any claims data. There's another way in which private insurers have proved less than supportive of ACOs and groups that are trying to reduce costs for the plans and the employers they represent.

Many commercial shared savings contracts, Daghestani says, let ACOs keep only 10%–20% of their shared savings; by comparison, the MSSP allows ACOs that contract for upside-only risk to retain a much higher percentage of their savings.[18] ARC is saving the state $8 million to $10 million a year, he notes, but earns back only $1.4 million of that.

"We understand that the health plan and the employer need to keep some of those savings, but an 80/20 or 90/10 split is an imbalance. It doesn't allow us to go all-in and invest aggressively in infrastructure," he says.

Wagar points out that it's also challenging for ACOs to sustain their level of income because their benchmarks keep changing from year to year. At one time, the MSSP used historical benchmarks, so an ACO always had to save more each year to see a return—a guarantee of failure for efficient groups. Now CMS blends that with regional benchmarks, which Wagar sees as a positive. But he notes that the MSSP's attribution of patients to physicians keeps changing, so that a patient may be in one ACO this year and in a different ACO next year.

"You've intervened with somebody who had a lot of visits to you a year and a half ago and closed their care gaps," he explains. "Now they have fewer or no visits to you, and they disappear into someone else's ACO [because of MSSP attribution rules]. That fouls up the risk pool." The only solution, he says, is for CMS to allow Medicare patients to pick the ACO they wish to belong to.

Meanwhile, the consolidation of the industry continues to be a challenge to some ACOs. Farias notes that RGVHA tries not to refer patients to employed specialists because hospitals are allowed to charge facility fees in addition to the professional fees for these visits. (CMS has changed this policy, but a federal court has struck down its new "site-neutral" payment policy.[19-20]) To make matters worse, she says, the local hospitals are hiring still more specialists out of independent practice, reducing the pool of cost-efficient doctors that the ACO can send patients to.

"That's why we need to take the next step as an ACO to incorporate specialists," she says. "Now that we have better data from our software vendor, we want to reach out and develop some preferred partnerships with independent specialists. That's the only way we're going to sustain savings in these specialty areas."

NEW DIRECTION FOR PHM

No matter how good a job an ACO or group does in managing population health, there's a limit to how much it can curb health spending. One reason is that healthcare accounts for only 10%–25% of the variance in individual health over time.[21] A far greater influence on health is exerted by the economic, social, and environmental factors collectively known as social determinants of health (SDOH). Just as primary care is upstream of specialty and hospital care, SDOH is upstream of primary care. Consequently, health plans and ACOs that manage population health are increasing their focus on these non-medical factors.

The next chapter will examine what's happening in this area and will consider the likelihood that SDOH can be addressed in ways that will cut health costs significantly.

CHAPTER 7

Addressing Social Determinants of Health

Jeremy Seals was once the kind of person known in the healthcare business as a "frequent flyer." In a single year, he visited the emergency department at Oregon Health & Science University in Portland 15 times and was admitted to the hospital 11 times, according to a report by Oregon Public Broadcasting. At the age of 40, his health was poor: he had had a heart attack when he was 35; he had congestive heart failure and terrible nerve pain in his legs.

What made his situation worse was that, because of his ill health, he was no longer able to hold a job. Then he became homeless and started living in his car.

"I basically lived at the emergency department," he told Oregon Public Broadcasting. "Ever since I'd had a heart attack, anytime my chest hurt, I'd either call the ambulance or go up to the hospital, and I think it was also out of desperation to just get out of my car and off the street."

Because of his frequent ED visits, Seals came to the attention of one of Oregon's coordinated care organizations (CCOs), which the state had created with federal funding to lower its Medicaid costs. The care manager assigned to work with Seals helped him schedule doctor appointments, get dialysis, and take his medications correctly. But that wasn't all. She also got him new boots (his old ones had holes in them) and a sleeping bag. She made sure he had passes for a local community center so he could shower. Eventually, she helped him land a spot in adult foster care so he had a place to live.

As a result of these and other interventions, Seals had only four ED visits and four hospitalizations the year after he entered the CCO program. Just averting a single hospitalization more than paid for the time his care manager had spent with him.[1]

Seals' case shows how addressing the "social determinants of health" can make a big difference in patient outcomes and health costs. Social determinants of health (SDOH) include a broad range of factors, such as socioeconomic status, race, environment, housing stability, food security, transportation, interpersonal violence, and alcohol and drug abuse, that influence a person's health.

Healthcare accounts for only 10%–25% of the variance in individual health over time, according to the World Health Organization. A much greater influence is exerted by genetic factors (up to 30%), health behaviors (30%–40%), social and economic factors (15%–40%), and physical environmental factors (5%–10%).[2]

Health behaviors are strongly affected by the other non-medical factors, so they are viewed as part of SDOH. And, as we'll see, mental health—which has an important influence on physical health—can be affected by social determinants such as poverty and violence. So, all these factors need to be considered together in devising a strategy to address SDOH as part of population health management.

Upstream from Primary Care

As explained in Chapter 4, good primary care is essential to any reform model that seeks to lower costs and improve outcomes because it is upstream from specialty and hospital care. But doctors have a much smaller influence on health behavior, which is upstream from primary care. Talk to any primary care physician and you'll get an earful about patients who don't follow their care plans and don't take care of themselves. Depending on the kind of population that the doctor treats, some of these people may have trouble paying rent or putting food on the table. They may be struggling with severe stress and/or depression. They may be victimized by intimate partners. They may not have transportation to go to the doctor's office or the pharmacy, and they may not be able to afford their medications.

According to a national survey, most physicians believe unmet social needs lead to worse health and that patients' social needs can have as big an impact on their health as their medical conditions do. However, 80% of the respondents said they didn't know how to deal with their patients' non-medical needs.[3]

In a fee-for-service environment, moreover, primary care doctors are not being paid for anything other than face-to-face office visits. They try to do the best they can by advising patients to quit smoking or drinking or leave boyfriends who beat them up. But behavior change is difficult, and physician advice alone has a limited impact on compliance.

"You can't make a patient better just by prescribing a pill," says Karen Handmaker, the healthcare consultant and former IBM Watson Health executive. "They might not be able to afford the pill or get the pill, or they might not be eating right. Addressing social determinants of health is going to have a cheaper, faster impact than healthcare alone. This is why there's a demand for community health workers, who can see what's going on in people's homes."

David Nash, MD, of the College of Population Health at Thomas Jefferson University, has a similar view. "Economically, focusing on the highest-risk patients is probably going to give the highest [financial] return in the short run," he says. "But the underlying reason that they're at such high risk is driven by the social determinants. For example, the homeless are among the highest utilizers [of healthcare]. But the core problem is the fact that they're homeless. So the answer to the riddle is to tackle the social determinants."

Widespread Social Issues

Research bears this out. Fifty-three percent of consumers who responded to a McKinsey & Co. survey said they were impacted by social determinants such as food, transportation, safety, housing, and social support. Those reporting higher ER and hospitalization rates were more likely to have unmet social needs.[4]

Similarly, a report on screening patients for SDOH said, "Individuals with unmet social needs are more likely to be frequent emergency department (ED) users, have repeat 'no-shows' to medical appointments, and have poorer glycemic and cholesterol control than those able to meet their needs."[5]

The impact of SDOH—and of increasing inequality—also can be seen in life expectancy. Better educated, more affluent Americans have a rising life expectancy, while the opposite is true for the poor and uneducated. In the 1970s, a 60-year-old man in the top half of the income distribution could expect to live 1.2 years longer than a man in the bottom half. By the turn of century, such an individual could expect to live 5.8 years longer than a less well-off man.[6]

A frequently cited 2002 article by J. Michael McGinnis, *et al.*, about social determinants found that about 60% of early deaths could be attributed to factors other than poor medical care and genetic predispositions. Clearly, SDOH interventions can promote health, the coauthors said. However, they added, "The cost-effectiveness of various interventions to improve population health is less clear."[7]

What has made SDOH interventions more cost-effective today, observers agree, is the growth of value-based care. Melinda Abrams, director and vice president of the Commonwealth Fund, says that the gradual shift to value-based payments has already changed the conversation about integrating healthcare with social services to address the needs of very sick patients.

In a recent report on SDOH, the National Academies of Sciences, Engineering and Medicine (NASEM) declared that the time has come for the nation to develop a program to make SDOH an intrinsic part of healthcare. The report said that SDOH data needs to be better integrated into healthcare delivery and that providers should make organizational commitments to addressing these factors.[8]

CURRENT SDOH INITIATIVES

In recent years, healthcare payers and providers have become increasingly aware of the importance of SDOH. To lower health costs, some organizations are trying to provide certain kinds of social support to high-risk patients or, more commonly, refer them to community resources. Health plans are leading this movement because they are most at financial risk. Risk-bearing ACOs and physician groups are also starting to get on board.

Some major hospital systems such as Dignity, Trinity and Northwell have launched significant SDOH initiatives, and 57 systems have invested a total of $2.5 billion in housing and other SDOH programs.[9] But most healthcare organizations are still just nibbling at the edges.

For example, a survey of Michigan emergency departments found that SDOH screening of super-utilizer patients is rare. There are several barriers to implementation of screening, including lack of financial support for programs that address social needs, the authors said.[10]

Another reason many hospitals are not paying much attention to SDOH is that better population health can actually cost them money. For example, Nemours Children's Health System in Jacksonville, Fla., started a home visit program to identify triggers of asthma. This program reduced ED visits and readmissions of children with asthma, but it hurt the healthcare system financially because fewer kids used hospital services.[11]

Most healthcare systems that intervene to help patients who lack adequate food, housing, and/or transportation, Nash says, have some type of financial exposure to the cost of care. "As the care delivery systems take on more risk on the road to value, they'll be more stimulated to participate in this process," he predicts.

Health Plans Step Up

Many private health insurers, meanwhile, have already ramped up SDOH initiatives. Kaiser Permanente, long a bellwether of national healthcare trends, is in the forefront of this movement. In January 2019, the big HMO announced it was investing more than $100 million in a multiyear initiative to address homelessness in the eight states where it has operations. The company also announced a new care network that will allow Kaiser providers to connect patients with community resources that address social needs such as housing instability and food insecurity.[12]

CVS and Aetna, its health insurance subsidiary, have launched a social network similar to Kaiser's. In partnership with SDOH software developer Unite US, the big pharmacy chain is helping Medicaid and Medicare/Medicaid beneficiaries covered by Aetna to more easily find and access aid from social service agencies in their communities. CVS is also investing $100 million in affordable housing for at-risk and underserved patients.[13]

UnitedHealthcare, the nation's largest private health insurer, is also taking on SDOH. Providers in United's Medicare Advantage plans made 560,000 referrals to social services in 2017 and 2018, the company said. Through a partnership with Mom's Meals, United also distributed over 2.5 million meals to its members in 2018.[14]

That same year, the Blue Cross Blue Shield Association founded the BCBS Institute, which is focused on social determinants. The institute has partnered with Lyft, enabling Blues plans to offer transportation to members who need it to access healthcare. The organization is also working with CVS and Walgreens to improve access to pharmacy services.[15]

Horizon Blue Cross Blue Shield of New Jersey has teamed with RWJ Barnabas Health to address the social needs of people who often visit EDs in Newark. Using community health workers, Horizon has targeted 1,000 frequent flyers and enrolled 40% of them in the program. Horizon reports that care costs for this population have dropped 25% as a result.[16]

The Geisinger Health Plan in Pennsylvania found that providing diabetic patients with fresh food had a greater impact on their health than medications did. After identifying people who were "food insecure," Geisinger enrolled them in a class on diabetes self-management, where a care team gave them "prescriptions" to a food pantry at a Geisinger clinic. After the program's first year, the plan's costs for these patients dropped by two-thirds. At the same time, their average HbA1c level—a measure of blood sugar—fell from 9.6 to 7.5.[17]

Government Initiatives

State Medicaid programs, Medicare Advantage plans, and traditional Medicare have also launched SDOH initiatives. In 2016, the Center for Medicare and Medicaid Innovation (CMMI) created the Accountable Health Communities Models, a five-year, $157 million demonstration project. Participating organizations are required to screen Medicare and Medicaid beneficiaries for health-related social needs and to refer patients to community-based services where it makes sense. Among the 30 organizations currently participating in the program are hospitals, HMOs, community health centers, city health departments, and a United Way chapter.[18]

The Centers for Medicare and Medicaid Services (CMS) has also given Medicare Advantage plans the green light to offer certain SDOH services. "For example, chronically ill beneficiaries enrolled in a Medicare Advantage plan can now receive meal delivery in more circumstances, transportation for non-medical needs like grocery shopping, and home environment services in order to improve their health or overall function as it relates to their chronic illness," a CMS news release said. "About 250 plans in 2020 will offer access to these types of supplemental benefits, reaching an estimated 1.2 million enrollees."[19]

However, a recent Urban Institute study found that Medicare Advantage plans are offering a narrow range of SDOH benefits and that none of them are doing so nationwide.

One reason is that CMS requires these benefits to be related to specific clinical criteria rather than letting the plans simply target frequent ED visitors. Also, the report said the plans don't want to shift supplemental benefits, such as vision and dental coverage, away from their members to fund SDOH services for a small percentage of enrollees.[20]

CMS has also approved Medicaid waivers to eight states (Alabama, California, Kansas, Massachusetts, New Hampshire, New Jersey, New York, and Texas) to enable them to reinvest federal Medicaid savings in care redesign programs.[21] The most notable of these Delivery System Reform Incentive Payment (DSRIP) programs is the one in New York.

In 2014, New York announced its plan to reinvest $8 billion in DSRIP money to overhaul its Medicaid program. The aim of the six-year program is to reduce avoidable hospital use by 25% while building the infrastructure required for value-based care.[22] New York has contracted with 25 performing provider systems (PPSs) that include both provider networks and community-based organizations (CBOs) led by safety-net providers. The participants have implemented various system improvement, population health, and clinical improvement projects.[23]

A survey of the participants, though, revealed that most DSRIP networks haven't robustly addressed social determinants of health. One reason for the limited focus on patients' unmet social needs, the stakeholders said, was "the dominance of hospitals in the governance and leadership of the PPSs." There was a "large cultural divide between most hospitals and CBOs," which had little experience working together and different business models.[24]

Initiatives in Other States

SDOH was a key component of Oregon's 2012 plan to bolster its Medicaid program. Under this scheme, the federal government gave Oregon $2 billion, to be paid back in future savings for its Medicaid program. The state used the money to create 15 coordinated care organizations (CCOs), which are locally governed networks of healthcare providers that deliver care to Medicaid recipients. The CCOs' goal is to save money by focusing on prevention and by reducing ED visits and hospitalizations. Part of their approach, as we saw in the case of Jeremy Seals, is to address social determinants of health for the sickest patients.[25] To date, the program has saved over $1 billion, according to one report.[26]

In Vermont, 85% of primary care practices participate in the Vermont Blueprint of Health, a state program that has organized community health teams (CHTs) to help practices deal with social determinants of health. These CHTs, which include nurse care managers, social workers, behavioral health counselors, dieticians, and health educators, help physicians care for complex patients who have significant social issues. Private insurers, Medicare, and Medicaid fund the Blueprint, including payments to CHTs and incentives for physicians to participate.[27]

Community Care of North Carolina (CCNC), a similar program, fields care managers who work closely with primary care physicians and a multidisciplinary team including physician assistants, psychiatrists, pharmacists, and community health workers. CCNC focuses on complex patients, especially those with multiple chronic conditions.[28] As part of North Carolina's current Medicaid overhaul, all Medicaid patients must be now be screened for SDOH, and providers are encouraged to use free software to refer patients to CBOs and follow up on them.[29]

WHERE PHYSICIANS STAND ON SDOH

As mentioned earlier, most physicians know how critical social determinants can be and wish they could do something about them. Among the most glaring needs that many patients have, in their doctors' view, are fitness programs, nutritious food, and transportation assistance. Urban doctors attach special importance to employment assistance, adult education, and housing assistance.

With nearly half of physicians employed by hospitals, those doctors' ability to respond to SDOH is circumscribed by their institutions' policies. Up to now, as noted previously, most healthcare systems have not been especially motivated to address patients' unmet social needs. Those that are doing anything on SDOH, such as Norton Healthcare in Louisville, Ky., tend to focus on supporting recently discharged patients so they don't get readmitted, says Handmaker.

Some at-risk ACOs and medical groups are going further. Rio Grande Valley Health Alliance, for example, has contracted with Uber and Lyft to ensure that patients can get to doctor appointments. In addition, the ACO directs patients who have insufficient food to food pantries. In some cases where people have had their electricity cut off because of unpaid utility bills, the ACO has even intervened to get the lights turned back on. If an elderly or disabled patient can't afford a walker, the ACO will pay for that.

The Heritage Provider Network, similarly, has long intervened to help patients with unmet social needs. Mark Wagar, president of Heritage Medical Systems, says this has been one of the keys to the organization's success.

Wagar is encouraged by payers' newfound interest in SDOH. "Some payers, including Medicare Advantage plans, are starting to provide resources for this. If you do these things the right way, you'll get paid for it," he says. "We were doing some of that already, but now we can be more aggressive on it when we know there's some return."

Doing the Right Thing

Not all of the doctors who see benefit in addressing SDOH are at financial risk. For example, Gregory King, MD, a partner in a small family practice in Bennington, Vermont, said the Vermont Blueprint for Health has helped his practice tremendously. Before the Blueprint came along, he told *Medical Economics* in 2017, he'd encourage patients with social needs to get in touch with various community agencies. But his office didn't have time to look up contact information or introduce the patients to the right people. So, his advice had little effect.

Now that he has access to a community health team, however, he can direct these patients to professionals who know how to get them the help they need, he said.

Montefiore Health System has an extensive care management program funded by New York's DSRIP program. Montefiore, based in the Bronx, employs about 600 care managers, including nurses, social workers, and health educators, who address the chronic diseases of high-cost patients and connect them with community resources if they have unmet social needs.

Asif Ansari, MD, medical director of one of Montefiore's physician practices, told *Medical Economics* that he wholeheartedly supported this program. Many of his and his colleagues' patients, he said, have trouble paying for medications and lack transportation and access to healthy food.

"Our physicians understand that we need this collaboration, this support and these resources to impact our patients' lives and their health," he said, referring to the social workers and other non-medical professionals at Montefiore. "When I compare practicing here 10 years ago and now, the difference in what I can do for my patients is significant."[30]

BEHAVIORAL HEALTH

Behavioral health may be impacted by an individual's environment and other social determinants of health. For these reasons, efforts to address social needs are often combined with an emphasis on behavioral healthcare.

Individuals with mental health and substance abuse conditions cost 2.5 to 3.5 times more to care for than do patients who have none of these issues.[31] When health-related productivity costs are combined with medical and pharmacy costs, in fact, the most expensive condition is depression, followed by obesity, arthritis, back/neck pain, and anxiety.[32]

Despite these facts, insurance companies still emphasize physical health more than behavioral health in their coverage policies. They cover behavioral health care to some extent, but generally pay therapists much less than other clinicians—except for psychiatrists, who mostly prescribe medications and care for people with severe mental illnesses.

More than a quarter of U.S. adults have some kind of mental disorder,[33] but only 43% of these people received any treatment in 2018.[34] From 10% to 20% of patients in primary care practices have mental health problems, and a much larger percentage of high utilizers do.[35] Primary care doctors, however, receive little training in behavioral health care and find it hard to counsel patients. So, they tend to prescribe medications and/or refer patients to psychologists, licensed clinical social workers or psychiatrists. But the patients often fail to follow up.[36]

Integration with Primary Care

Behavioral health care is more effective when behavioral health professionals practice alongside primary care doctors. For example, integrating depression treatment with medical care has been shown to be twice as effective as traditional depression care.[37]

The National Committee on Health Assurance (NCQA), as a condition for patient-centered medical home recognition, requires that practices support patients' behavioral health and collaborate with behavioral health professionals. However, it doesn't mandate the colocation of behavioral health providers in primary care practices.[38]

The Patient-Centered Primary Care Collaborative (PCPCC), in contrast, strongly supports the integration of behavioral health and primary care.[39] The PCPCC points to studies that document the decreased costs associated with this kind of integration. One of these studies showed that depression treatment in primary care resulted in a cost savings of $3,300 per patient over four years, returning $6.50 for every dollar spent.[40]

Nevertheless, few primary care practices—whether or not they're medical homes—include behavioral health professionals. According to a Commonwealth Fund report, "Behavioral health integration is still rare, and the integration of substance abuse services [is] even rarer, in part because there's been little or no financial incentive or administrative advantage to bringing what are now standalone medical and behavioral health operations together."[41]

SCREENING FOR SDOH

Physicians and their staffs have long asked patients about their social and family histories, and many doctors also inquire about patients' tobacco and alcohol use. But to identify patients who need help with their social determinants of health, more extensive screening is required.

A recent study examined the percentages of U.S. physician practices and hospitals that screened patients for food insecurity, housing instability, utility needs, transportation needs, and interpersonal violence. Only 16% of practices and 24% of hospitals reported screening for all five SDOH factors. Interpersonal violence was the social determinant most often screened for by both physician practices (56%) and hospitals (75%). About 30% of practices and 40% of hospitals screened for food insecurity; 28% of practices and 60% of hospitals screened for housing instability. [42]

Practices that served disadvantaged patients, including federally qualified health centers, reported higher screening rates. So did patient-centered medical homes and practices that participated in ACOs or bundled payments. Nearly half of academic medical centers screened for all five social determinants, and critical access hospitals and those with large Medicaid populations also screened at above-average rates.

Respondents cited lack of time and financial resources as the main barriers to screening. The relatively low level of screening can also be attributed to the limited evidence of a link between SDOH screening and better outcomes or lower spending, as well as "steep barriers to addressing social needs within clinical care," the researchers noted. The higher incidence of screening in hospitals, they added, may be related to the fact that they have greater resources than physician practices do.

Screening Tools

Several standardized instruments are available to screen patients for social needs. The best-known of these tools is the Protocol for Responding to and Assessing Patients' Assets, Risks, and Experiences (PRAPARE). Developed by the National Association of Community Health Centers, this tool includes eight of the 12 domains recommended in 2014 by the Institute of Medicine (IOM), plus several other questions.[43]

Health Leads has also created a social needs assessment based on the IOM domains, and CMS has developed a screening tool for its Accountable Health Communities. In addition, the American Academy of Family Physicians (AAFP) has devised long- and short-form screening tools for family practices.

Patients may be asked to fill out screening questionnaires in waiting rooms or on portals, or medical assistants may ask them the questions after they room the patients. In either case, the goal is to have the answers in the electronic health record (EHR) by the time the physician enters the exam room. With this information in hand, the doctor can ask the patient about concerning items and discuss how to address them.

EHR Integration

The IOM recommended that 10 patient-reported SDOH domains and one neighborhood/community-level domain be documented in EHRs.[44] However, the integration of SDOH screening tools with EHRs is still in the early stages. In addition, little is known about how to implement these tools within clinical workflows.

Both Epic and Cerner, the biggest EHR vendors, have begun integrating new SDOH screening tools into their systems, and it's a good bet their competitors will follow suit. Cerner's tool requires patients to answer questions on a portal or a practice staffer to enter data into the EHR. Cerner says it also enables providers to refer patients to social services.[45]

Nash is skeptical, however. The big EHR companies, he says, "have been talking about this for five years," and he doubts they will ever have effective SDOH modules. "They can't, they won't. It's not their core business."

That's why the market for SDOH software is still dominated by third-party vendors such as Innovacer, Zeomega, and MDClone, he says. Other significant players in this field include Healthify, NowPow, and Unite US.

The software developed by Unite US, for example, combines screening, decision support, electronic referral management, assessment and care plan management, and outcome tracking. The company helps providers develop "coordinated care networks" and engage community partners.[46] Among its customers are Kaiser Permanente,[47] MVP Health Care in Albany, N.Y.,[48] and Norton Healthcare in Louisville, Ky.[49]

SDOH INTERVENTIONS

As the New York DSRIP survey indicated, healthcare and social service providers have very different perspectives. In a 2016 book entitled *Provider-Led Population Health Management*, Ronan Rooney, the founder of an SDOH software firm, explained the difference between how doctors view their patients and how social workers look at their clients. The provider would think about prescribing a drug, for example, and the social worker would try to figure out how the client could locate and get to a pharmacy where he could buy the medication at low cost, Rooney said.[50]

To combine these contrasting perspectives into a truly person-centered approach, Rooney advocated forming multidisciplinary teams that include both clinical and social service professionals. Such a team ideally would be big enough to deal with 12–15 high-risk people at a time, he said. Helmed by a primary care physician, the team might include a care coordinator, a nurse, a behavioral health specialist, a social worker, a transportation coordinator, a pharmacist, and an attorney. The team members could be drawn from multiple offices, facilities, and business entities and could communicate with one other online.

This team model recalls the one that primary care expert Thomas Bodenheimer has proposed, in which primary care "teamlets" are supported by extended care teams (see Chapter 4). It also has much in common with a different model for integrating medical, behavioral, and social services in the treatment of very sick and frail elderly patients. In their paper on the latter approach, experts at the Commonwealth Fund said, "Multidisciplinary teams of clinicians, case managers, and patients working together can better tailor treatment plans to address medical needs by managing behavioral health conditions such as severe depression and non-medical issues such as unstable housing."[51]

Melinda Abrams of the Commonwealth Fund strongly supports this team approach. She also believes that non-physicians should carry most of the load, since doctors already have too much on their plates. In her view, physicians just need to have the right information about a patient's social determinants served to them at the right time, so they can discuss it with patients and make the appropriate referrals.

"You don't need a ton of doctors, you need midlevel people, and you bring in doctors when necessary," she says. "You also have to change the payment and incentive structure."

Bring in Social Workers

Handmaker suggests that primary care practices hire social workers, as some have already done. "Social workers are the highest level of this type of person who might go into the home, deal with behavioral health issues, counsel family members, and so on," she says. "Some social workers can actually provide therapy. They can help coordinate care across the social services spectrum. They might also manage others such as community health workers. The latter might be the lowest-paid but provide the highest value. They might have some training. But they're often in entry level jobs and field jobs—feet on the street jobs."

A Medicaid-managed care plan in her area has care coordinators doing exactly this kind of thing, Handmaker notes. "They go to healthcare clinics and community health centers, talk to plan members, help coordinate care, and see what's going on in their homes. They're the ones who can see there's no food in the cupboard or there are leaks in the roof. They can see if old people need more social services or social interaction. They can see that an asthmatic child lives in a house with lots of allergens and mold or that the rug is a fall risk for an older person."

Home health aides can also do some of this work, since they're already in the home, she adds. Right now, this is not strictly part of their job description, but it could be under value-based care. "Home health agencies could have different revenue streams by coordinating for other services. If they go into the home to take care of an older person, they could see the patient doesn't have food or has other challenges."

Population Health Management and SDOH

From a public health perspective, addressing social determinants of health is foundational to population health management. As at-risk physician groups and ACOs see it, however, PHM is mostly about healthcare for a defined population. While the groups that are more experienced with PHM increasingly emphasize SDOH, it's still secondary to the main task of improving health through care coordination, patient engagement, and better preventive and chronic care.

Organizations involved in PHM, as explained in Chapter 6, must decide how much emphasis to place on managing care for various population segments. Smaller organizations and those that are new to PHM tend to focus on high-risk and rising-risk individuals. But the overriding goal of PHM is to optimize the health of all patients to prevent them from getting sick or sicker.

The budgets that at-risk groups must manage within are designed to cover healthcare, not SDOH interventions. Those interventions, whether they be referrals to community resources or the delivery of certain services by the healthcare organization, may reduce health costs and help the at-risk entity succeed financially. But the cost of the infrastructure to execute on SDOH must also be considered, and there is a limit to how many people can receive SDOH-related services from the organization.

So, one issue that confronts any group or ACO that takes on SDOH is how much of its patient population to include in its SDOH initiative. To some extent, that depends on whether the organization primarily is referring patients to housing agencies, food pantries, legal aid, and the like, or whether it also delivers some services, such as free transportation or home visits to assess patient living conditions. But ultimately, the decision comes down to whether SDOH interventions can reduce health costs enough to guarantee the organization a return on investment.

Considered in that perspective, helping high-risk, high-cost patients with health-related social services is a no-brainer. But it's unclear how far down in the population risk hierarchy an organization should go. Should it also provide such services to rising-risk patients? Should a diabetic, overweight patient who isn't an ER frequent flyer also be included, for example?

"Probably, and that probably makes it difficult to afford it," Abrams says. "In addition to identifying those who have the greatest needs and are at greatest risk, you have to identify those who are amenable to change. Another way of doing it is to start with the highest-need, highest-cost patients, because that's where you're going to see the greatest savings. And with those savings, you can invest not just in the top 1% or 5% [of high-cost patients], but also in the top 10% or 15%."

COMMUNITY COLLABORATIONS

Another challenge, Abrams notes, is to ensure that the community-based organizations that provide most social services are adequately funded, especially as the demands on them from healthcare organizations increase. The majority of social services are provided by local governments, public health agencies, and nonprofit agencies. None of these entities has been adequately funded in their work with the poor, and the situation has worsened under the Trump Administration.

The money available to CBOs "has decreased as part of the war on the poor that's being waged," Nash declares. "It makes no economic sense whatsoever. It's counterproductive. Although health is derived from these investments, we're actually decreasing these investments, and continuing to pour money into bricks and mortar facilities, doctor training and super-subspecialization. The system is upside down and backwards."

The news is not all bad. As a 2017 report on SDOH partnerships noted, "a broadening recognition of the critical role of the social determinants of health is forging increasingly common ground for providers of healthcare and human services." As a result, more partnerships between healthcare organizations and CBOs are emerging across the U.S.[52]

However, the report said, "most commonly, partnerships provided services to impact immediate-term clinical needs, such as reducing hospital admissions or length of stay." This was usually because the participating healthcare systems had financial incentives to do these things.

Community Benefit

Among those incentives is the "community benefit" that not-for-profit hospitals must provide to justify their tax exemptions. Two not-for-profit hospitals in Spokane, Wash., for example, pay for beds in shelters that provide homeless patients with a safe place to stay after hospital discharge so they can heal better and more quickly.[53] The hospitals' investment comes out of the funds that they must invest in the community to keep their tax exemption. Unfortunately, few other healthcare systems have a similar conception of community benefit.

Not-for-profit hospitals—nearly 80% of all U.S. acute care facilities—have always been required to supply a community benefit in exchange for their exemption from federal, state, and local taxes. The Affordable Care Act added new requirements to the section of the Internal Revenue Code that governs hospitals' tax-exempt status. Among other things, hospitals must now produce an annual community health needs assessment with an accompanying implementation strategy. But they don't have to spend a certain percentage of revenues on helping communities meet those needs.[54]

In a 2015 report to Congress based on 2011 data, the Treasury Department stated:

> In aggregate, private tax-exempt hospitals provided less than 10 percent of their total expenses as community benefit, consisting of about 2 percent charity care, 3 percent unreimbursed Medicaid and others means-tested programs, and 4 percent other community benefits, *of which less than 0.5 percent was for community health improvement services* [emphasis added].[55]

In Abrams' view, health systems can't be expected to fund social services for a large portion of an area population, including many people who are not their patients. However, she says, "One way we can help to support the community-based organizations and build the community infrastructure is if large hospital systems use their community benefit dollars to work with those partners to upgrade their capacity: help them update their IT systems, develop workflows to exchange information with them, work with them on their business acumen, and develop measures that are meaningful for both sides."

In Louisville, Norton Healthcare is collaborating with the community to build the United US platform connecting healthcare providers with social services, Handmaker says. "The city and the school system are paying some money into it. And the unique thing about Louisville is that the Unite US platform is not emanating from a health system or a health plan. It's a community asset that we want all the payers and health systems to participate in. And we're making progress in that direction, which I think helps to spread the risk and encourages providers to spend money on infrastructure."

CONCLUSION

The growing recognition of social determinants' role in health is a very positive sign. Driven by the transition to value-based care, it has sparked a movement that, in Nash's view, is here to stay. "I think it's the spearhead of a major shift, and it makes economic sense."

Nevertheless, the new emphasis on SDOH raises a question that Ashok Rai, MD, the president and CEO of Prevea Health, put to me: "Where does the provider responsibility end and the society's responsibility begin?"

Nash replies, "That's the $64,000 question. Society, the way we're currently funded, has abrogated this question and turned the responsibility over to the healthcare system. Because politically, it's supercharged."

Abrams believes that society is ultimately responsible for addressing social determinants of health. "The provider's responsibility, in my view, is not necessarily to solve and manage and address every problem, but it is to identify, recognize and coordinate the response to those problems. It's not realistic or desirable for a primary care provider to take on food insecurity for every single one of his or her patients. But it's important to assess it and to identify partners in the community and work with them to address it together."

It's unclear, though, how much society is willing to spend to ensure that social determinants of health are addressed. "Changing social inequalities and even investing tax dollars in social and community programs always represent zero-sum activities where those with more resources need to share with those with few resources," the McGinnis paper concluded. "It takes more than just evidence that social change would improve health to convince the general public that such redistributive investments should be undertaken. These choices are very much about ideology and social values."[56]

CHAPTER 8

Physician-Led Healthcare Reform

As noted earlier in this book, we cannot control health costs without greatly reducing the endemic waste that plagues our system. Moving to a single-payer, Medicare for All system would greatly reduce one part of that waste—administrative costs—but would have little effect on the waste in care delivery. The drop in administrative costs would occur only once, after which health spending would resume its inexorable rise. Price controls, the only other cost-reduction mechanism in the Medicare for All proposals, would harm many providers if their incomes were cut to the levels that those schemes necessitate. This is a self-defeating approach. Unless physicians can be engaged in the reform process, it is doomed to failure.

To make Medicare for All work for all stakeholders, it must give healthcare providers a strong incentive to cut the amount of waste in the system; but that isn't as simple as just having doctors practice more efficiently in return for a share of the savings. The entire system needs to be restructured from top to bottom to provide the optimal conditions for physicians to deliver high-quality care in the most efficient manner. Primary care doctors must be placed in charge of the system, and they must form groups large enough to take financial risk so that they can be paid for value rather than volume. By reducing waste and improving outcomes, high-performing physicians—both primary care doctors and specialists—could take better care of patients while maintaining or raising their own incomes.

Like other people, most physicians are wary of change. Under a restructured system, they'd have to make major changes in how they practice. They'd have to practice in groups different from any they've ever known, in many cases with physicians they don't know. The financial incentives underlying their business would be turned upside down. Why should they do this?

To understand why, physicians must recognize that some kind of fundamental change is inescapable. The current fee-for-service system, like Soviet communism in 1989, cannot continue for long. The American people are crying out for change because they can no longer afford healthcare. This is the number one issue for voters, and politicians—at least on the Democratic side—are responding to this widespread popular discontent.

Whatever physicians may think about Medicare for All, it's coming, probably on the wings of a public option.

If the government adopted a long-term transition strategy, as outlined in Chapter 1, more and more people would join a public plan that would probably pay physicians at Medicare rates. Private insurance would continue to pay more, but it would shrink as a percentage of their business. As a result, doctors would be faced with a painful choice: either remain as they are and see their incomes decrease, or participate in physician-led healthcare reform that allows them to recapture their lost revenue by taking financial risk.

Managed Competition

Besides risk, the other major component of this physician-led reform model is competition between providers. That may come as a surprise to those who believe that a single-payer, tax-financed system would necessarily squelch free enterprise and result in the government making all decisions on healthcare, but this doesn't have to be the case.

In the 1990s, it will be recalled, the Clinton Health Plan relied largely on Alain Enthoven's theory of "managed competition." Under this legislation, health plans with standardized benefits would have competed for enrollees under very strict government regulation. The physician-led reform model does something similar, but with a major difference: Instead of managing the competition between health plans, it sets the conditions for competition between large primary care groups. This approach places the competition where it should be, between the providers who are best situated to reduce waste without stinting on necessary care.

Such a model would be difficult if not impossible to implement under a multi-payer system. The primary care doctors must be financially at risk for all their patients to align their incentives; under the current system, in contrast, they are constantly whipsawed between the incentives of fee for service and value-based arrangements of various kinds. Additionally, as long as profit-making health plans take primary insurance risk or administer the plans of self-insured employers, they will try to interfere in care management. As doctors know well, that micromanagement is not good for them or their patients.

Instead, care management should be directed by primary care physicians. As I've pointed out several times in this book, PCPs are best-suited to manage care because they are upstream of the major cost drivers: hospitals, specialists, ancillaries, and post-acute care providers. Through their treatment and referral decisions, PCPs influence the cost of a case and the patient's outcome. They can appropriately manage many patients who have chronic conditions without referring to a specialist. They can coordinate care across care settings, and they are well placed to interface with community-based organizations that address patients' unmet social needs.

Ideally, during the decade-long transition to Medicare for All, the care delivery system would be transformed along the lines described above. Primary care groups capable of taking financial risk would be incentivized to deliver high-quality care at the lowest possible cost. They'd refer to and collaborate with specialists who were committed to the same goals. Overall spending growth would slow and possibly reverse, yielding the extra money required for universal, comprehensive coverage while allowing healthcare providers to thrive as well.

This rosy scenario, however, cannot become reality without concerted action by the federal government. The corporate gigantism that has overtaken healthcare—in care delivery, health insurance, and pharmaceutical manufacturing—is too big for the free market to tame. The states are unlikely to agree on the regulations needed to rein in enormous healthcare organizations that often cross state boundaries, so any proposal to fundamentally restructure healthcare will require federal legislation.

NATIONAL ALL-PAYER LAW

As hospital systems become larger and employ more physicians, healthcare prices will continue to rise and independent doctors will find it harder to remain independent. Hospitals will never fully embrace value-based care as long as it threatens their primary business model, which is to fill beds and generate outpatient revenues. To create a viable, sustainable healthcare system, the market power of hospitals must be eliminated.

Federal antitrust policy is not adequate to handle this task. Even if the Federal Trade Commission had more latitude to deal with mergers among not-for-profit entities, the industry is already so consolidated that the FTC would have to break up health systems involving thousands of hospitals. Such a gargantuan effort would be practically and legally unfeasible.

All-payer Systems

The government could curtail health systems' market power without breaking them up. For example, either states or the federal government could adopt "all-payer" models similar to those in Maryland and West Virginia. Under the Maryland model introduced 40 years ago, every insurer, including Medicare, Medicaid, and private health plans, pays uniform hospital rates negotiated between the state and the hospitals.

It would be difficult for other states to replicate this approach because commercial rates are now so much higher than Medicare and Medicaid rates, said Paul Ginsburg, chair of the medicine and public policy department of the University of Southern California and a fellow of the Brookings Institution, in 2016 testimony to the California Senate Committee on Health. A more feasible approach, he said, would be to emulate West Virginia, which sets only commercial insurance payments to hospitals.[1]

In either case, however, an all-payer system would eliminate the ability of dominant health systems to extract very high rates from private payers.

Before Maryland implemented its all-payer model in 1977, the average cost of a Maryland hospital admission was 26% above the national average. In 2007, the average cost per case was 2% below the national average. However, in 2000, after the state eliminated payment adjustments based on the volume of hospital admissions, those admissions began to increase rapidly.[2] Consequently, in 2014, Maryland started setting a global annual budget for each hospital in the state. Hospitals bill payers per admission (for inpatient care) or per service (for outpatient care) but are now expected to raise or lower their prices to remain on budget.[3]

In the first three years after this program was fully implemented, Maryland hospital spending rose only 1.4% annually, well below the CMS target of 3.6%. Acute care admissions and gross hospital spending fell 2.7% and 2.3%, respectively, between fiscal years 2015 and 2016. Moreover, quality improved: Maryland saw a 6.1% reduction in readmissions and a 43.3% drop in hospital-acquired conditions over the three-year period.

As might be expected, providers responded to global budgets by shifting more care to the ambulatory and post-acute care sectors. Consequently, non-hospital spending in Maryland grew by 4.2% in 2016, greatly exceeding the national rate of 1.9% and offsetting the decrease in hospital spending.[4]

Renewed Interest in States

A few decades ago, several other states used all-payer rate setting, but they all abandoned it for various reasons. Most of these laws fell prey to gaming by providers and to political infighting within the states.[5] Today, however, other states are following the path blazed by Maryland. In 2019, for example, Washington enacted a law under which the state will contract with private insurers to offer low-cost, tightly regulated plans on its ACA exchange. These plans will pay hospitals no more than 160% of Medicare rates. While this is much higher than the law's proponents had hoped for, it was the best they could do to get the program enacted.[6]

It's unlikely that most states will go in this direction; however, the federal government could adopt a national all-payer rate system. Early in the transition to Medicare for All, Congress could pass legislation requiring all private insurers and self-insured employers to pay the same rates to hospitals, with adjustments for charity care and rural needs. Such rates would have to be negotiated by the government, which would continue to pay current Medicare rates; current state Medicaid rates would also remain in place until Medicaid was folded into Medicare during the transition period. Eventually, after private insurance disappeared, hospitals would be paid at negotiated rates across the board.

If the concept of a national all-payer system seems quixotic, no less an authority than Donald Berwick, MD, former acting administrator of CMS, recently proposed limiting hospital charges to 120% of Medicare rates across the board. "This is enough revenue to offset Medicaid underpayments and should provide appropriate pressure on hospitals to become more productive," Berwick and Robert Kocher argued in a *Health Affairs Blog* post. The authors also recommended that future hospital price increases be limited to the annual increase in the consumer price index.[7]

Ginsburg supports the idea of unified administered pricing for hospitals. As quoted in my previous book, *Rx For Health Care Reform*, he noted that with universal coverage, states would no longer have to funnel money to inefficient hospitals to subsidize charity care. If all hospitals received the same risk-adjusted payments for the same procedures, he said, the inefficient ones would be likely to cut their costs or go out of business. On the other hand, he pointed out, the government would have to make allowances for special circumstances. For example, CMS would still have to subsidize teaching hospitals and trauma centers, he said.[8]

DIVESTING PRACTICES

Even under all-payer rate setting for hospitals, healthcare systems that employ a lot of physicians would still have bargaining power. To eliminate their ability to raise costs by negotiating higher rates for their employed physicians, the government could simply prohibit hospitals and other non-physician-owned entities from hiring doctors or owning their practices.

There are several good reasons for doing this. Besides raising costs, hospital employment of doctors can reduce the quality of care by forcing physicians to admit patients to lower-quality facilities.[9] Hospital-owned practices have more preventable admissions than do physician-owned practices, as noted in Chapter 3.[10] And, as Aledade CEO Farzad Mostashari, MD, observed earlier in this book, burnout is more prevalent among employed physicians than among independent doctors because the former lament their loss of autonomy.

The reluctance of healthcare systems to embrace value-based care must also be considered. Compared to independent practitioners, employed physicians have less incentive to restrain hospital utilization, so the divestment of owned practices would liberate physicians who are now "aligned" with hospital business strategies to pursue value-based care under a different set of financial incentives. Hospitals' divestment of their practices is thus a cornerstone of the physician-led reform model I'm proposing.

Corporate Practice of Medicine Laws

Many states already have "corporate practice of medicine" laws that bar corporations from employing physicians. These statutes were enacted to avoid conflicts of interest between physicians' duty to provide the best care for their patients and their employers' dictates—exactly the kind of conflict in which many doctors find themselves today. Most states with such laws allow hospitals to hire doctors, however, since they're also in the business of medicine.[11]

The sole exception is California. That state's corporate practice of medicine law prohibits any non-professional organization except for a public hospital, a narcotics treatment program, or a nonprofit medical research firm from directly employing physicians. Unfortunately, the California corporate practice of medicine law has not had the intended effect. Instead of hiring doctors, private hospitals and health systems simply lease their services from "foundations" that stand in for professional corporations.

The federal government could enact a stronger law that prohibits hospitals from directly or indirectly employing doctors. The statute should be written so that it also applies to insurance companies that employ doctors, such as United/Optum and Anthem. The venture capitalists that have recently been snapping up physician practices to turn them over for a profit[12] should be forced to divest those practices as well.

It's unclear how much it might cost the government to compensate insurers and private equity firms for divesting their practices. Optum's recent $4.3 billion purchase of the giant DaVita Medical Group might be a marker for that expense; but however much it costs, corporations cannot be allowed to buy physician practices and use them for their own purposes. Healthcare is a public good, and its overriding goal must be to improve individual and population health.

Hospitals' Objections

Hospitals would not have to be compensated for returning physicians to private practice. As we've seen, it's unclear whether most hospitals would be worse off economically if their medical staffs were independent rather than employed. Considering the losses that hospitals incur on practice management, some hospitals would benefit financially from divesting their owned practices. The hospitals' main concern would be to prevent competitors from controlling their referring doctors. If no health system could employ physicians, that wouldn't be a problem.

Nevertheless, many hospitals would undoubtedly file lawsuits—or a class action suit—against the government. They might claim they were being unlawfully deprived of revenues that their employed physicians generated in excess of what those doctors would generate if they could refer to other hospitals, but this might be a hard case to make in court. Government attorneys would point out that hospitals cannot legally require employed doctors to refer to them. They could also observe that hospital employment of doctors has driven up health costs and, in some cases, resulted in inferior or unnecessary care.

The hospitals might also argue that they were being forced to divest their practices without compensation for their intrinsic value. Most hospital-owned practices, however, were acquired for little more than the value of their hard assets (equipment, fixtures, etc.) and receivables. Since most of these practices are losing money, it would be difficult to maintain that the hospitals should be compensated for giving them up.

Certain kinds of physicians should continue working for or exclusively contracting with hospitals because they are indispensable to inpatient or ED care. Among these are radiologists, anesthesiologists, pathologists, emergency department specialists, and critical-care physicians. Hospitals should also be allowed to employ hospitalists, who can increase the efficiency of care; however, as discussed in the next chapter, at-risk physician groups should also have their own hospitalists.

Hospitals would continue paying members of faculty practices for teaching and supervising residents, but the clinical practices of these physicians should also be divested.

PRIMARY CARE GROUPS

Under the physician-led reform model, hospitals would lose their market power and divest their physician practices near the beginning of the transition to Medicare for All. All other changes in care delivery follow from these two fundamental changes, and nothing else is possible without them.

The next step in this project would be to establish incentives for primary care physicians to join or form groups of a certain size, which I call "statutory groups." As mentioned earlier, these groups would be designed to take financial risk and compete with one another. The incentives to form such groups would increase over time. At first, they might include government loan guarantees and the ability of these groups to participate in the Medicare Shared Savings Program (MSSP), but this would be only be the beginning. As an increasing number of people joined the public plan and a growing percentage of physician reimbursement was paid at Medicare rates, PCPs would see their incomes fall. To earn more, they would have to join one of the statutory groups. By doing so, they'd have the opportunity to make at least as much as or potentially much more than they do today (see Chapter 11).

In lieu of forming statutory groups, doctors in small practices could establish or join networks of the requisite size. This wouldn't be a big change for the many doctors who belong to network ACOs or IPAs today; but over time, physicians would likely recognize that integrated groups offered them the best chance of financial success. This is partly because physicians who take financial risk together must be clinically integrated and follow clinical guidelines that all of the doctors approve. This is harder to do in a network than in a group; moreover, physician networks that use multiple EHRs are less efficient than groups that use a single system.[13]

During the transition to Medicare for All, primary care physicians would have several options to raise their incomes by delivering value-based care. They could be part of an ACO that held value-based contracts, contract directly with Medicare Advantage plans that offered bonuses for reducing costs, or set up a direct primary care practice that didn't take insurance. As the conversion to a single-payer system neared completion, however, all of these alternatives would be eliminated. After that, the only way primary care doctors could earn more than Medicare rates would be to join a statutory group or network.

While this might seem like an excess of central planning, the government must step in forcefully to accelerate the move to value-based care across the board. As discussed earlier, fee for service still dominates U.S. healthcare, and health costs are anticipated to grow much faster than GDP or wages in the next decade and beyond, so a way must be found to bend the cost curve in the near future.

In 2018, the MSSP's net savings were only 2% of the annual increase in Medicare spending,[14] and there's no indication that value-based contracts have significantly lowered private expenditures. Medicare Advantage plans are popular with beneficiaries and physicians, but their upcoding of case severity has resulted in overpayments by Medicare.[15] Global capitation is not a realistic option for most physician groups. Thus, something else is needed. I believe that a single-payer system coupled with the physician-led reform model is the alternative most likely to rein in costs.

Assembling PCP Groups

The building blocks of the statutory primary care groups already exist. To start with, there are more than 1,000 accountable care organizations (ACOs), of which 42% are physician-led.[16] Within the MSSP, 61 ACOs, or 11% of the total, consisted mostly or wholly of primary care doctors in 2018. The median size of ACOs in the MSSP was 315 physicians; commercial ACOs tended to be bigger.[17] So hundreds of ACOs include enough PCPs to form groups of the requisite size.

Large multispecialty groups could also give birth to statutory primary care practices. In 2018, about 27.5% of physicians practiced in groups of more than 30 doctors.[18] Many of these groups were owned by hospitals. If the hospitals divested these practices, they could form the nuclei of many primary care groups of the desired size.

The American Medical Group Association (AMGA), which represents primarily large groups, has 440 members. The median number of doctors in these groups is 180.[19] Assuming that a third of these physicians are primary care doctors, on average, at least 220 AMGA members include enough primary care physicians to form one or more statutory groups of the size needed.

Overall, it appears that at least 1,000 statutory groups could be created out of the box. That's far short of the number of competing groups that would be required under the physician-led reform model, but nearly half of practicing physicians are employed by hospitals, and the majority of doctors participate in ACOs.[20] Therefore, it's likely that the actual number of PCPs already working together in groups or networks of the requisite size is larger than appears on the surface.

The Great Separation

For the reasons enumerated below, the non-primary care specialists in these groups would have to separate themselves from the primary care doctors, or vice versa. Either the specialists or the primary care physicians could leave these groups and form their own practices. In multispecialty ACOs, however, the primary care doctors would stay, because a specialist-only ACO would not be able to manage care or control costs.

While the reform law would not require multispecialty groups or ACOs to split up, most of them probably would do so because their primary care physicians could earn more by taking risk in statutory groups as fee-for-service payment rates fell. If the ACOs wanted to remain as they were, perhaps at some point multispecialty ACOs would no longer be allowed to participate in the Medicare Shared Savings Program. There are a number of different ways in which the government could induce PCPs and specialists to part and go their own ways.

In some cases, there would not be enough PCPs left in a group or an ACO to reach the size threshold for the statutory groups, but these organizations would probably attract other primary care doctors because of their prebuilt infrastructure and/or group culture.

The primary care doctors in the statutory groups would include internists, family physicians, pediatricians, and med-peds (doctors board-certified in internal medicine and pediatrics). Because each of these primary care specialties addresses different needs and demographic groups, it would be desirable to have a specialty mix in each group, but that might not be possible in some geographic regions.

Obstetricians/gynecologists would not be considered primary care doctors in this model, because they don't handle a wide enough range of conditions and most of them perform procedures. Non-hospital-employed hospitalists and geriatricians, however, would fit naturally into the primary care groups.

Why Specialists Must Leave

There are two reasons the competing groups in the physician-led reform model must be primary care only. First, specialists are not distributed equally across the United States. In less-populated areas, there are relatively few specialists; even in larger markets, certain specialties may be in short supply. If there is to be fair competition between primary care groups, they all must have equal access to the specialists. Scattering some specialists across the primary care groups would impede that access, because the specialists would be less available for referrals from other groups than they would be to referrals from doctors in their own practice. A primary care group that didn't have access to all necessary specialties would probably not be in business for long.

The other reason for excluding specialists from the primary care groups is that those groups would be taking financial risk. If a statutory practice included specialists, there would be a natural incentive for the primary care doctors to refer to those physicians. That would be fine if the specialists were the highest-quality, most efficient doctors in the area, but there's no reason to suppose that this would be so in all cases, or even in most cases. For the primary care groups to be successful in bearing financial risk, they must refer patients to high-performing specialists as much as possible.

Many high-functioning multispecialty groups exist today. Mayo Clinic, Cleveland Clinic, Intermountain, Geisinger, Partners Healthcare, Baylor Scott & White, Kelsey-Seybold, Summit Medical Group, Everett Clinic, Ochsner, Advocate Aurora . . . the list goes on. What happens to those groups in this restructuring? The primary care physicians in the groups—whether they or the specialists left to form their own practices—could still refer to their former colleagues and collaborate with them via the electronic systems discussed in Chapter 10.

The hardest challenge would be the Kaiser Permanente groups, some of which include thousands of doctors. Each of these groups might spin off dozens of primary care practices in their regions. These groups could refer to the remaining Kaiser specialists, although some of those might have to split into smaller practices also, if they were too dominant in a market.

It may be argued that dividing up multispecialty groups in this manner would increase the fragmentation of healthcare providers. On the other hand, virtual integration of care teams, which will be explained later, could get all the providers caring for a patient on the same page.

What Kind of Risk?

Over the decades since the first wave of managed care, U.S. physicians have shown themselves to be markedly risk averse. That's understandable: In the 1990s, insurance companies tried to jam the HMO style of practice down the throats of doctors across the country. They made primary care physicians into gatekeepers, which both doctors and patients hated. Some primary care doctors took full professional risk before they knew how to manage care and lost their shirts. On top of it all, a significant drop in capitation rates in California, the birthplace of HMOs, wiped out some physician groups.

Primary care capitation, which is much more common today than prepayment for all professional services, carries far less financial risk for primary care physicians. However, it doesn't motivate most doctors to practice differently if only a minority of their business is prepaid. In addition, it can incentivize some doctors to refer out to specialists more frequently than they'd do otherwise.

Some groups accept global capitation that prepays them for all healthcare, including hospital care. Such contracts are rare, though, and the groups that hold them are usually very large and experienced in population health management.

Many ACOs and group practices have shared savings contracts with commercial and/ or government payers. As explained earlier, these arrangements may involve upside risk only or upside and downside risk. For example, in the "enhanced" risk track of the MSSP, ACOs take upside and downside risk for the total cost of care for their attributed Medicare patients. These ACOs receive up to 75% of the shared savings; if they spend more than their benchmark amount, they must pay a minimum of 40% of the overage back to CMS. The upside can't exceed 20% of the benchmark, and the downside can't exceed 15% of it.[21]

While the MSSP has some drawbacks, especially in provider attribution and benchmarking, it has gained considerable traction. In 2018, 37% of the 548 participating ACOs—including those taking upside-only and two-sided risk—received $739 million in shared savings from the program. Significantly, ACOs in the two-sided risk track saved $96 per Medicare beneficiary, while those without downside risk saved just $68 per beneficiary.[22]

In 2018, only 18% of MSSP participants were in risk-based tracks,[23] but a recent analysis found that nearly 30% of ACOs took two-sided risk under either Medicare, Medicaid, or commercial contracts. Among physician-led ACOs, 32% accepted downside risk.[24]

Another report on risk-taking ACOs in the MSSP noted:

> Approximately two-thirds of physician-based ACO respondents reported that they were likely to remain in the program if required to accept downside risk, compared with only about one-third of hospital-based ACOs. . . . This reflects the fact that physician-based ACOs have performed better, and a higher proportion of these ACOs have earned shared savings, than hospital-based ACOs. Physician-based ACOs have generated substantial savings by reducing spending for both inpatient and outpatient hospital services, which has not been true for hospital-based ACOs.[25]

What this reveals is that doctors in many physician-led ACOs have become comfortable with and adept at cost and quality management. Coupled with the fact that more than half of physicians now belong to an ACO,[26] the success of doctor-led ACOs suggests that the incentive to lower the total cost of care through shared savings is acceptable to many physicians. While ACOs bearing downside risk are still in the minority, the ability of many ACOs to manage costs within a budget predicts continued success for physician-led ACOs as they take on more risk.

The groups in our model, however, are smaller than most ACOs and are primary care only; consequently, they will need a transitional payment model to help them learn how to manage risk. One method of doing this would be to adopt something like CMS's Comprehensive Primary Care Plus (CPC+) program (see Chapter 2). To recap, track 2 of CPC+ pays primary care practices a monthly, risk-adjusted care management fee, along with performance-based incentives that include downside risk. Practices continue to receive a reduced amount of fee for service to counterbalance the performance-based incentives up to a certain level.[27]

This carrot-and-stick approach, which retains some fee for service, could be one way to wean primary care doctors from pay for volume. Ultimately, however, the groups should be prepaid for primary care, which would provide the flexibility they need to manage population health. Primary care capitation would also reduce the administrative burden on the practices by eliminating billing-related work.

Prepayment for primary care wouldn't incentivize the doctors to refer out because they'd also be taking a portion of the risk for the total cost of care. If they didn't do as much as they could for patients and work them up properly before referring them, more of their budget would go to high-cost specialists.

Unlike the MSSP risk tracks, which cover only Medicare Parts A and B, the total costs in the physician-led reform model would also include drug costs. On the other hand, the groups in our model would take less downside risk as a percentage of revenues than do the MSSP ACOs. The groups would also be supported by the infrastructure vendors discussed in the next chapter.

Group Size

The statutory groups must be big enough to take financial risk of the kind described above. In addition, they must have the human and technological resources required for population health management. However, they can't be too large, or the groups won't be able to compete on an even playing field.

In my earlier book, Lawrence Casalino, MD, now of Weill Cornell Medical College, said that groups of between 10 and 30 physicians could assemble the infrastructure to do disease management and measure performance. Managed care companies have fielded risk-taking groups with 20 to 80 doctors each,[28] and the Rio Grande Valley Health Alliance has shown that a group of 20-odd primary care doctors can successfully take two-sided risk in the MSSP.

Practice sizes would also vary by region. In large metropolitan areas, where there are far more doctors, the competing groups would be larger than they would be in smaller cities and exurban areas. In rural areas, there might be only enough primary care doctors—or physicians in general—to form one or two groups. Therefore, competition could not exist in those areas, but the groups could still take financial risk.

To figure out how many physicians should be in a primary care group, both the size of the local population and the ratio of primary care doctors to that population must be weighed. For example, New York City has an estimated population of 8.4 million. In contrast, 219,000 people live in Spokane, Wash., and 390,000 reside in its metropolitan area.[29-30] There were 114 primary care physicians per 100,000 people in the New York metro area in 2006, the latest year for which I could find data.[31] In 2014, by contrast, there were 79 primary care physicians per 100,000 in Washington State.[32]

Taking these factors into account, along with the size of the average PCP's patient panel, it can be estimated that groups of 50–100 primary care doctors would be the right size in the New York area if it were are subdivided into about 20 regions. In smaller markets like Spokane, groups of 25–50 physicians would suffice.

Assuming the average group included 50 full-time-equivalent primary care doctors, between 3,000 and 4,000 statutory groups would be required to care for the entire U.S. population.[33] Midlevel providers such as nurse practitioners and physician assistants would also have to be counted, so the numbers of physicians in these groups might be lower. If so, there could be more competing groups; however, there would still have to be enough practice owners in each group to take financial risk.

Specialists would form their own groups, but the size of these practices would also have to be limited. Under the reform model, specialists would be required to see patients referred by any primary care physician. If most of the specialists in a market or in a specialty field belonged to the same group, however, it would be difficult for the primary care doctors to secure their cooperation in reducing waste and coordinating care. No matter to which specialist in that group they referred, the practice would benefit financially. Taking business away from a noncooperating specialist in that situation would not have much sting.

In general, specialists would have a strong incentive to collaborate with PCPs because the latter would steer patients to the highest-performing, most-cooperative doctors. Aside from building referrals, the specialists would also aim to garner bonuses. Their base pay, like that of the primary care doctors, would not be much higher than Medicare rates as private insurance faded out; but primary care groups that netted shared savings would be required to pay part of that to the specialists who helped them hold down costs. The minimum percentages would be set by law, but the primary care groups could give their best specialists more.

MANAGED COMPETITION

There's an old adage that all healthcare is local. Most people, unless they're in a rural area, see a doctor whose office is fairly close to where they live. If a patient has to be admitted to the hospital, their doctor will generally send that person to the hospital with which they're affiliated, or to a specialist who has admitting privileges at that facility. Tests are done at local labs or imaging centers, and prescriptions are filled at local pharmacies. Hospitals discharge patients to home or to local skilled nursing facilities.

Because of the local nature of healthcare, it would make sense to administer Medicare for All on a region-by-region basis. There is a precedent for this in the regional health authorities that administer national health insurance in Canada and the United Kingdom.

Under the physician-led reform model, a similar regional health authority would supervise healthcare in each area with a population of a certain size. This body would not be a government agency, but an independent executive council. Its members would represent consumers and employers—who would pay federal health taxes—and healthcare providers, who would be paid out of those taxes. Since each of these stakeholder groups has somewhat different interests, the opportunity for all of them to provide input into the decision-making process should help clarify the issues. The authority's supervision would also guarantee a degree of local control over the single-payer system.

Large metropolitan areas would have to be split into multiple districts, each with its own regional health authority. For example, New York City might have 20 districts, compared to just one in Spokane.

The regional health authorities would delegate much of their responsibility for managing the local healthcare system to "health utilities." Similar in some ways to electric utilities, health utilities are private companies—possibly former health insurers—that would run the day-to-day operations of the single-payer system and manage the competition between physician groups. The health utilities would be highly regulated, and their fees and functions would be strictly limited by federal law. Health utilities would not take insurance risk—the government would do that. Each regional health authority would contract with a health utility for a specified period of time—say, three years. At the end of that period, the council would look at the health utility's performance and decide whether to renew the agreement.

Regarding the competing groups, the main functions of the health utilities would be to enroll patients in particular primary care groups, process and pay claims to other providers, measure the performance of the groups, and post the scores online. The health utility would have claims data for most of the services provided to patients, and a national claims database would be automatically cross-checked to pick up out-of-the-area claims. Thus, the health utility would be able to calculate a group's total cost of care for its patients and compare that to its risk-adjusted benchmark, but the health utility would play no role in utilization or quality management. That would be up to the primary care groups themselves.

Neither the regional health authorities nor the health utilities would be established until near the end of the transition to Medicare for All. As explained earlier, the conversion from a system of competing insurers to one based on competing providers could take place only after private health plans had been phased out for the most part. Once that happened, the field would be cleared to place the competition where it belongs: between those who actually deliver care.

PROVIDER REPORT CARDS

The competition between the primary care groups would be driven by the consumers who received that care, using provider report cards posted on the health utility's website. Before selecting a primary care doctor in one of the competing groups, consumers could compare the groups on quality, total cost of care, and patient experience. Depending on which group they selected, their federal health tax—a payroll tax deducted from their gross pay—would be higher or lower. If they picked a lower-cost group, they would pay less in taxes.

Overall, an individual's or a family's income and their choice of a primary care group would be the only factors determining the amount of their tax. People who didn't earn enough to pay a health tax would not be penalized for selecting a doctor in a higher cost group. Other incentives could be found to get these individuals to pay attention to quality scores.

The publication of group quality scores would be a check on any group that might try to cut corners on care. In addition, the groups would have to meet a certain quality threshold to share in savings, as ACOs do in the MSSP.

There have been numerous attempts over the years to enlist consumers in improving quality by publishing provider "report cards." Health insurers, employer coalitions, multi-stakeholder community groups, and the federal and state governments have all published ratings in the hope that consumers would choose higher-quality, lower-cost physicians and hospitals.

Most of these efforts have to come to naught. For the past two decades, studies have consistently found that consumers were largely uninterested in these report cards and rarely used them to pick providers. Here's what RAND researchers found in 2002:

> Although evidence from surveys and focus groups suggests that consumers want more information about the performance of their health care providers, few individuals are apparently influenced by the information in their decision making. According to the surveys, consumers' choice of

hospitals relied more on anecdotal press reports of adverse events than on the comparative assessments that were available.[34]

Similarly, a 2012 paper based on a survey of and interviews with experts on report cards stated, "Public reporting to date has been disconnected from consumer decisions about providers."[35] A 2014 consumer survey by the Kaiser Family Foundation found that about 10% of Americans said they had seen comparative quality information on hospitals or doctors. But of those who had viewed the information, just 4% used it to select a hospital and 6% to choose a doctor.[36]

A 2018 study of provider ratings found that in 2015, there were only 5.3 million unique page views on Medicare's Physician Compare and only 3.7 million unique page views on Hospital Compare. These were small numbers in relation to the number of Medicare beneficiaries. Other public report cards also had relatively low viewership, the researcher found.[37]

Websites on which patients rate their physicians, like Healthgrades and Vitals, are much more widely used than objective report cards, the paper noted. In 2012, 65% of U.S. adults knew about physician review sites and one in four had consulted one when picking a PCP. Only 5% of the sample, however, had ever rated a doctor online themselves.[38]

More objective doctor report cards are also available in some places. California, Pennsylvania, and New York publish heart surgery outcomes and provider ratings. Consumers' Checkbook and ProPublica rate surgeons based on Medicare data.[39] CMS is supposed to post quality scores of all doctors who participate in its Merit-Based Incentive Payment System (MIPS); but today, Physician Compare includes MIPS quality ratings on only some doctors.[40]

Some physician report cards measure the quality of groups rather than individual doctors. For example, the California Department of Managed Care's website posts quality and patient experience ratings of physician groups and IPAs.[41] Physician Compare also has begun posting quality data for some groups participating in MIPS.[42] The Wisconsin Collaborative for Healthcare Quality posts detailed quality information for group practices and health systems in Wisconsin,[43] and Minnesota Community Measurement, a private, nonprofit organization, rates clinics, medical groups, and hospitals.[44]

Why Report Cards Aren't Used

Observers cite several reasons for the public's unenthusiastic response to provider report cards. First, many people are simply unaware that they exist. Second, patients tend to trust their own doctors to refer them to the best specialists and hospitals. Third, even when consumers do look at comparative data on physicians and hospitals, they often find them hard to understand, inconsistent, and lacking the pertinent information they need to make decisions.[45]

The literature on this topic suggests that most consumers don't have a compelling reason to look at report cards. One obvious reason is that most people are healthy at any point in time. Sick people, being vulnerable, tend to depend on their doctors' guidance. Also, since most provider scorecards don't include out-of-pocket costs for particular services or procedures, there is no financial incentive for consumers to use the report cards.

There are a couple of hints that cost information might move this needle. One recent study found that, when presented with a combination of cost data and easy-to-understand quality data, consumers were more likely to choose lower-cost, higher-performing providers than higher-cost, lower-performing providers.[46] And in the 2012 paper based on interviews with experts, representatives of consumer and quality organizations said that cost data should be included in provider report cards.[47]

While much needs to be done to improve these report cards, consumers would be much more likely to use them if they had financial skin in the game. From that viewpoint, making the level of health taxes partly contingent on consumers' selection of a physician group would provide a strong incentive for them to study the online group rankings. But to spur groups to improve quality, it would be also be important for consumers to factor that into their decisions.

QUALITY MEASUREMENT

A big problem with today's quality measures is that they're more about processes than outcomes. In other words, doctors are being judged on measures like the percentage of their diabetic patients who got annual eye exams rather than how well the patients controlled their blood sugar as a result of following the regimen prescribed by their doctor.

Process measures don't reveal much about the quality of care and don't capture whether patient symptoms were improved; therefore, they shouldn't be used in the public report cards used to compare the competing groups. Nevertheless, some process measures might be valuable for internal quality improvement and for identifying outlier physicians.

Measures of intermediate outcomes reveal more than process measures about how well patients fare as a result of treatment or preventive care. Examples of such measures include the percentage of diabetics with a value of 8% or less on an HbA1c test or the percentage of patients with hypertension who have their blood pressure under control. A lowering of cholesterol levels, a reduction in alcohol consumption, smoking cessation, and a reduction in asymptomatic pre-cancer abnormalities (e.g., colonic polyps) are other intermediate indications that can be linked to future health outcomes.[48] However, intermediate outcomes measures are available for only some chronic conditions and may not reflect patients' current symptoms.

Outcomes measures like mortality and hospital readmissions are important, but they depend on a number of factors that may or may not be under a physician's control. Physiological measures such as the sustained virologic response in a patient with hepatitis C or HIV can show how well a treatment has worked within a certain time frame; however, the patient perspective provides a more holistic interpretation and a more comprehensive assessment of a patient's long-term outcomes.[49]

To obtain this perspective in a usable form, some healthcare organizations rely on patient-reported outcomes measures (PROMs) that "use validated questionnaires to turn a symptom into a numerical score." PROM surveys, which can be general or disease-specific, measure functional status, health-related quality of life, symptoms and symptom burden, personal experience of care, and health-related behaviors such as anxiety and depression.[50]

While some physicians may be skeptical of PROMs because they're based on patients' subjective feelings, many validated functional status surveys exist. Organizations such as Partners Healthcare have found them to be useful in tracking recovery after procedures and the response of cancer patients to radiation therapy. Partners also uses angina and dyspnea surveys to measure patient outcomes after cardiac catheterizations. By having patients fill out surveys on the patient portal, which is connected to Partners' EHR, the group has reduced the administrative burden of these measures and has made the outcomes data available at the point of care.[51]

Based on the studies cited above, it appears that people are going to have a hard time understanding group scorecards unless they're fairly simple and address the issues that matter most to patients. These might include the risk-adjusted percentage of patients who visited the ER or were hospitalized in a given time period. They also might encompass scores comparing the intermediate outcomes of patients who have certain chronic conditions.

PROMs could also be summarized on a disease-specific or a procedure-specific basis. These would include the overall patient-reported outcomes of the specialists selected by the primary care groups. If these numbers were easy to grasp and relevant to patients' lives, many more people might look at the groups' quality scores and not just at their cost rankings.

A REAL-WORLD PROOF OF CONCEPT

To see a physician-led reform model in action, we'd have to go back to Minneapolis/ St. Paul in 1996. That was when the Buyers Health Care Action Group (BHCAG), a coalition of large, self-insured employers in that market, began contracting directly with provider groups known as "care systems." For nearly a decade, this experiment showed that direct contracting could lower costs for high-quality care while lifting the burden of health plans off employers, consumers, and physicians.[52]

In 2005, this daring experiment ended when Medica, one of the three dominant health insurers in the market, acquired Patient Choice, the direct contracting program that BHCAG's member companies offered their employees. Patient Choice had already lost nearly half of its enrollees because some BHCAG employers had been lured away by the major health plans' loss-leader prices. In addition, Patient Choice had never been able to sell its insurance to small and medium-sized businesses that were not self-insured. To do so, Patient Choice would have had to obtain a state insurance license, which required large financial reserves.

Nevertheless, at its peak, Patient Choice had about 150,000 enrollees. Participating employers benefited from the cost savings created by the program. In 1998, two years after the provider groups started competing with one another for patients, the average cost to companies for employees who enrolled in Patient Choice was 20% below the average commercial rate of Minnesota HMOs. Cost increases for the BHCAG employers from 1997 to 1999 were 5%–6% a year. That was far below the cost increases of 6%–13% for plans in the state employees' health system during the same period. From 1999 to 2003, Patient Choice's annual price hikes averaged about 6% a year—two points below the market average.

Ann Robinow, the director of Patient Choice before it was acquired by Medica, told me that the program performed better than conventional health plans for two reasons: First, its administrative costs were only 5%, compared to an average of 15% for commercial insurers, and second, employees responded to financial incentives to choose doctors in the more cost-efficient care systems.

Physicians also liked Patient Choice, even though it supplied only about 5% of their revenues, on average. "Patient Choice tried to get everyone's incentives aligned appropriately," said Rolf Skogerboe, MD, a member of the 80-doctor Columbia Park Medical Group in Minneapolis, when I interviewed him in 2005. "And you have to applaud that, because the incentives of a health plan are typically not aligned with either the patient's or the doctor's incentives. They're at cross-purposes to both, so they make everybody mad. This was an honest attempt by employers whose interest was to do the best job they could for their employees."

How Patient Choice Worked

While Patient Choice used third-party administrators to enroll employees and pay claims, BHCAG's members—including such companies as General Mills, Honeywell, Pillsbury, and 3M—were the entities contracting with 16 physician groups and IPAs. The ratio of primary care doctors to specialists in these groups varied; however, the primary care physicians in each group were central to the program. When an employee signed up with Patient Choice, he or she chose a primary care doctor in one of the groups. The total cost of the employee's care was attributed to that group, regardless of which specialists or hospitals were used.

Each care system was required to submit a budget that would cover all care provided to its Patient Choice enrollees in the following year. However, the groups had no way of knowing in advance how sick the patients who enrolled with them that year would be. In a significant departure from customary health plan practice, BHCAG used a new risk-adjustment model from Johns Hopkins University to adjust payments to each group based on the differences between the diagnoses of their patients and the acuity of their conditions.

Using analyses of the claims data from its members, BHCAG assigned the care systems to either low-, medium-, or high-cost categories. In addition, the groups' quality, service, and patient satisfaction were measured. The employer coalition disseminated these comparative ratings to their workers, along with the cost tiering of the groups.

The employees in Patient Choice could use this information to select a doctor; however, since there was no data available on individual physicians, they were actually selecting a group. If they picked a care system that was in a higher cost tier, they had to pay a higher percentage of the insurance premium. The difference in cost to the employee between the high- and low-cost groups ranged from $30 to $60 a month for a single person.

In a survey, three-quarters of Patient Choice members said they used information about the care systems provided by their companies. That isn't surprising, considering that money was at stake. In 1998, the four lowest-cost clinics scored the biggest enrollment gains, ranging from 15% to 57%. One mid-cost group with high quality ratings attracted 30% more members. A group in the high-cost tier lost 20% of its Patient Choice enrollees.

By 2005, about 70% of Patient Choice members belonged to care systems in the low-price tier, which had grown as groups in other tiers had reduced their costs. Robinow and other observers said that additional providers would have improved their performance, too, if Patient Choice had represented a larger share of their business.

Virtual Capitation

BHCAG companies couldn't legally prepay the care systems because they lacked insurance licenses. So, they opted to pay "virtual capitation" to the groups. If their risk-adjusted cost of care fell below their budget in a given year, BHCAG raised their fee-for-service reimbursement rate the following year. If a group's costs exceeded its budget, the opposite happened.

This is not the same as the payment methodology used in my physician-led reform model, but it has some similarities. As in the proposed model, the Minnesota doctors did not take insurance risk directly; the self-insured employers did. Virtual capitation also bears some resemblance to the group bonuses and paybacks in the physician-led reform model, and the cost performance of the groups in this model would be measured in relationship to an annual benchmark, similar to the budget of each Patient Choice care system.

One big difference is that the Minnesota care systems set their own budgets each year. Under the proposed model, in contrast, the health utilities would calculate each group's benchmark at set intervals, following government rules. This makes sense because the physician groups would be taking financial risk for all patients, not just 5% of the market; if they erred in their budget projections, they could get into serious trouble. It would be safer to base group budgets on some combination of historical and regional benchmarks, as explained in the next chapter.

The main lessons of the Minnesota experience—that competition between provider groups can reduce costs, that patients can drive the competition if they have the right financial incentives, and that physicians will support this approach—demonstrate that physician-led reform can produce the results we want in a restructured health system. Obviously, though, healthcare has evolved in many ways over the past quarter of a century. The next two chapters show how the physician-led reform model would change the current practice environment and how it could be achieved.

Building the New Delivery System

The physician-led reform model would require a lot of change, but that change would evolve from what's going on right now in value-based care. While the transition to value would be greatly accelerated, the roots of the new model are growing under us today.

Because the restructuring of healthcare delivery is so closely tied to the evolution of ACOs, much can be learned from those organizations. The comparison is limited: Most ACOs are larger than the statutory groups would be, a minority of ACOs have risk contracts, and they're operating in a very different payer environment than Medicare for All. Nevertheless, their experience contributes much of the background for this chapter.

From the viewpoint of physicians taking back control of the healthcare system, ACOs are an obvious starting point. According to the National Association of ACOs (NAACOS), 42% of ACOs are physician group-led, 27% are hospital-led, and 31% are led by both.[1] An earlier survey found that physicians were the decision makers in 78% of ACOs, whether physician- or hospital-led.[2]

Although more than half of physicians already participate in ACOs, fewer than a third of those ACOs are taking two-sided risk. The reform plan would require the many physicians who have little or no experience with this kind of risk to learn a whole new way of practicing. So, while it would be possible to gather most primary care doctors in statutory groups over a decade, it would certainly take longer to complete the transformation of clinical care. Some groups would be ready for this new way of practicing out of the box; others would be slower to adapt to value-based care and financial risk.

Despite the many challenges involved in restructuring the system, primary care physicians would be the biggest winners in the end. Being in charge of the system, they'd have much greater influence over patient care than they do today. Their business model, which is failing under fee for service, would be significantly improved under value-based care. And, while they'd have to take some downside risk, their potential upside would be substantial. Primary care doctors in very successful groups might be earning incomes similar to those of specialists today.

This chapter explores the nuts and bolts of assembling the statutory groups, the infrastructure they'd need and how they'd obtain it, how they'd manage population health, and how the groups would select and collaborate with specialists, hospitals, and post-acute care providers.

Before we get into these details, however, the essentials of forming groups and networks of the requisite size must be explained.

GROUP FORMATION

As noted in the last chapter, many of the statutory groups could be formed from the current ACOs and hospital-owned groups. But thousands of primary care groups and networks would have to be built from scratch or created by practice mergers. These groups would be composed of doctors who were not used to working with one another, let alone taking financial risk together.

There would be a natural tendency for physicians to pursue other options until forced to comply with government regulations. But the foresighted practices would see the writing on the wall early on. They'd begin to form larger groups and build the infrastructure they'd need to take financial risk.

Practice Mergers

When practices merge, they generally have different amounts of net worth that must be equalized. The main ingredients of practice net worth are hard assets (equipment and fixtures), accounts receivable, and "goodwill," which is the value of intangibles such as location and reputation. But over the past 15–20 years, the goodwill value of primary care practices has declined radically as hospitals have snapped them up for little more than the value of hard assets and receivables. So, no money typically changes hands in these kinds of practice mergers.

Nevertheless, mergers are not without cost. To start with, consultants, accountants, and lawyers are involved in mergers; their services are also needed to set up clinically integrated networks and ACOs. For example, an ACO requires an operating contract that sets forth its corporate structure and other aspects of the agreement among its member practices, notes Robert Shaw, a partner in the law firm Smith Anderson in Raleigh, N.C. Such an operating agreement might specify physicians' responsibilities, their consent to follow practice guidelines, and how they are to be paid out of the ACO's shared savings.

In a statutory group or network formed under the physician-led reform model, practices could keep their own EHRs or could collectively buy a new EHR, which would create significant efficiencies. A pre-existing group might already have a single EHR; a newly formed group would have to purchase one to become fully integrated.

While EHR costs vary widely, a 2011 study of how much it cost a primary care network in North Texas to buy and implement a midlevel EHR system provides a marker—albeit one that must be updated for inflation. For an average five-physician practice in the network, EHR implementation—including hardware and software costs, hosting, and technical support—cost about $162,000, plus $85,500 in maintenance costs in the first year. That came to nearly $50,000 per physician.[3]

Many practices today pay monthly fees for cloud-based electronic health records (EHRs). There is no upfront cost for the software, but there are still hardware, implementation, and maintenance costs. Experts say that the five-year costs of on-premise and cloud-based EHRs are roughly similar.

Big Infrastructure Costs

Beyond the costs of merging or forming networks and putting EHRs in place, an ACO or a statutory group that plans to take financial risk needs an infrastructure that includes data aggregation and analytics capabilities. Human resources such as care managers, social workers, and other nontraditional care team members also are needed to keep patients out of the hospital and other expensive care settings (see Chapters 6 and 7).

The average cost of launching an ACO in 2016 was $1.6 million, according to a NAA-COS survey. Annual operating expenses were in the same range.[4] Farzad Mostashari, the CEO of ACO management firm Aledade, estimates that the number is probably closer to $2 million today, and that doesn't include the financial reserves needed to take downside risk, which will be discussed later.

Shaw says that wealthy physicians or doctors with outside financial backing provide the bulk of the initial investment in many ACOs. These founders own the majority of the ACO's equity and take half of any shared savings that the ACO earns. It's unclear whether this arrangement incentivizes the other ACO members to work hard to reduce costs and improve quality.

A study of physician-led ACOs in the upside risk-only track of the MSSP found that they had a variety of funding sources, including physician contributions, loans, venture capital, and investments by founders. ACOs not financed by larger companies, the study found, had a limited ability to make upfront investments in health IT, and their data analytics infrastructure was very basic. As a result, these ACOs depended mainly on Medicare data to manage care, and they received very little clinical information from outside of their member practices. Also, they didn't form specialty referral networks and had difficulty getting timely data from hospitals.

"Clinical and functional integration (e.g., information exchange) with specialists and hospitals were not among the initial priorities for the first years of an ACO's existence, and, as a result, were generally poor," the researchers stated.[5]

Most of these physician-led ACOs were not set up to take two-sided risk. They evidently just tried to coordinate care well enough to garner some shared savings under upside risk-only contracts. But that is not to say that they couldn't have expanded their infrastructure at a later stage of development. This same pattern might be seen among the statutory groups in our reform model as they cohere and gain more experience in population health management.

Government Financing

One approach to financing the infrastructure of the statutory groups would be to have the government fund it by setting primary care capitation payments high enough to cover the cost. The government could recoup its investment over time from its share of the groups' savings.

The Health Care Payment Learning & Action Network (LAN), a collaborative network of public and private stakeholders established by the Department of Health and Human Services, advocated a similar approach in a recent white paper on primary care payment models (PCPMs). In their recommendations on how to transform primary care, the LAN authors said:

> Prospective payments [i.e., capitation] should be in excess of historic primary care payment amounts to support the infrastructure of the clinical team that will be held accountable for greater coordination of services and for bending the total health system cost curve. . . . PCPMs should use prospective payment to fund the necessary investments by primary care organizations in practice infrastructure to result in more efficient delivery of health care.

The report's authors envision that payers' additional spending on primary care will be recouped through "savings from reductions in the utilization of unnecessary care outside the primary care setting. . . . In return for accepting increased payment rates, primary care teams will create additional value for the healthcare system, consumers and purchasers."[6]

Infrastructure Vendors

While the government doesn't plan to implement this strategy, many ACOs have found another way to finance their infrastructure. Instead of borrowing money or relying on funds from member practices, they have turned to private companies to provide the financing. Generally, these firms—some of which are backed by venture capital or trade on the stock market—charge a monthly fee for each attributed patient or receive a portion of the ACOs' earnings off the top.

A wide spectrum of companies offer various combinations of population health management software and services. They include firms that sell infrastructure packages to any ACO and others that provide support services to a group of ACOs that they manage. The accompanying sidebar lists some of these companies and what they do.

LEADING INFRASTRUCTURE VENDORS

Evolent Health integrates data from multiple EHRs and provides analytics, automation, standardized workflows, and risk stratification models, along with care managers and medical directors that work with ACO practices. The publicly traded firm also supplies prebuilt clinical and financial reports that can be customized by ACOs.[7]

Lightbeam's product line includes data aggregation and analytics that measure care gaps, stratify the population by health risk, and track cost, financial risk, and productivity. Lightbeam also offers a health information exchange, referral management, automated patient messaging, and care management software, but the firm does not supply care managers or other personnel.[8]

Privia Health, an Arlington, Va., firm that manages ACOs in four states and Washington, D.C, furnishes population health management infrastructure to its ACOs. It also performs billing and collection functions for the ACO groups, most of which use the same EHR and practice management system. Privia is backed by private equity investors, but all the practices in Privia ACOs remain independent.[9-10]

Aledade, which was described in Chapter 4, not only provides population health management software but also delivers a range of on-the-ground services, including practice transformation coaching and contracting.[11] It places care managers in some ACO practices but prefers that they hire their own. Aledade also draws on venture capital investments.

Lumeris operates a Medicare Advantage plan and helps launch provider-sponsored plans. The company advises providers on population health management strategies, aggregates and analyzes clinical and organizational data, and offers population health services, including infrastructure development.[12]

Arcadia features "population health for the enterprise." The firm aggregates and analyzes clinical and claims data, identifies care gaps, does patient outreach, provides reports on quality and utilization, coaches providers, measures performance, negotiates contracts, and advises ACOs on care management and other aspects of population health management.[13]

Caravan works predominantly—but not exclusively—with health system-led ACOs. Besides the usual menu of data analytics and reporting and population health management, the vendor promises to limit ACO risk in the MSSP by covering any losses after the first 1 percent.[14]

Mostashari calls what Aledade does "population health as a service." Because the firm takes 40%-50% of its ACOs' shared savings, however, Shaw regards the company as a management services organization (MSO). Some ACOs have an even closer relationship with MSOs. Partners in Care (PIC), a New Jersey-based ACO and clinically integrated network (CIN), is majority-owned by an MSO called Continuum Health.[15]

MSOs have a long, checkered history in managed care. Back in the 1990s, some MSOs funded by private equity rebranded themselves as "physician practice management companies," or PPMCs. Companies like Phycor, MedPartners, and PhyMatrix bought practices, often partly or wholly for stock, with the aim of pumping up their valuations and going public. But their business model was faulty; even with capital infusions, they weren't able to increase practice revenues enough to justify their management fees. Eventually, eight of the 10 largest PPMCs went bankrupt, leaving their physician investors with worthless stock.[16]

Today's infrastructure vendors, however, are a different breed than the PPMCs of yesteryear. To begin with, they're not run by venture capitalists, even if they have private equity backing, and they're not interested in buying practices. Their financial interest lies in ensuring that their ACOs save money and generate shared savings that they split with the vendor. Aledade, for example, manages and supports the population health management activities of its ACOs. It shares in the ACOs' earnings but not in the other revenue streams of member practices.

Practice Sales Must Be Banned

Nevertheless, it's important to remember the lessons of the PPMC apocalypse. Although private equity is vital to providing the capital for the infrastructure vendors, investors should never again be allowed to buy and sell physician practices. So, not only must venture capitalists divest their current practices, as discussed in Chapter 8, but the statutory groups in our model should not be allowed to sell themselves. To prevent business collapses and ensure they can pursue their healing mission, they must always be under exclusive physician ownership.

In the physician-led reform model, the competing groups would have their choice of infrastructure vendors. Depending on their financial resources and their stage of evolution, they might require more or fewer of the services these companies offer. The big advantage of this approach is that instead of each group having to reinvent the wheel and find the capital to pay for its infrastructure, they can benefit from the expertise and the resources of companies that have already figured it out.

Partners in Care (PIC), the large New Jersey CIN and ACO, has developed its own homegrown data warehouse and analytics over many years and is now looking to replace these applications with off-the-shelf software. But an ACO starting up today should contract with an infrastructure vendor, advises David DiGirolamo, executive director of PIC.

"The physician organization should consider buying an operational package that includes services and [software] solutions," he says. "They should have a partnership that allows them to make decisions and direct operations, but not have to get into the nitty gritty details. Building the infrastructure yourself would take years, and your business would be three years behind you before you could build it."

FINANCIAL RISK

The statutory groups would have to learn how to handle financial risk and how to protect themselves from insolvency. Even primary care capitation can be a risk if utilization isn't managed, but the risk is limited to the services of the physicians themselves. Therefore, every group, as soon as it was fully organized, could be prepaid for primary care. Upside risk for the total cost of care, similarly, doesn't threaten groups with insolvency. If they don't reduce healthcare spending enough to garner shared savings, they are only on the hook for the cost of their infrastructure. If they're splitting profits with an infrastructure vendor, their upfront share of that cost would be fairly minor.

But taking two-sided risk for the total cost of care is completely different. While not as perilous as global capitation, which transfers 100% of the downside risk to the provider group, a far lower amount of downside risk can threaten a group or ACO with insolvency if they don't have financial reserves or insurance. The statutory groups might be at risk for only 10%–15% of their budgets. Nevertheless, one or two catastrophic cases could throw a group's finances into a tailspin even with the lower risk limit.

For this reason, CMS requires ACOs in the MSSP's two-sided risk tracks to maintain financial reserves equal to 1% of total per capita Medicare Parts A and B spending for the beneficiaries assigned to them. The repayment mechanisms for ACOs may include any combination of

- Funds placed in escrow with an insured institution.
- A line of credit as evidenced by letter of credit.
- A surety bond issued by a certified surety bond company.[17]

The government would certainly require the statutory groups to have similar reserves or equivalent reinsurance under the physician-led reform model. How large those reserves would have to be and where the groups would obtain the funds are the questions we now turn to.

How Much Risk Is Too Much?

Paul Keckley, a healthcare strategic adviser and a former Navigant and Deloitte executive, says that CMS's 1% reserve requirement is insufficient. If an ACO or group is taking a significant portion of risk for the total cost of care in the MSSP, he estimates, it should maintain reserves of between 1% and 4% of total annual spending.

Under Medicare for All, the patient population of each group would include people of all ages, the majority of whom would have a lower risk profile than current Medicare beneficiaries. According to CMS, per capita personal healthcare spending for the 65 and older population is more than five times higher than the cost per child and almost three times higher than the spending per working-age person.[18] So the total cost per capita under Medicare for All would be far lower than it is in the MSSP.

Let's stipulate that the proper reserve percentage for a population with an average risk profile is 2%. In 2018, the average cost of personal healthcare was approximately $10,000 per person.[19] Based on that figure, a primary care group with 100,000 patients would need reserves equal to 2% of $10,000 times 100,000, or $20 million.

The median MSSP ACO includes about 300 physicians. ACOs of that size "probably have the financial reserves" they need to take financial risk, says Terri Welter, a principal with ECG Management Consultants. "For smaller groups, it's a problem. They probably need a lending mechanism or should decide not to take on as much risk."

Aledade funds the reserves for its small ACOs with venture capital, Mostashari notes. But Keckley cautions that some infrastructure vendors may not remain stable in the long term. So ACOs should perform due diligence on their vendors before letting them provide reserves. The same would apply to the statutory groups in our model.

Another approach taken by some ACOs is to gradually fund the reserves out of shared savings from upside risk contracts. The physicians in Privia's Virginia ACO, for example, have put aside a reserve of 2% of total annual health costs so they can take two-sided risk in the MSSP. But Privia is still considering the possibility of buying reinsurance, says Mark Foulke, the firm's executive vice president.

"The question is what is our risk tolerance," he says. "Because in the enhanced track of MSSP, we can lose 15% of our benchmark, which for us is $125 million in the worst-case scenario. We think that's highly unlikely. So, we're working with the physicians and our actuaries to understand what is our realistic risk tolerance if we were to exceed that 2% loss rate, and what we need to meet that rainy day requirement. We're deciding what else we need to do to meet our risk tolerance and risk threshold. We can either do that by increasing contributions to the reserve fund or by evaluating reinsurance."

Reinsurance, also known as stop-loss insurance, kicks in when an insured entity's losses pass a certain amount, known as an attachment point or trigger. The lower the attachment point, the higher the cost of the stop-loss insurance. Generally, ACOs have found that reinsurance is too expensive when their population is fairly small and therefore unpredictable. But as the population grows, Welter notes, the cost of reinsurance falls as a percentage of total spending.

Keckley regards a population of 100,000 as the tipping point where reinsurance starts to make economic sense for a risk-taking ACO or group. However, he notes, the likelihood of incurring catastrophic losses varies by region; it's much higher, for example, in an inner-city area or in rural Appalachia than in an upper middle-income suburb. "100,000 is a good starting point if you had a normal distribution or risk—but that's the big if," he says. A particular reinsurance contract, he adds, should cover a period of at least three years to be affordable.

From the foregoing, it's clear that the statutory groups would have a range of options to fund their reserves. But larger groups would be in a much better position to do that than smaller groups or networks in less-populated areas. Therefore, the government might consider stepping in to backstop groups that might not be able to finance reserves on their own.

KEY MEASUREMENTS

Patients must be attributed to individual primary care physicians in order to determine which group is responsible for their care. Attribution is the prerequisite for calculating the total cost of care, as well as for risk adjustment and benchmarking.

Until recently, the MSSP retrospectively attributed patients to ACOs based on claims data. At the end of the year, CMS would decide which patients belonged to a particular ACO and then reconcile the payments to that ACO against the cost of caring for the patients who were attributed to it. This approach created problems for ACOs because they didn't know which patients were assigned to them until the end of each performance year.[20]

Starting in January 2020, CMS began offering ACOs the choice of prospective or retrospective attribution; the agency also gave Medicare beneficiaries the option of enrolling in an ACO. Whichever method an ACO selects, CMS provides a preliminary prospective list of enrollees at the beginning of the year.[21]

Not all ACOs have chosen the prospective method. Privia, for example, has decided to stick with retrospective attribution because it believes it will do better financially under that method. But Welter predicts that most ACOs eventually will embrace prospective attribution, which gives them more control. Keckley says CMS's approach to ACO assignment is improving, but that more must be done to address what he calls the "volatility of populations."

Under the physician-led reform model, most people would choose a primary care physician in one of the statutory groups; if they didn't, they'd pay the maximum health tax for their income level. Typically, consumers would choose or elect to stay with a doctor prior to the start of each calendar year. The enrollment process, which would be conducted by the health utilities, would be similar to the process of enrolling in a health plan today. The system would have to keep track of people who signed up for the first time in the middle of the year or died during the year. Nobody would be able to switch groups until the next year's enrollment period.

With these restrictions in place, the question of prospective vs. retrospective attribution would become moot. Patients who enrolled with a particular group would be attributed to that group.

Risk Adjustment

Capitation payments and benchmarks for the total cost of care must be risk-adjusted for each patient's health status. CMS and private payers have developed sophisticated risk-adjustment techniques that depend on claims data.

To risk-adjust an ACO's historical benchmark, the MSSP employs the CMS-HCC prospective risk-adjustment model, which is also used in the Medicare Advantage program.[22] ACOs have complained about this approach because it caps risk-adjustment increases for an ACO population to 3% during a contract period. Not only do some ACOs regard that as insufficient, but CMS's shift from a three-year to a five-year contract period in the MSSP has magnified that inadequacy.

Keckley and Mostashari agree that the 3% cap is unrealistic. "Those numbers came from actuaries and consultants, but they don't make a lot of sense," Keckley says.

The physician-led reform model should use the best available risk-adjustment methods to level the playing field across the competing groups and to reimburse them appropriately for primary care. There should be no arbitrary limits on upward risk adjustment, but the health utilities should keep a close eye on the groups to guard against unjustified case-mix changes. In addition, social determinants of health should be incorporated into risk adjustment so that groups with different kinds of populations are scored fairly.

Benchmarking

Benchmarking is the key to the equitable payment of shared savings for the total cost of care. Supported by patient attribution and risk adjustment, benchmarks can be based on the historical claims experience of an ACO, the experience of other providers in the region, and/or the national experience of ACOs.

Under the historical benchmarking method, efficient ACOs are punished because their performance is compared to their own previous claims experience; therefore, they have to work harder than inefficient ACOs to generate savings. In the MSSP, the disincentive to low-cost ACOs has been further compounded by rebasing their benchmark at the beginning of each contract period. But lengthening the MSSP agreements from three to five years has mitigated the negative impact of that policy.

CMS now combines historical with regional benchmarking, which makes the benchmark of a particular ACO partly contingent on the performance of other ACOs in the same region. Thus, if the ACO is more efficient than its peers, its benchmark is raised to somewhere between its own claims experience and that of the other ACOs in the area. This makes it easier for the ACO to achieve shared savings in relation to the benchmark.[23]

Mostashari is happy with the new approach. "I think they've hit the right balance between incentivizing improvements and rewarding and sustaining attainment," he says.

Similarly, Mark Foulke of Privia Health says, "Generally speaking, we're very favorable to what CMS is doing. It allows physicians to find a balance of comfort for them."

Keckley points out that the hybrid benchmarking method is too new to evaluate. "I like the regional approach for a lot of reasons," he says, "but I can't evaluate it without a baseline from which I can normalize the data and make the comparisons." He estimates it will take three years to see whether the approach works.

The verdict on benchmarking will clearly be in long before our reform model could be implemented under the best of scenarios. So, for the time being, it seems like a safe bet to follow CMS's lead in setting benchmarks for the statutory groups.

HEALTH UTILITIES' ROLE

As explained in Chapter 8, the health utilities would manage the competition among the statutory groups in each region. They would handle enrollment of patients in the groups, the measurement and public reporting of group performance, and the processing of claims by healthcare entities other than the primary care practices. They'd also provide the claims data that the groups would need to take financial risk.

The health utilities would also play a crucial role in the stability of the system. To begin with, they'd ensure that the statutory groups met size requirements; when groups became too big, they would reassign some of their doctors to smaller practices. These physicians would not have to leave their offices; they'd simply belong to a different group or network. Doctors would always be able to switch groups as long as the group they selected was willing to accept them.

The opposite problem would exist with groups that lost doctors and became too small. This could happen for a number of reasons, including retirement, mismanagement, and the loss of physicians to other groups. The health utilities could not reassign doctors to these groups; however, if the practice became too small to compete or take risk, and could not recruit more doctors, the health utility would help it shut down and would work with the other groups to absorb its remaining physicians.

When a new group or network was formed—something that would happen frequently in the early years of the model—the health utility would supervise the induction of that group into the region's managed competition system. Although the health utility would not finance or build the group's infrastructure, it could provide some guidance to the group to increase its likelihood of success.

The health utilities would have to follow national regulations for the measurement of cost, quality, and patient satisfaction. The regional health authorities would ensure that the health utilities adhered to those rules.

In addition, the health utilities would calculate the benchmarks for their region's groups and would determine how much they had saved and should be paid, or how much they owed if they'd exceeded their budgets. But the federal government would authorize the payments and would rigorously audit the health utilities to ensure they were calculating them properly.

POPULATION HEALTH MANAGEMENT

Earlier in the book, I discussed the technological capabilities and human resources that are required for population health management (PHM). To recap briefly, information is the life blood of PHM. The infrastructure vendors hired by the statutory groups would aggregate, normalize, and analyze clinical and claims data to provide timely, actionable information to physicians and care teams. This actionable data would include risk stratification, care gap identification, and reports on the utilization of services at both site and individual provider levels. The groups would also receive reports on the utilization and quality of specialists, hospitals, and post-acute care providers.

While the entire patient population should be managed at some level, most ACOs focus on intervening with high-need, high-cost individuals. In a recent survey of ACOs, 85% of the respondents reported implementing a program to address these patients' needs. Eighty percent of the ACOs had transitional management programs to facilitate the movement of patients between care settings, such as from hospitals to skilled nursing facilities. Seventy-seven percent had nurse care coordination programs, with the nurses either embedded in practices or centrally located. Many ACOs used their patient-centered medical homes to intervene with this population, and about half of them had a post-acute care/SNF program.[24]

In the statutory groups, the care managers would work mainly with these high-need, high-cost patients in conjunction with physicians. Other members of the care team would educate and support rising-risk patients to prevent them from getting sicker and potentially being hospitalized. Automation software could be used to alert patients of the need to obtain necessary preventive and chronic care and to suggest how they might maintain their health, given their risk factors. While some groups might start out managing only the sicker patients, the goal would be to eventually take care of the entire population on a more or less continuous basis.

An ACO of 50–75 doctors needs about 15 care managers, each of whom is part of a three-to five-physician practice, Mostashari says. PIC has one care manager per 25,000 members in commercial contracts and one per 10,000 Medicare beneficiaries in the MSSP, notes John Breault, CEO of PIC and senior VP of payer strategy for Continuum, its corporate parent .

Extended Care Teams

Besides care managers and clinicians, the groups' care teams might include behavioral health specialists, disease educators, nutritionists, pharmacists, and other ancillary providers. To address social determinants of health, the care teams might also include social workers and/or community health workers. In the earlier-mentioned survey, 72% of the ACOs said they'd hired social workers.

In a study cited in Chapter 4, Thomas Bodenheimer, professor emeritus of family and community medicine at the University of California San Francisco, described advanced primary care teams that include a core team or "teamlet" and an extended team. The core team consists of a physician or a midlevel practitioner and one or more medical assistants. The extended team may include any of the ancillary clinical and social work professionals mentioned above. These professionals work with all the providers, and patients receive care from the teamlets and the extended teams. Everybody works to the limit of their license: Medical assistants may provide routine diabetes services, for example, and RNs can change medication doses within standing orders.

In another study, Bodenheimer and his colleagues explored the implications of a delegated team model of primary care for determining appropriate panel size. The researchers first estimated the amount of time it would take for a primary care physician to provide all recommended preventive and chronic care services. Then they looked at how much of this work could be automated or safely delegated to lower-level clinicians in an advanced care team. The researchers concluded that with maximal delegation, primary care doctors could provide high-quality care to more than twice as many patients as they could if they tried to do all this work themselves.[25]

This study has significant implications for the statutory groups. First, the use of advanced care teams such as these could make the groups more efficient. Second, it would allow them to provide higher-quality care. And third, at a time when the primary care shortage continues to worsen, it would help them stretch their physician resources. The same kind of delegated care model could support a nurse practitioner or a physician's assistant, making it possible for these midlevel practitioners to be counted as primary care providers in the groups.

A word is in order here about the alternative primary care settings mentioned earlier in the book. The physician-led reform model can accommodate retail clinics that employ only non-physician clinicians. In fact, these alternative settings would help support the primary care groups by increasing access. However, the providers in these settings would be required to coordinate care with each patient's primary care physician. To better align incentives, they might be paid out of each group's primary care budget at rates set by the government.

COLLABORATING WITH SPECIALISTS

As stated earlier, primary care efforts to better coordinate care are often stymied by the limited cooperation of specialists and other residents of the medical neighborhood. Under fee for service, the siloed, fragmented nature of healthcare makes it difficult, if not impossible, to organize and plan care across care settings for optimal results.

Under the physician-led reform model, in contrast, specialists would be financially dependent on primary care physicians. If they refused to play ball with the primary care groups, they'd be paid at Medicare rates. But if they cooperated with the groups, they'd get far more referrals and would participate in the primary care doctors' shared savings.

Like many ACOs today, the groups would carefully select their specialists, based partly on performance data. The PIC ACO, for example, has data on specialists from all of its major commercial insurers as well as Medicare, Breault says. Half of the ACO's 500 doctors are specialists, and PIC has selected the specialists in its larger clinically integrated network.

Privia Health also uses data to select specialists, but has found there are limits to what the data can reveal about them. "You also have to engage the docs," says Privia executive Sam Starbuck. "We use data-driven forms of decision and then sit down with our PCPs and ask them for quality information about specialists. When you get into rural areas, it's 'who do I sit next to at church and play golf with.' But using the data to inform those conversations helps. And often we find that some high-cost specialists don't understand why they're flagged that way. It may be easy to change that classification simply by educating them about their use of high-cost imaging facilities."

When a primary care group is trying to deliver value-based care, the relationship between primary care physicians and specialists changes. Under the proposed reform model, many PCPs would feel empowered to provide services that are within their scope of practice but that they currently refer to specialists. They might freeze off warts, do colposcopies, set minor fractures, and/or take greater control of medication management. They also would tend to work up patients further before referring them to increase the appropriateness of referrals.

Moreover, specialists would be incentivized to help train primary care doctors and midlevel practitioners in tasks that they could perform without referring the patient out. In the fee-for- service system, specialists' incentive is to increase referrals, although they prefer them to be appropriate. But with PCPs holding the key to their incomes, specialists would be likely to do free consults with generalists when asked.

Project ECHO

A much-praised program called Project ECHO has transferred knowledge from specialists to rural primary care doctors for many years. Founded in 2002 by Sanjeev Arora, MD, at the University of New Mexico Health Sciences Center in Albuquerque, Project ECHO uses telemedicine to enable specialists to collaborate with primary care physicians so that patients don't have to travel long distances to visit the specialists. Using inexpensive videoconferencing technology, the specialists train rural healthcare providers to supply services that the specialists normally would provide themselves.[26]

One study of the program showed that among hepatitis C patients of participating providers, the virus could not be detected in 58% of them 24 weeks after their treatment by local primary care doctors. That was nearly identical to the percentage of sustained viral response in patients seen in person at the academic medical center in Albuquerque.[27]

A report on Project ECHO by the Robert Wood Johnson Foundation said the approach has wider potential. Although Project ECHO began in rural areas, the paper said, "It can be used as well in underserved urban communities. In these settings, community-based health clinics and primary care clinicians are called upon to provide specialized medical care to low-income, often uninsured patients who present with complex, chronic conditions."[28]

The Veterans' Health Administration launched a similar project in 2011, eventually spreading it across the country. In this program, specialists use telemedicine to train PCPs in treating chronic pain, diabetes, heart failure, hepatitis, chronic kidney disease, and women's health.[29]

Collaborative Relationship

As previously noted, the physician-led reform model could increase the fragmentation of care by dividing primary care physicians from specialists. But this need not be the case. With the help of the latest information technology, economically aligned PCPs and specialists could work together more closely than they usually do today (see Chapter 10). Their main locus for collaboration would be chronic-disease management, using methods that have had good success in some multispecialty groups and healthcare systems.

The Chronic Care Model, for example, was first developed at Group Health Cooperative, a group-model HMO in Seattle, more than 20 years ago. While the model has evolved since then, it still aims to "reduce fragmentation while at the same time improving health outcomes at an acceptable cost to the healthcare system." The core elements in the Chronic Care Model are "mobilizing community resources, promoting high-quality care, enabling patient self-management, implementing care consistent with evidence and patient preferences, effectively using patient/population data, cultural competence, care coordination, and health promotion."[30]

Studies of the Chronic Care Model have shown consistently positive results for patients with conditions such as diabetes, asthma, chronic obstructive pulmonary disease, depression, and HIV.[31-32]

For the purposes of this discussion, let's focus on the Chronic Care Model's care coordination piece. According to the Group Health Cooperative Institute, "Referrals and transitions work best when all parties—patients, primary care providers, and consultants—agree on the purpose and importance of the referral, and the roles that each will play in providing care."

The issues and expectations that should be included in agreements between patient-centered medical homes (PCMHs) and specialists, the Institute says, include the following:

- Types of patients referred—many specialists have developed criteria for the patients they prefer to see
- Information provided at time of referral
- Notification of the PCMH of ER visits and hospitalizations
- Testing to be completed prior to referral—if PCPs complete a specialist's preferred laboratory testing prior to the referral, it increases the value of the consultation and reduces possible duplicate testing
- Availability for "curbside consults"
- Consultation report content and timeliness
- Post-ER or post-hospitalization care expectations
- Specialist-to-specialist referrals—many PCPs do not want specialists to refer their patients to other specialists without first consulting with the PCP.[33]

In a multispecialty group that has adopted the Chronic Care Model or another disease management approach, the PCPs and specialists must agree on the practice guidelines they will follow. As noted in Chapter 5, it's not easy for providers to agree on clinical protocols, even if they're in the same specialty and the same group. Yet the PCPs in statutory groups could get specialists to sign on to nationally recognized guidelines that both parties have tweaked, if those protocols would result in better care.

It also would be wise to follow the lead of OptumCare by using physicians in the same specialty to educate their colleagues about new evidence-based guidelines that a statutory group has adopted. In fact, the best way to overcome physicians' resistance is to have their peers talk to them about the reasons for practice changes.

Under the physician-led reform model, however, the specialists would face additional challenges related to the competing groups. If each group had its own set of practice guidelines, the specialists would have the same problem that doctors now have with multiple insurer guidelines and quality measures. Therefore, it would be advantageous for the primary care groups in a particular region to sit down with specialist representatives and agree on the guidelines they wanted to use. A precedent for such a regional concord is provided by the Institute for Clinical Systems Integration in Minnesota (see Chapter 5).

Modified Gatekeepers

Another point of contention between PCPs and specialists is the "gatekeeper" role that some health plans have assigned to primary care doctors. The requirement of HMOs that patients see a primary care physician before going to a specialist—and the consumer backlash it sparked—was one of the reasons for the failure of the first managed care wave.

Today's HMOs cover 24% of enrollees with employer-sponsored insurance and many seniors in Medicare Advantage plans. Typically, they require PCPs to approve referrals to specialists, as their forerunners did. A 2018 study of commercial HMOs and PPOs in Massachusetts found that HMO insurance was associated with lower rates of new specialist visits than PPO insurance, which usually had wider networks and fewer restrictions on specialty care.[34]

As noted, the physician-led reform model would require consumers to choose a primary care doctor in a statutory group. But patients wouldn't be prevented from choosing out-of-network specialists. Their PCPs would encourage them to see one of their group's favored specialists and might show them that doctor's quality scores. If a patient insisted on being referred to a different physician, however, the PCP would accommodate him or her. In that case, the patient would either have a higher copayment or pay some other fee if there were no copayments under Medicare for All. Poor people would pay nothing to see a specialist.

HOSPITALISTS AND POST-ACUTE CARE

A quarter century ago, a new type of specialist known as a hospitalist emerged on the scene. Usually general internists, hospitalists follow patients in the hospital and coordinate their care. There are more than 50,000 hospitalists in the United States today.[35] Many of them work directly for hospitals or for hospitalist groups that contract with hospitals. They practice in over 80% of hospitals that have more than 200 beds.[36]

Primary care doctors may refer patients to hospitalists, but few of them follow their own patients in the hospital anymore. After initial opposition to the concept, PCPs recognized that hospitalists were economically beneficial to them. The ambulatory care doctors were spending a lot of time traveling to the hospital to round on their relatively few hospitalized patients. Meanwhile, the pressures of managed care were forcing them to see more patients in the office, and they weren't necessarily adept at inpatient care. In a survey in the early 2000s, 85% of physicians rated hospitalist care of their patients as excellent or good.[37]

Hospitalists have also been a boon to hospitals, partly because they have reduced patients' average length of stay. Since hospitals are paid prospectively for episodes of care, getting patients out sooner boosts hospitals' bottom lines.

Because most hospitalists are directly or indirectly employed by hospitals, they tend to support the strategies of their institution. However, in a single-payer system where the government negotiated payments with hospitals, the hospitals' financial incentives would not necessarily be aligned with those of independent physician groups taking risk for the total cost of care. Consequently, hospitalists' incentives would also be different.

For example, a hospitalist might want to discharge a patient sooner than his or her primary care physician might consider appropriate. An earlier discharge would not reduce the cost of the hospitalization, but it might cost a statutory group more in the long run if the patient bounced back to the hospital. The hospital, in contrast, would get paid for the readmission—although it might be penalized by the government if its readmission rate was excessive.

Some ACOs have found it advantageous to hire their own hospitalists. "The more sophisticated groups usually have their own hospitalists or they have a close tie to the ones who are there," Welter says.

Mostashari says it would make sense for Aledade's ACOs to hire hospitalists, although they haven't done so up to now. "Our philosophy is that we don't have hospitals in our ACOs. So, the strategy we use is to keep patients out of the hospital. Once they're in the hospital, we lose the ability to help the patient until they get discharged. So, we reduce the inflow and also reduce the chaos that happens when the patient is discharged. But if we had the opportunity to influence the care during hospitalizations, I'm sure a lot could be done to improve that."

Considering that hospitals generate such a large percentage of health costs, it's understandable that some ACOs hire their own hospitalists if they can afford them. Alternatively, Welter suggests that ACOs place discharge coordinators in the hospitals they work with to make sure patients are discharged to an appropriate care setting with the support they need.

The statutory groups could take either or both of these approaches, but they'd be better off if they had the capability to influence the course of inpatient care. This might be even more important if hospitals were paid significantly less than today and had more of an incentive to game the system.

Post-Acute Care Providers

Post-acute care providers are not financially aligned with ACOs for a variety of reasons. Home health agencies may have alliances with or be owned by physicians who prescribe more home care than patients need, as the Rio Grande Valley Health Alliance discovered. And the PIC ACO has found that New Jersey nursing homes try to hold onto their Medicare patients for the maximum number of days that CMS will cover.

Also, patients may not receive the care they need in skilled nursing facilities (SNFs) or from home care nurses. The first step toward ensuring that the care is appropriate, Welter says, is having a discharge coordinator in the hospital who will guide the patient to the right setting. "It's also about having relationships with the SNFs and home health agencies so that they're going to follow consistent guidelines. But it's really about getting patients to the right setting and following up with them to make sure they don't end up back in the hospital. We see a lot of activity in that area."

In Welter's experience, most hospitals give patients a list of facilities they can go to, and they send them to the one the patient selects if they have an available bed. ACOs may have their own list of preferred SNFs that they try to get patients into.

Privia Health, for example, has established compacts with certain nursing homes that are willing to collaborate with its ACOs and do "clinician-to-clinician case reviews," Starbuck says. These involve regular calls between the SNFs and Privia's team "to review current status and the planned discharge date and ensure we're facilitating smooth transitions back to the primary care physicians. That process is one we apply to many of the post-acute care providers."

Some hospitals are more cooperative than others about discharging patients to Privia's preferred SNFs and home care agencies, Starbuck adds. The ACO manager provides data to the hospital to identify Privia's patients when they visit an ED or are admitted.

"In some other facilities where we're viewed as a competitor, it's more challenging," he notes. "It's about continuously trying to remove all the noise around the C-suite and get down to the folks who are providing the care, and tell them who our preferred providers are for discharge."

SNFists, Pro and Con

The reader will recall that Prevea Health (no relation to Privia) in Green Bay, Wisc., had some of its physicians, called "SNFists," round on its patients in skilled nursing facilities.

Mostashari approves of this approach, although Aledade hasn't adopted it. "We do have several doctors who are old fashioned and still round on their patients in the hospital and the nursing facility," he says. "Those patients get better care and improve faster. So that's a good thing."

The PIC ACO tried SNFists for a while, Breault says, and it didn't work. The main problem, he says, was that long-term-care patients were wrongly attributed to the SNFists, harming the ACO's risk profile in the MSSP. The SNFists were supposed to follow only the patients discharged to short-term rehab, who had much lower health risks.

In the wake of that experience, he notes, PIC decided to embed nurses in SNFs rather than have doctors round there. "Our care managers are actively supporting the outcome of treatment in those facilities and also ensuring there isn't overutilization of the SNF."

Choosing the Right Care Settings

Physician groups at financial risk must learn how to manage both the utilization of services and the cost of those services. To keep spending down, it's vital to choose the lowest-cost high-quality providers, whether those are hospitals, SNFs, labs, imaging centers, or ambulatory surgery centers (ASCs). Otherwise, the costs attributed to a group will be higher than necessary.

For example, notes Mark Wagar, president of Heritage Medical Systems, "Somebody might be admitted to a hospital when the procedure could be done in an outpatient setting to avoid hospitalizing the patient."

Ken Cohen, MD, chief medical officer of New West Physicians and senior medical director of OptumCare, points out that many ASCs provide quality equivalent to that of hospital outpatient departments (HOPDs) at a lower price. "Assuming they can provide equal outcomes and equal service, why would our healthcare system be responsible for paying more?" he says.

This issue has come to the fore of late because United Healthcare recently began requiring prior authorizations to have certain procedures done in HOPDs rather than in ASCs.[38] Why the big national insurer is doing this is in no mystery: HOPDs charge 25%–39% more than ASCs do for the same procedures, according to the Medicare Payment Advisory Commission (MedPAC).[39]

Now that I've explained the nuts and bolts of assembling the statutory groups and ensuring they can function in the physician-led reform model, the next step is to give them the health IT tools they need to perform at a high level, be measured fairly, and engage with patients better than most practices do today. Those topics are the subjects of the next chapter.

Taking Advantage
of Health IT

Information technology has already transformed healthcare, as it has changed every other industry. To begin with, healthcare providers have become computerized. Most hospitals and physicians have moved from paper to electronic health records (EHRs)—a transition that took place primarily during the past decade. More and more consumers are using smartphone apps, coupled with add-on devices and wearables, to track their efforts to improve their health and manage chronic conditions. Home-based remote monitoring systems are making it increasingly possible for patients to be discharged from hospital to home. And a growing number of consumers are participating in video telehealth visits with healthcare providers using their mobile phones, tablets, and home computers.[1]

As noted in Chapter 6, population health management (PHM) depends largely on health IT. By aggregating and analyzing data from multiple sources, PHM software can supply actionable information to providers and care managers so that they can intervene with individual patients at the right time and in the right place. Moreover, timely data on resource utilization and population health enables risk-bearing groups and ACOs to take appropriate actions so they don't exceed their budgets.

Despite physicians' justifiable issues with EHRs, there is reason for optimism about the long-term potential of health IT. EHRs will become more usable and useful. Interoperability between EHRs will become real as technical barriers fall. Online collaboration among providers caring for the same patients will improve chronic care. Telehealth and remote patient monitoring will eliminate geographical distance and patient mobility as obstacles to high-quality, timely care. Mobile health apps will enable providers to track chronically ill patients continuously. And artificial intelligence will expand the boundaries of what is possible in healthcare.

All of this is on the horizon or starting to happen already. By the time we have Medicare for All and the physician-led reform model could conceivably be implemented, the building blocks of the technological future described above will be in place. At that point, these health IT tools can be expected to have an enormous impact on care delivery and the resources required to manage population health.

This chapter discusses the current state of health IT, where the technology is going, and how it might impact the restructuring of healthcare proposed in this book.

EHR USABILITY

Electronic health records have hampered many physicians and reduced their productivity. On the other hand, EHRs have also digitized healthcare information so that it can be analyzed and used to improve quality and manage population health. This is the tradeoff at the heart of the EHR debate: Healthcare transformation requires data, but EHRs must be transformed to make them easier to use and more effective in patient care.

The current situation is appalling. Primary care physicians spend only 27% of a typical day in direct contact with patients, according to a 2016 study. Almost half of their day is consumed by administrative activities, and 37% of physician time in the exam room is spent on EHR and desk work.[2] Another study found that family physicians spend twice as much time on EHR tasks as they do on direct patient care. They also work in the EHR at home an hour or two each day.[3]

Both in studies and in my conversations with physicians over the years, EHR documentation has been singled out as particularly grueling. The standard EHR comes with numerous templates that, in essence, program the doctor to follow certain processes and ask particular questions, often to satisfy the billing requirements of Medicare and private payers. These templates include dropdowns with boxes that must be checked off at every step. Documentation by exception is possible in some areas, such as the review of systems. Also, physicians dictate some portions of the note, often with the aid of voice recognition software. But overall, data entry is challenging. It competes with doctors' thought processes, limits their engagement with patients during physical exams, and reduces the amount of personal time available to them.

EHRs also generate text that is often difficult to read, making it challenging for doctors to locate relevant information. In addition, some physicians pull past notes into current notes to speed up documentation. That adds to the "note bloat" that so many doctors have decried because it produces overlong and opaque notes.

Payer requirements to measure quality have added to the burden on clinicians and their staffs. According to a 2017 survey of nearly 1,500 practices, mandated quality reports under the federal government's EHR incentive program—popularly known as "Meaningful Use"—didn't necessarily support quality improvement, but they did increase work. "Practices reported numerous challenges in generating adequate reports," the researchers noted.[4]

Fixing EHRs

Many proposals have been made to improve the usability of EHRs. In a *Harvard Business Review* article, Robert Wachter, MD, a professor and chairman of the department of medicine at the University of California at San Francisco, and Jeff Goldsmith, a health policy expert, said that for EHRs to become truly useful tools, a "revolution in usability" is needed. Patient care, rather than billing, should be the central focus, they argued.

EHR should become "groupware" for the clinical team, enabling continuous communication among team members, Wachter and Goldsmith said. All team members should be able to add their own observations of changes in the patient's condition, the actions they've taken, and the questions they are trying to address. It should be easy for clinicians starting shifts or joining the team as consultants to see what's going on.[5]

Similarly, the American Medical Association and the RAND Corp., in a 2014 study of EHR usability, proposed that EHRs be redesigned to support team-based care and promote care coordination. Their other six recommendations were that EHRs

- Enhance physicians' ability to provide high-quality patient care.
- Offer product modularity and configurability.
- Reduce cognitive workload.
- Promote data liquidity.
- Facilitate digital and mobile patient engagement.
- Expedite user input into product design and post-implementation feedback.[6]

Despite these and other proposals, however, there has been little discernible progress in improving EHRs. One reason is the continuing dominance of fee for service, which requires the documentation of each service provided. Innovation has also been hampered by the need of EHR vendors to comply with regulatory requirements. During the Meaningful Use era, for example, software development focused on meeting government certification criteria.[7] More recently, the Office of the National Coordinator for Health IT, as a condition of EHR certification, has begun requiring developers to integrate an application programming interface (API) based on the Fast Health Interoperability Resources (FHIR) standard.[8]

On the positive side, CMS recently changed its documentation requirements for evaluation and management (E&M) coding.[9] When this rule change takes effect, physicians potentially will be able to spend less time checking off boxes in their EHRs.

Applying New Technology

Health IT experts have long called for the development of software that would allow physicians to speak to computers and have their dictation automatically converted to structured data in the EHR. Voice recognition software is incapable of performing this task. Certain kinds of natural language processing (NLP), aided by machine learning, have been used to mine medical concepts from unstructured text.[10] But, partly because of the multiplicity of medical terms for the same concept, NLP software still can't translate speech into discrete data that can be slotted automatically into EHR fields.

EHR companies and third-party developers recently have focused on combining voice recognition and artificial intelligence in "digital assistants" that can help physicians document in EHRs using voice commands. "Macros" triggered by voice commands are available in some speech recognition programs, but AI-based digital assistants can do more.

For example, a digital assistant called Suki has been piloted by the American Academy of Family Physicians (AAFP). After analyzing the practice patterns of a particular doctor, Suki understands what that physician intends, not just what he or she says, according to Suki founder Punit Soni. For example, the digital assistant could machine-learn how a particular doctor prefers to document a normal review of systems and generate that part of the note automatically, Soni told *Medscape Medical News*.[11]

In some family medicine practices that tested Suki, this approach cut EHR documentation time by more than 50%, says Steven Waldren, MD, vice president and chief medical informatics officer of the AAFP. This time savings increases the amount of time that physicians can spend with patients, he adds.

However, Peter Basch, MD, senior director for IT quality and safety, research, and national health IT at MedStar Health in Washington, D.C., is not impressed by Suki. In his view, the digital assistant is a "shortsighted" approach that's tackling "yesterday's problem," especially in light of CMS's new rules on E&M documentation.

"Focusing on a digital assistant rather than on how you're managing the patient is the wrong way to go," he says. The EHR must not only be able to reduce the burden of billing-related documentation, he argues, but it must also break away completely from the "checkbox mentality" to help doctors and care teams improve patient care.

The Smart EHR

What Basch envisions is a "smart" EHR that would help him manage his entire patient panel and draw his attention to the most pertinent issues of each patient he sees.

"The EHR of tomorrow would have a screen that says, 'show me how my patient is doing' with particular focus on using visualization techniques," he says. "It would also show me who's in trouble or who's likely to be in trouble, based on whether they're getting sicker or are likely to be admitted or readmitted to the hospital."

Basch says he'd like to have an EHR that places patient information in context. "When I look at a lab result for liver function, I don't just want to see prior results, I want to look at other things if they're elevated," he says. "For example, show me the meds that the patient is on that could possibly impact liver function. Or show me imaging studies. Because right now I do that manually.

"Let's say people come to see me with abdominal pain, and I'd normally pull up lab results, consults, or imaging studies. Just like Amazon does, the application sees that in other cases, I've asked for the sonogram, not a CT study. It could be a little smarter [than current EHRs] and learn from experience."

Waldren is looking in the same direction. "Two things may help us realize EHRs' potential," he says. "One of them is the alignment of the business forces—the move toward value-based care and payment. Everybody wants to develop the IT tools to deal with that. Also, the technology we have today is still pretty dumb when it comes to understanding clinical terms and clinical content. With the revolution around machine learning and AI, the business will now have the technology to make EHRs much smarter."

The workflow features in EHRs will also have to change to support value-based care, Waldren notes. "But when you try to create workflows, there are a lot of decision points on which path should you follow." There are too many of these decision points in each workflow to preprogram rules for all of them, he points out. "Whereas if we can use machine learning to look at the data and predict what people are going to do, it can predict what that next piece of work is likely to be, based on the clinical scenario."

The idea of using machine learning to create a context-based EHR was proposed in a 2012 paper. Such an EHR would standardize, annotate, and contextualize information from the patient record, improving access to relevant parts of the record and informing medical decision making, the authors said. Instead of simply providing a clinical summary on an EHR screen, it would "synthesize fragments of evidence documented in the entire record to understand the etiology of a disease and its clinical manifestations in individual patients."[12]

Recently, Google Health announced it was piloting a context-sensitive clinical documentation tool at Ascension Health, one of the largest healthcare systems in the United States. This tool reportedly provides an improved method of navigation that allows users to jump around in an EHR to search for particular pieces of EHR data and identify related medical concepts. An earlier Google patent application would use its "deep learning models" to guide predictions of future health events and contextualize patient data to highlight pertinent past events in an EHR.[13]

Going beyond usability, EHRs still fall short in the area of population health management, as noted earlier. They're not designed for use by care teams or care managers, and they can't aggregate or analyze data from outside sources. PHM software vendors—as well as the infrastructure vendors that serve at-risk ACOs and groups—currently help fill this gap. But to coordinate care effectively for individual patients, the primary care groups in our model need a care collaboration platform that would enable greater interoperability among EHRs.

INTEROPERABILITY

Ever since President George W. Bush launched a nationwide campaign to computerize healthcare in 2004, interoperability—the ability to share patient information across disparate EHRs—has been one of the government's key objectives. Yet, 16 years later, full interoperability is still far from being achieved.

In 2017, only 10% of physicians could send and receive data, locate data, and integrate data from outside sources into their EHRs, according to a government survey. That was up only one percentage point from 2015. Similarly, the percentage of physicians who were able to simply send and receive data remained flat at less than 40%, and the percentage of doctors who could integrate data actually dropped from 31% to 28%. The only domain in which interoperability improved was in the ability to locate outside data, which jumped from 34% to 53%.[14]

Hospitals and health systems, which have greater resources and IT expertise than do independent medical practices, reported far greater interoperability than did physicians. The percentage of hospitals that engaged in all four forms of interoperability jumped from 26% in 2015 to 41% in 2017. Moreover, six in 10 hospitals said their clinicians used outside data in patient care.[15]

However, a recent survey by the Center for Connected Medicine found that only 37% of hospitals were very successful in sharing data with outside providers. Nearly a third of hospitals had trouble sharing data within their own healthcare system. The majority of hospital leaders reported that they were moving to a single systemwide EHR to address these challenges.[16]

Steps Toward Interoperability

The backbone of health information exchange today is still the lowly fax—although in recent years, that has been upgraded to computer faxing. For many medical practices and hospitals that are not on the same EHR, faxing remains the standard method of referring patients, sending consult reports, sending and receiving discharge summaries, and exchanging other clinical documents.

The next step up from faxing is Direct secure messaging, a healthcare-specific form of email that a public-private consortium created several years ago. All government-certified EHRs are capable of exchanging Direct messages through "health ISPs" similar to the companies that consumers use for conventional email. Providers often attach standardized clinical summaries known as Continuity of Care Documents (CCDs) to these Direct messages.

DirectTrust, which created the trust framework needed to authenticate Direct messages, reported that nearly 251 million Direct messages were exchanged in the second quarter of 2019. That number represented an increase of 53% over the prior quarter and almost 400% over the same period in 2018.[17] David Kibbe, MD, the former president and CEO of DirectTrust, attributes much of the increased traffic to growing uptake by hospitals.[18]

However, not many physicians see Direct as an advance. Some primary care physicians have told me that when they use Direct messaging to request a consult with a specialist, they also fax the same request because they're not sure whether the specialist will see the Direct message. Moreover, they say, specialists send back reports via Direct only sporadically.

Some providers use regional and statewide health information exchanges (HIEs) to move certain kinds of data. There are roughly 100 of these entities, which typically enable hospitals to send practices care summaries, test results, and admission-discharge-transfer (ADT) alerts. The number of HIEs hasn't grown in several years, however, and some experts believe that newer network services that include EHR vendors will eventually supplant the exchanges.[19]

Documents vs. Discrete Data

Even if these methods of data exchange were more widely used, they would allow healthcare providers to trade information only at the document level. Document exchange is not true interoperability, because physicians need to be able to find the data they're looking for quickly. When they have to wade through a document and then copy the piece of information they need into an EHR field, the data exchange is too slow and laborious to be effective.

A small amount of progress has been made on this front. For example, the Epic EHR is able to extract problem, medication, and allergy lists from CCDs and deposit them in the correct fields. But Basch notes that he has to accept or reject these lists in total. "When the same person makes three visits to an orthopedist and we get a 20-item problem list and a 10-item med list, and we've already looked at the information once and it shows up again, it's like going through your junk emails, and it's cumbersome," he says.

The most promising method for discrete data exchange is Fast Health Interoperability Resources (FHIR), a standards framework that allows information to be exchanged without customized interfaces. But there are still technical and business challenges to overcome before FHIR can be used to exchange structured information between disparate EHRs. The two main use cases for FHIR today are external apps that expand EHR functionality and the ability for patients to download their own records from patient portals.

How FHIR Works

In essence, FHIR uses snippets of data known as "resources" to represent clinical entities such as medications and diagnoses. FHIR APIs enable FHIR-based apps to plug into EHRs and use the data in the EHR database for a particular purpose. For example, a consumer can use the Apple Health app's FHIR-based Health Record feature to download his or her records from multiple providers and assemble them into a single personal health record on his or her iPhone.

Other software developers have designed FHIR apps for providers. Examples include pediatric growth charts, calculators for cardiac and atrial fibrillation stroke risk, a chest pain application, a tool for comparing medication prices, and an app that assists in medication reconciliation.

Some EHRs, including those from Epic, Cerner, Meditech, Allscripts, athenahealth, and CPSI, are already FHIR-enabled. Other EHR companies are expected to add FHIR APIs in the near future to meet government certification criteria. The leading vendors have already made available hundreds of FHIR-based apps, according to Nathan McCarthy of ECG Management Consultants. These third-party apps are designed for a particular EHR or can be used with multiple types of EHRs, he says.

Few physicians are using FHIR-based apps yet to expand the functionality of their EHRs, partly because they're so new. Another reason, Waldren suggests, is that the EHR vendors are not allowing FHIR-based apps to "write back" to their software. "There are a lot of technical and security challenges to being able to write back to an EHR's database," he says. "But you've got to have that for these apps to be successful."

Although FHIR apps can pull individual data elements from EHRs, they cannot be used yet for two-way EHR interoperability at the discrete data level. In an interview with *cio.com*, John Halamka, MD, then executive director of the Health Technology Exploration Center of Beth Israel Lahey Health and former CIO of Beth Israel Deaconess Medical Center in Boston, attributed this partly to the write-back issue.

John Kravitz, CIO of Geisinger Health in Danville, Pa., agrees. "Right now, FHIR integration is mostly outbound," he told *cio.com*. "There's just one area that's inbound, and those are text-based documents. Discrete data inbound via FHIR is not occurring right now."[20]

CARE COLLABORATION PLATFORM

As noted in the last chapter, the physician-led reform model depends heavily on care teams. Within a primary care group, care team members could communicate through secure texting and an enhanced EHR that allowed documentation by care managers and other non-physician clinicians. To ensure proper care coordination across the medical neighborhood, however, primary care doctors, specialists, other providers, and patients would need a different kind of mechanism to exchange information and discuss treatment plans.

This would be especially important for patients who have chronic conditions. Today, these patients are referred out as needed, and specialists send reports back to primary care doctors. However, PCPs don't always receive these reports and they don't even necessarily know whether their patient saw the specialist. Moreover, the referral includes notes from the primary care doctor but not the care manager who might be working with the patient.

Under the physician-led reform model, as explained earlier, primary care doctors and specialists would be in separate practices. To counter the increased fragmentation of care that would inevitably result, it would be imperative for all the physicians caring for a patient to communicate electronically. In addition, population health management requires continuous care for people with chronic conditions; while care managers do the bulk of this work, there must be a way to keep all treating providers in the loop.

Beyond Interoperability

Interoperable EHRs could support this kind of collaboration. But, as we've seen, we're still a long way from full interoperability. What's needed is a care collaboration platform that could use current and emerging health IT to support care coordination across care settings and business boundaries. Such an online platform, which could be launched directly from EHRs, would allow treating providers and their care teams to collaborate with one another in the care of particular patients.

Functioning as a kind of FHIR app, the platform could be used to pull in relevant data on a patient from disparate EHRs without the need for interfaces. As a result of the increasing standardization of EHR data, which should be well along a decade from now, this information could flow into a single, updatable record available to all users. Until write-back from FHIR apps to EHRs is available, however, only documents such as consultant reports, updated care plans, and CCDs could be sent back to the EHRs.

If each primary care group in an administrative region used a different care collaboration platform, this would present a challenge to the specialists in the groups' networks. The simplest solution would be for the groups in the region to agree to use the same platform. The cloud-based technology would allow each group to collaborate with specialists in their own way without compromising patient privacy or revealing their methods to competitors.

Among the EHR data elements and documents that could be exposed to the care collaboration platform are referrals, recent visit notes, consultant reports, test results, diagnoses, allergies, and medications. Data on a patient's care management and social determinants of health would also be available. And there would be up-to-date information on the patient's condition between visits, whether it came from care managers, self-reports, or remote monitoring.

The most important component of the care collaboration platform would be a longitudinal care plan that would follow a chronically ill or recovering patient through their healthcare journey. This care plan would also be the locus for communications among the participants. Any of the patient's providers of record could update the plan with the consent of the patient's primary care doctor. Each time the plan was updated, it would be automatically transmitted back to the participants' EHRs. In addition, the platform would send alerts to care teams whenever a patient had a significant event.

Observers' Comments

A care collaboration platform such as this one could help improve care across care settings, say some experts.

"That's one of the core pieces of technology that's needed: a semantically rich platform that is not tied to any particular practice or doctor but is patient-centered and is pulling things together," Waldren says. "It's semantically rich so you can share knowledge and share tasking. There's one care plan for the patient and everyone contributes to that care plan. That way, the PCP knows exactly what the cardiologist is doing, and the cardiologist knows about the other specialists and what the primary care doc is doing, and it's all coordinated together. You also allow the patient to be part of the care team and contribute."

Waldren's allusion to a "semantically rich platform" refers to the need for "semantic interoperability" between the medical terminologies used in different EHRs and different healthcare organizations. Many of these terms have not been mapped to standard codes and therefore cannot be represented as FHIR resources, Halamka told *cio.com*.[21]

Micky Tripathi, director of the Argonaut Project, a consortium of providers and technology vendors that has played a key role in the development of FHIR, says that a FHIR-based care collaboration platform could be built in the next decade. It would be predicated, he says, on the ability of EHRs themselves to function as platforms that can query and retrieve specific data elements from other EHRs through FHIR APIs. He doesn't dismiss concerns about semantic interoperability, but says that this challenge will be overcome gradually as more and more data elements are added to the FHIR catalog.

One of the first use cases for a care collaboration platform, Tripathi says, would be alerts about changes in a patient's health condition. For example, if a patient's asthma worsened significantly, his or her doctor would want to communicate that immediately to specialists and care managers who are co-managing the patient.

Today, he says, an EHR could not consume that alert, because it isn't part of the standardized common data set that every certified EHR must include. EHRs are able to extract problems, medications, allergies, and immunizations from the standardized Continuity of Care Document (CCD) and not much else. But FHIR includes resources for all 22 elements in the CCD.

These common clinical data elements are part of the U.S. Core Data for Interoperability (USCDI), he explains. The Office of the National Coordinator for Health IT is rapidly adding new USCDI data elements, all of which will be expressed as FHIR resources, he says. Eventually, these new standard data elements and corresponding

FHIR resources will be available in all EHRs. "So, we'll keep getting better at semantic interoperability because of the USCDI," he says.

Today, FHIR resources cover about 80% of what physicians commonly do, including most of the care they provide for chronic conditions such as diabetes, asthma, and hypertension, Tripathi says. "What is missing is a lot of the care management things, which are very rudimentary and ill defined. A care plan is required for EHR certification, but it's unstructured. You just have to list the care team, health concerns and patient goals."

The Argonaut Project is also working on a "subscription resource" that should be available by 2021, he notes. By using that FHIR utility, he says, a care collaboration platform could specify in advance what kinds of data it wants pushed to it automatically from participating EHRs.

TELEMEDICINE

The rapidly evolving field of telemedicine promises to have a major impact on healthcare in general and primary care in particular. The growth of value-based care and risk contracting is expected to boost telemedicine, and vice versa. In addition, the COVID-19 pandemic has greatly accelerated the use of telemedicine in the United States. For the physician-led reform model, the ramifications of this technology are huge.

The terms "telemedicine" and "telehealth" are often used interchangeably. In some contexts, telehealth or "connected health" connotes a larger set of technologies that include remote patient monitoring and mobile healthcare. For the purposes of this discussion, I'll use the term "telemedicine" to describe virtual encounters of any kind between clinicians and patients. These encounters encompass asynchronous communications such as secure texting and email, as well as video "visits" that take place on smartphones and computers. In addition, telemedicine includes physician-to-physician virtual consults, which some groups use to speed care delivery.

Long Evolution

Telemedicine began many years ago, long before smartphones were invented. Rural doctors used teleconferencing equipment in their offices to consult with specialists located in metropolitan areas, usually with the patient present. This approach, which is still in use, has spared many patients from having to travel long distances to see specialists.

Over the past decade, telemedicine services such as American Well, Teladoc, and Doctor on Demand have offered consumers virtual consults with doctors, either telephonically or through video visits on their smartphones and computers. In the past few years, many healthcare systems and large groups have begun to provide remote consults using their own physicians. In some cases, these are the patients' own physicians; more commonly, the groups have cadres of physicians who host virtual visits as a regular part of their work.

In telemedicine's initial stage, few insurance companies covered it; those that did reimbursed physicians at a lower rate for virtual visits than for office visits. This discouraged physicians from participating because they didn't want virtual visits to cannibalize higher-paid in-person encounters. Today, 31 states require private health plans to reimburse virtual visits at the same rate as office visits, and two other states have partial parity laws. In addition, Medicaid covers telemedicine, to varying extents, in all 50 states.[22]

Medicare has been slower to cover telemedicine. For many years, CMS paid only for telemedicine visits initiated in physician offices in rural areas.[23] Later, the agency liberalized its policy in two ways: It allowed virtual "check-in visits" from any location to determine whether a Medicare patient needed to come into the office,[24] and it permitted Medicare Advantage plans to offer telemedicine as an extra benefit.[25] For the duration of the coronavirus pandemic, CMS has largely lifted its restrictions on the use of telemedicine.[26]

Slow Uptake

While private insurance claims for telemedicine services have increased rapidly in recent years, this growth started from a very small base.[27] A 2019 survey found that only one in 10 consumers had used telemedicine in lieu of a doctor's office visit, urgent care visit, or ER visit in the previous 12 months. The report attributed this low rate of virtual visits partly to a lack of consumer awareness about their access to telehealth services. Nearly half of the respondents also said they believed that the quality of care received in a telehealth session is poorer than that in a doctor's visit.[28]

Employers and insurers jumped on telemedicine early in the hope of reducing costs. But in 2016, although 85% of insured people had access to doctors hired by telemedicine companies, just 2%–3% of them were availing themselves of the service. At that time, two reasons were given for the low uptake: The remote consults were mostly telephonic, and there was a lack of continuity with the patients' own physicians.[29]

In an interview with *Medical Economics*, Jerry Penso, MD, president and CEO at AMGA, said there are inherent limits to the approach of having patients consult remotely with doctors hired by outside services. These doctors don't know the patients who consult them, and they rarely coordinate care with the patients' regular physicians, he noted. "The critical piece is to make sure the care is coordinated."[30]

Even before the pandemic, larger groups and health systems began offering telemedicine services directly to their patients. For example, the Austin Regional Clinic uses an outside telemedicine platform that allows video, voice, and text messaging. After sending a text about his or her problem, the patient is quickly connected to a doctor. A group of 20 clinic doctors handles these requests 24/7. Some do it on their own time for extra money; others fit video visits between in-person clinic visits.

Kelsey-Seybold, a multispecialty group in Houston, uses the virtual care platform in its Epic EHR for both video visits and "e-visits" based on online messaging through the EHR's patient portal. When a physician encounters a patient in a scheduled video visit, the doctor sees the patient on one side of the screen and views the EHR on the other side.[31]

Until the COVID-19 crisis, only 3 percent of Kelsey-Seybold's visits were virtual, and the telehealth doctors at the Austin Regional Clinic handled only about 30 virtual visits a week. Even at Kaiser Permanente, only a small percentage of patients made video visits,[32] although the big HMO allowed patients to request telehealth encounters with their own doctors.

"A new patient would typically have a physical exam face to face," explains Richard Isaacs, MD, CEO and executive director of the Permanente Medical Group. "After that, they could ask for a virtual visit. First, they'd send their provider a question through secure messaging, then there would be a response and maybe a request for more information. The patient could also send a picture. Based on all of that, a virtual visit could be initiated or the physician might ask the patient to come into office."

Acute vs. Chronic Care

Outside of rural telehealth and the Veterans Health Administration (VA) system, telemedicine is used most often to diagnose and treat minor acute problems such as influenza, low back pain, conjunctivitis, and urinary tract infections.[33] Given that the doctors hired by telehealth companies don't know their patients, this is understandable; even physicians who do virtual visits with their own patients are reluctant to diagnose or treat remotely anything that might be a serious problem.

In recent years, however, the focus of telehealth has begun to expand. Some groups, including those of Kaiser Permanente and Kelsey-Seybold, are using video visits for post-surgical follow-ups. And some groups employ telemedicine to do follow-up visits with patients who have chronic diseases, as well.

"Virtual health has been great for my diabetic patients," Kelsey-Seybold's Donnie Aga, MD, told *Medical Economics*. "I know them really well, and they can go to the lab at any time; fasting is not an issue. For routine follow-ups on diabetes, it's very well done."

Virtual visits with behavioral health providers have become widespread. Mental health professionals at Summit Medical Group in Summit, N.J., for example, regularly do remote therapy and medication management sessions with patients who have difficulty getting to the office, according to James Korman, Psy.D., chief of behavioral health and physician wellness. Primary care physicians can consult with therapists or do video visits with patients.

The VA has taken the lead in the more inclusive approach to telemedicine. A VA program that encompasses both remote monitoring and videoconferencing reached nearly 120,000 veterans in 2012 and generated annual savings of $1,999 per patient. Hospital admissions decreased by 38% compared to the previous year; inpatient bed days of care decreased by 58%; and patient satisfaction was 85%.[34]

The Virtual Future

Large groups that hold risk contracts value telemedicine because it supports population health management, according to Richard Trembowicz, a principal with ECG Management Consulting. The AMGA's Jerry Penso, similarly, told *Medical Economics* that for groups taking financial risk, telemedicine can make care more effective and efficient.

Some experts interviewed for this book went further, predicting that eventually, the majority of patient visits will be virtual. However, Jonathan Weiner, professor of health policy at the Johns Hopkins Bloomberg School of Public Health, says this will happen only if small-practice doctors are given a financial incentive to do virtual visits with their patients.

Waldren expects a "significant amount of growth with the technology we have today, but there will have to be better technology to extend the ability to do the physical exam remotely." To do telemedicine right, he says, "you need remote monitoring and some kind of analytic capacity to watch the signal and see whether there's something there that requires intervention."

If that happens, he says, "The majority of interactions with patients will be virtually done. So, you may have four visits a year from your diabetic patients, but you may have weekly or monthly interactions with them to keep tabs on everything."

Basch agrees that "micro virtual visits" between physician encounters will become normal in healthcare. However, he says, we first have to get beyond the notion that virtual visits are just for minor acute problems.

"A bigger bang for the buck is going to be bundling it with visit-based care for management of chronic illnesses," he says. "The idea that the primary market for telehealth is sore throats and sprains and colds is stupid. It's convenient for patients, but it's not using technology to its utmost. Instead, it's creating virtual urgent care. That's useful for some people, but doesn't make a big dent in healthcare spending."

After speaking with his colleagues at MedStar Health, Basch estimates that between 10% and 70% of patient encounters with primary care physicians could be done via telemedicine. "There are visits that are necessary—new patients, people with new episodes of a condition, or who have belly pain or chest pain. But what fills up most of my days as an internist are routine follow-ups for hypertension and diabetes and so forth. I need to see your BP and your blood sugar, and if there's a question, come in."

eConsults with Specialists

Chapter 9 explored Project ECHO and other telehealth programs that enable PCPs to get remote training from specialists. In addition, some primary care doctors are able to consult with specialists about particular cases online or through videoconferencing.

In California, Community Health Center Network (CHCN), a coalition of community health centers in Alameda and surrounding counties, offers econsults to its primary care physicians. Doctors send questions with relevant patient histories to a specialist network, and an appropriate physician responds within four hours. If his or her advice resolves the case, the primary care doctor doesn't have to refer the patient out.

In a study of CHCN econsults, the researchers found that 25% of virtual visits were resolved without requiring an in-person visit to the specialist. In cases where a referral was required, the econsults decreased the average wait time for a specialist visit by 17%. More than half of the primary care doctors reported increased job satisfaction resulting from the use of the platform, and 82% said that the econsults improved their patients' quality of care.[35]

Kaiser Permanente's northern California region uses a smartphone platform to link PCPs with specialists via videoconferencing. "It's all about care without delay," Isaacs says. "If you have a primary care physician who's connected immediately to a specialist via smartphone technology, that drives a lot of efficiency."

For example, he notes, when a patient comes into the office with a skin lesion, the PCP can evaluate it and send a secure text message with an image of the lesion to a dermatologist during the visit. The dermatologist responds as soon as possible.

"It's almost impossible to do tele-dermatology unless you're in an integrated system like Kaiser Permanente," Isaacs notes. "The dermatologist would never provide telephone advice in the fee-for-service world. Under fee for service, there would be no way for the specialist to generate a bill for that. But in Kaiser, a doctor can get this expertise when it's needed."

REMOTE MONITORING

The other major branch of telehealth is remote patient monitoring, which includes home and mobile monitoring. Both kinds of monitoring can be used for chronic-disease management, but the vast majority of mobile health apps are wellness and fitness programs.

The evidence so far doesn't show an improvement in the outcomes of people who use the latter kinds of apps on their smartphones. But there is some evidence of benefit for chronic-disease apps and for home monitoring. Because of this technology, some observers believe, an increasing number of patients will be discharged from hospitals to home rather than to SNFs or rehab facilities.

In addition, many homebound seniors will be able to manage their chronic conditions at home with the help of remote monitoring, patient education, and virtual and in-person visits from care teams, predicted E. Ray Dorsey and Eric J. Topol in a 2016 article. For people with chronic conditions, including the 2 million elderly people who are homebound, "the patient-centered medical home will increasingly be the patient's home," they wrote.[36]

The best evidence on home monitoring comes from studies of patients with congestive heart failure (CHF). Several years ago, Geisinger Health Plan, based in Danville, Pa., reported that home monitoring for patients with CHF cut readmissions by 44% compared to a control group.[37]

In another study, more than 3,000 CHF patients at Partners Healthcare received in-home monitoring of weight, blood pressure, heart rate, and pulse oximetry. These data were uploaded daily, and decision support software identified the patients who needed attention. As a result of this approach, hospital readmissions dropped by 44% as compared to usual care, the study found. The program generated cost savings of more than $10 million in a three-year period.[38]

In a 2018 report, the eHealth Initiative, a nonprofit research and advocacy firm, argued that remote patient monitoring can improve outcomes. "By continuously tracking the routine and biometric measurements of people with chronic conditions, providers are empowered to intervene earlier in disease progression, which helps prevent complications that can result in unnecessary in-person or hospital visits."[39]

Moreover, the report said, remote patient monitoring (RPM) can help clinicians track patients' health conditions after hospital discharge.

> RPM improves outcomes in post-acute care by helping patients and doctors manage short-term care after in-person treatment with remotely-collected data. Programs educate patients on their condition, recovery needs, and pain management while providing regular reminders, early interventions, post-discharge information, or medication adherence tracking. With the information garnered from PGHD [patient-generated health data], providers are able to evaluate the effectiveness of treatments and customize care plans between patient visits.[40]

'Fear of the Bad Event'

Waldren expects the use of remote monitoring equipment to result in an increasing number of people being discharged from the hospital to home. But he thinks there will be some resistance among physicians who fear that recently discharged patients could get into trouble at home.

"There's the fear of the bad event—not that they couldn't manage the condition at home, but that they don't catch something and it spirals out of control with remote monitoring."

Then there's the question of accuracy. Home monitoring equipment is not manufactured to the same specifications as the monitoring equipment used in hospitals. Joseph Kvedar, MD, vice president of connected health for Partners Healthcare, says RPM's accuracy will always be limited because more accurate home and mobile monitoring gear would cost too much.

Kvedar, a big proponent of telehealth, has long maintained that a better screening method to "separate the noise from the signal" in monitoring data is needed before most providers will pay attention to home device data. Some progress has been made in this area, he says, but screening remains a challenge for physicians. "We have to be able to analyze these data streams and report insights," he notes.

Basch agrees. "To monitor patients with certain conditions, I don't need to see their blood pressure every five seconds. I don't need to see their weight seven times a day. We don't need vast streams of monitoring data. We need to start smaller and increase as we need it."

mHealth Apps Proliferate

Back in 2012, only five years after the advent of the iPhone, there were between 20,000 and 30,000 mobile health apps on the market.[41] By 2015, there were 165,000 mHealth apps available in the iTunes and Android app stores.[42] In 2017, the number of these apps had almost doubled to 318,572, according to IMS Health.[43]

Consumers are interested in very few of these apps. In 2015, just 12% of mHealth apps accounted for 90% of consumer downloads, and 36 apps generated nearly half of downloads.[44]

Of the top 25 apps downloaded, 80% had at least one positive observational study demonstrating clinical efficacy, IMS Health reported.[45] But a randomized controlled trial of multi-sensor apps found no short-term benefits in health costs or outcomes for patients monitoring their glucose, blood pressure, and heart rhythm with connected devices.[46] Moreover, apps that track a patient's diet or symptoms don't necessarily lead to behavior change, and patients tend not to stick with chronic-disease apps for more than a few months.[47]

As noted earlier, the overwhelming majority of mHealth apps are designed for healthy people who want to quantify their health and keep fit. Of the apps aimed at people with chronic conditions, the most numerous programs are those that focus on rheumatoid arthritis, Parkinson's, Alzheimer's, mental health, walking and gait, epilepsy, and migraine.[48]

Some mHealth apps are part of programs that help patients with a particular disease, such as diabetes. For example, Livongo Health sells a program that gives diabetic patients a blood glucometer, free test strips, and a software application that offers coaching and tracking based on the patient-generated data. Welldoc's FDA-cleared BlueStar system for diabetes management analyzes patient data, compares the data to past trends, and sends analytics to the patient's healthcare team. It also features behavioral coaching and educational content for the patient. Both companies claim significant cost savings from the use of their apps.[49-50]

Meanwhile, the market for mHealth apps is growing. According to a recent consumer survey by Stanford Medicine and Rock Health, an investment research firm, 42% of respondents now track some aspect of their health digitally, up from 18% in 2015. One in three respondents owns a wearable monitoring device, such as a Fitbit or an Apple Watch, and one in four wearable owners uses it to manage a diagnosis.[51]

But there's a disconnect between this burgeoning consumer interest and the response of healthcare providers to date. A 2014 study by Manhattan Research found that a third of doctors had recommended mHealth apps to patients in the previous year; however, only a small percentage of doctors prescribed particular apps, and most of those were fitness and diet applications.[52] In 2018, a spokesman for IMS Health said those numbers hadn't changed much.

Eric Topol, who has written extensively about mHealth, said in a 2014 article that many physicians are not adopting the technology because they're resistant to change, don't want to be drowned in data, and are concerned about potential liability. Also, he said, there weren't enough good studies on the accuracy of the apps.[53]

While recognizing that doctors have good reasons to be cautious about prescribing mHealth apps, Topol was optimistic about the future of this technology. So is Waldren. The combination of remote monitoring with video visits, he says, might improve care for chronic diseases, but to really move the needle on chronic care, he notes, "there will have to be better technology to extend the ability to do the physical exam remotely."

Because of the inherent problems of reimbursement for remote monitoring in a fee-for-service world, it's likely that the technology will blossom only after U.S. healthcare transitions further to value-based care. Speaking of telehealth in general, Topol and Dorsey noted that closed systems like Kaiser Permanente, the Department of Defense, and the VA system all encourage the use of telehealth to improve health and reduce costs. The rise of bundled payments and ACOs, they said, offers opportunities for further experimentation with telehealth.[54]

Kvedar, in a paper cowritten with Molly Joel Coye and Wendy Everett, also viewed telehealth as a vehicle to make healthcare more efficient and effective.

> This approach facilitates remote diagnosis and treatment, continuous monitoring and adjustment of therapies, support for patient self-care, and the leveraging of providers across large populations of patients. Because these technologies improve the sharing of data and tasks among teams, they allow team members to practice at their highest levels of skill and training. Physicians and nurses can then work more efficiently by allocating their time to the patients who most need attention.[55]

Outcomes Measurement

Kvedar believes that remote patient monitoring could also help improve outcomes measurement. As mentioned in Chapter 5, process and intermediate outcomes measures have limited utility, especially when applied to chronic conditions. Some organizations, as noted, use patient-reported outcomes measures (PROMs) based on surveys about functional status, health-related quality of life, and so forth. The challenge is the subjective nature of this data.

Aspects of a patient's functional status can be measured more objectively with smartphone apps. A 2016 study of an mHealth app that measured functional mobility in the elderly, for example, found that the app was as accurate as a lab-based reference condition.[56]

Kvedar is enthusiastic about the potential for using remote monitoring to measure long-term outcomes. While many doctors doubt that patient self-reports are valid, he says, home monitoring and mHealth apps could be used to supplement patient surveys.

"We've seen evidence of that over the years in various projects we've done and research endeavors we've been part of," he says. "The majority of the model isn't quite there yet, however. PROMs are a big step forward, but objective information coming from mobile devices and wearables should not only supplement, but even supplant, patient reports."

Kvedar admits that it's difficult to measure pain in any way other than asking patients about it. "Pain may be the exception and there may be others. But increasingly, we'll be able to get good objective data about you from passive data collection."

Outcomes measurement aside, telehealth technologies are starting to have a major impact on how care is delivered. If these technologies were more fully developed and were applied within the context of value-based care, they could enable physicians to provide better care to more patients at lower cost. But much more than health

IT will be required to bend the cost curve by reducing waste significantly. The next chapter summarizes how physician-led healthcare reform could achieve this goal. It also explains how doctors could increase their incomes if this model were adopted under Medicare for All.

CHAPTER 11

The Payoff

The previous three chapters have discussed how a physician-led reform model could be built, how it would function under Medicare for All, and the new health IT tools that could contribute to its success. Now it's time to consider how all of this could help physicians eliminate waste, which is the key to curbing health costs.

How much waste could physicians safely jettison? As noted in Chapter 5, the Institute of Medicine in 2010 calculated that approximately 30% of total healthcare costs—$765 billion in that year—was wasted. Of that amount, the portion that physicians could affect directly included unnecessary services ($210 billion), inefficiently delivered services ($130 billion), and missed opportunities for disease prevention ($55 billion).[1] Together, those components added up to $395 billion, or more than half of the total. So, doctors could, in theory, reduce total health costs by at least 15% without harming care.

A recent paper, based on published studies and government reports, found that 20%–25% of U.S. health spending is wasteful. The authors estimated that the cost of this systemic waste ranges from $760 billion to $935 billion, based on current healthcare spending. They calculated that providers could eliminate $191 billion to $282 billion of this waste, or 5%–7.5% of total healthcare costs, by reducing low-value care, delivering more recommended care, and better coordinating care.[2]

There is no intrinsic reason to believe that this new study is any more accurate than the earlier ones, including the IOM report and the Berwick and Hackbarth paper cited earlier. So perhaps we should split the difference and assume that physicians could cut enough waste to reduce total spending by 10% over time.

PHM Alone Won't Cut It

Some health policy experts say that we can't expect much of these savings to come from population health management (PHM). In a commentary in the *Journal of the American Medical Association*, Ashish Jha, MD, professor of global health at Harvard, said the few studies of PHM effectiveness have shown some health benefits, but no cost reductions. "Although some interventions may be cost-effective, they are almost never cost-saving," he argued.[3]

Jha cited an article on the cost-effectiveness of preventive care and disease management. According to this paper, by Louise B. Russell of Rutgers University, hundreds of studies have shown that preventive services, such as cancer screening, usually cost more than they save because they have to be applied to large populations. Similarly, the accumulated costs of treating hypertension are greater than the savings because some people who take blood pressure medications would never develop heart disease or suffer a stroke.[4]

Of course, that shouldn't deter healthcare providers from providing these potentially life-saving drugs to their patients. Moreover, PHM can reduce the odds that patients with serious chronic diseases will be hospitalized and generate high costs. Preventive care can also save money in some cases, depending on how it's done. Russell noted that "careful choices about [screening] frequency, groups to target, and component costs can increase the likelihood that interventions will be highly cost-effective or even cost-saving."

Intensive Primary Care

Some primary care models that feature aspects of PHM have been shown to save money. As discussed in Chapter 4, intensive primary care for patients with chronic diseases can reduce ED visits and hospital admissions. Advanced primary care, as embodied in the patient-centered medical home (PCMH), also has been shown to lower the cost of care, and ACOs built on the foundation of PCMHs tend to have better results than those that lack this critical building block.

It's also important to remember that 5% of patients generate around 50% of health costs. When an ACO or group closely manages these high-risk patients, it can make a big difference. The Cornerstone medical group, for example, used this approach to cut costs for patients in four high-risk categories by nearly 13% in a single year (see Chapter 6).

Many groups and ACOs have succeeded under financial risk contracts with similar strategies. For example, Heritage Provider Systems (HPN) focuses less on population-wide outreach than on managing the top 10%–20% of healthcare utilizers. "You want to get to them, because they're the ones who could head downhill quickly," says Mark Wagar, president of HPN affiliate Heritage Medical Systems.

The availability of accurate, timely data is essential to identify these patients and intervene with them, he notes. Moreover, Heritage uses data to measure performance and provide feedback to providers on their quality and utilization. It picks the most cost-effective specialists and hospitals and uses hospitalists to coordinate inpatient care. It finds out immediately when patients have been admitted or discharged and tries to ensure they go to the most appropriate post-acute care settings. All of these policies—as well as attention to high-risk patients' unmet social needs—have contributed to Heritage's ability to manage global capitation, Wagar says.

New West Physicians in Denver has taken a similar route to success. In essence, New West Physicians has thrived under risk contracting by carefully selecting specialists, hospitals, and ancillary services, keeping people out of the hospital, focusing population health management on high-risk patients, and eliminating the use of low-value care as much as possible.

Rio Grande Valley Health Alliance, the successful south Texas ACO, has combined population health management with several other techniques to reduce costs. Among other things, it has lowered home health costs by persuading outside doctors to increase the appropriateness of their orders; has used field nurses and care managers to work with high-risk and rising-risk patients; and has collaborated with Medicaid and community services to help patients with their socioeconomic issues, including lack of transportation.

Many risk-taking entities are starting to address social determinants of health, as described in Chapter 7. These efforts can cost more than they save if not carefully tailored to the patients who are most at risk. Evidence is still scarce about the long-term cost impact of such initiatives; however, to judge by the significant increase in social determinants of health-related investments by payers and providers, there's a widespread belief that it eventually will cut health costs.

Groups experienced in managing risk have reduced costs substantially while providing high-quality care. Using methods similar to those outlined above, for instance, the Aledade ACOs saved Medicare more than $69 million in 2018, while achieving an average quality score of 96%, according to the company. The ACOs reduced stays in skilled nursing facilities by an average of 17% and hospitalizations, by an average of 6%.[5]

The lesson to be drawn from these organizations' experience is that significant money can be saved through a variety of approaches that include but don't depend solely on population health management. To improve outcomes over time, it's essential to apply proven PHM techniques to the whole population. More targeted interventions can save money in a shorter time. But PHM is only one of the tools used by successful ACOs and groups to lower costs.

Reducing Underuse

All the studies on waste reduction cite the problem of underuse—that is, the failure to deliver care that could have obviated the need for more costly interventions later on. Despite the spread of value-based care, there is still a huge gap between the national guidelines for recommended preventive and chronic care and what is actually delivered. A major reason is that primary care physicians simply don't have time to provide all that care.

Primary care doctors are already overburdened, and it has been estimated that it would take 21.7 hours a day to provide all recommended acute, chronic, and preventive care for a panel of 2,500 patients. Obviously, that's impossible. But in their previously cited 2012 paper, Justin Altschuler, David Margolius, Thomas Bodenheimer, and Kevin

Grumbach figured out that, by delegating a portion of preventive and chronic care services to non-physician team members, practices could provide all recommended care "with panel sizes that are achievable with the available primary care workforce."[6]

Depending on the degree of task delegation (50%–77% of preventive care and 25%–47% of chronic care), the researchers calculated, a primary care team of this kind could provide high-quality care to panels of between 1,387 and 1,947 patients. That range is similar to the U.S. distribution of one primary care physician to 1,500 people.[7] It also matches the range of panel sizes within large integrated systems like Kaiser Permanente and the VA system.[8]

Decline in Office Visits

It's unclear whether this degree of delegation is practical or feasible under today's conditions. If not, is there enough primary care to meet the requirements of the physician-led reform model?

As noted in Chapter 4, there is currently a primary care shortage in the United States. However, a large study recently showed that from 2008 to 2015, the average number of PCP visits per person dropped by 20%. Specialist visits didn't increase in that period.[9]

There could have been several reasons for the decline in visits to primary care doctors. For one thing, the study didn't look at visits to nurse practitioners or physician assistants, who delivered more care during this period. Retail clinics and urgent care centers were also proliferating, and deductibles were rising. Those trends could have contributed to the drop in the number of office visits, David Nash, MD, of Jefferson University observes in regard to a similar study.

The authors of the primary care visit paper cited two other possible factors: The average visit time was lengthened by 2.4 minutes during the study period, and patients received more services and procedures in each appointment; and physicians offered more non-face-to-face care, such as secure messaging and virtual visits. The study pointed out that it was no longer necessary for patients to come in for lab results in most cases.

Health IT and Patient Demand

This raises the question of how much health IT has already reduced the demand for in-person primary care and how much more of an effect it might have in the future. As discussed in the previous chapter, experts predict that someday, the majority of patient encounters will be virtual. But it's still unclear how health IT might affect demand for physicians, or how that might be impacted by the increased delegation of care that health IT could support.

In a 2013 paper, Jonathan Weiner and Susan Yeh of Johns Hopkins and David Blumenthal, president of the Commonwealth Fund, attempted to answer these questions.

Their crystal ball was a bit foggy, to put it mildly. But they raised some important issues that reverberate today.

At a time when under half of physicians used basic EHRs, the coauthors tried to imagine a future in which a large percentage of physician practices had "comprehensive health IT" systems. These systems included interoperable EHRs, electronic clinical decision support, provider order entry, and secure messaging between doctors and patients. In this "digital practice milieu," the physician would be part of a multidisciplinary virtual team. Consumers would have personal health records and would interact with practices on patient portals.

Health IT, new economic incentives, and the increased availability of NPs and PAs, the authors predicted, would enable physicians to delegate much more care to other care team members than practices with less-capable IT systems could. At the same time, specialists would be able to use electronic communications to delegate more to PCPs.

As a result, they said, efficiency gains from health IT would enable physicians to meet the demands of 8%–15% more patients than they could without comprehensive health IT. Overall, they calculated, delegation empowered by digitalization might contribute to a 5%–12% decrease in demand for all physicians and a 3%–8% reduction in demand for specialists.[10]

Future Scenarios

So far, this study's conclusions have not been borne out. EHRs have reduced, not improved, efficiency in most practices. Moreover, interoperability between EHRs has not reached the point where it raises efficiency; in fact, to the extent that providers can receive outside data electronically, it often increases the clutter in their EHRs.

Asked why the paper's scenario hasn't come to pass, Steven Waldren of the American Academy of Family Physicians replies, "What EHRs do today is automate the business of healthcare, not the business of healthcare delivery. The studies said EHRs would help improve quality of care, and what we saw was more voluminous documentation and charge capture. Also, in 2013, there were no studies of the administrative burden of EHRs."

As for the delegation of duties supposedly made possible by health IT tools, Peter Basch of MedStar Health says, "I think it's close to zero, except when it's intentionally done in a closed system like Kaiser."

However, he doesn't rule out that something like this could happen in the future. "When you intentionally build in something that promotes delegation to make better use of resources, instead of continuing the hamster wheel of the visit-based patient relationship, and when we make more use of other things like secure texting, secure email, and fully connected IT—a lot of that has not penetrated for a host of reasons. So, we can't really say it works or it doesn't work."

It's likely that primary care groups would make better use of health IT if they were prepaid, as the Kaiser Permanente groups are. "I think the benefit of all these applications is magnified in a prepaid model, because it allows the physicians to use the appropriate tools at the appropriate time," says Richard Isaacs, MD, CEO and executive director of the Permanente Medical Group. "You're driving a more effective utilization, which is where the value comes in. There may be incentives to do more technology-based visits because it's convenient, but maybe they're not appropriate. We use the technology to drive effective care."

CUTTING WASTE

Physicians in all specialties contribute to the wasteful use of healthcare resources. As shared earlier in this book, Kedar Mate of the Institute of Healthcare Improvement said he sometimes sees patients unnecessarily admitted to the hospital. Specialists also sometimes order low-value or unnecessary tests or do low-value or unnecessary procedures. But primary care doctors also provide low-value care in certain cases.

For example, a recent study established that from 2003 to 2013, national PSA screening rates hardly changed: They were 17.2% in 2003, 22.3% in 2008, and 18.6% in 2013. The slight drop in the latter year followed the publication of two systematic reviews showing that PSA screening did not significantly reduce prostate cancer or overall mortality. After weighing the evidence, the U.S. Preventive Services Task Force said there was a small net benefit for men aged 55 to 69 years, but that the balance of benefits and harms in men remained close.

The study also found that in some areas, men over 75 were screened at *higher* rates in 2013 than in 2003. PSA tests for men of that age do more harm than good, the study authors noted.[11]

The researchers wondered why the evidence and guideline on PSA screening "has done so little to reduce low-value care." They suggested that some busy primary care doctors are likely to continue ordering the test rather than take the time required for shared decision making with patients.

Getting Specialists Onboard

Each year, U.S. healthcare systems perform nearly 6 billion lab tests that cost nearly $70 billion. About 30%–50% of these tests are unnecessary, according to a study in the *International Journal of Clinical Chemistry.*[12]

Since hospital tests are ordered principally by specialists, it would make sense for the primary care groups in our reform model to ask their specialists why there's so much waste in the hospital and how much of it could be cut back. The specialists would likely cooperate, since their financial incentives would be aligned with the PCPs'.

The attitude of specialists toward all kinds of low-value care would probably change if referrals and bonuses controlled by the primary care groups generated the majority of their income. The specialists might even ask their medical societies to include more high-volume, low-value tests and procedures on the lists they gave to the Choosing Wisely initiative (see Chapter 5).

The reform model probably would mold physician behavior in ways similar to the mindset of doctors in large, prepaid multispecialty groups. At Kaiser Permanente, for instance, where the medical groups are prepaid and quality and cost are constantly measured, physicians are incentivized to provide care that produces the best outcomes for patients, Isaacs says.

"For example, with elective knee replacement surgery, we've proven that patients recover better in the home setting. But in the fee-for-service system, there's no incentive to do surgical home recovery. We [at Kaiser] have moved away from hospital utilization except for when it's indicated. That's a clear quality benefit and a cost reducer."

Restructuring Impact

As pointed out earlier, the Medicare Shared Savings Program (MSSP) has reduced Medicare's net spending by a relatively small amount. So why should the physician-led reform model, which uses a similar payment method, achieve better results?

For one thing, only a small percentage of ACOs in the MSSP are taking downside risk, and ACOs that assume two-sided risk save more money than those that don't. At a more fundamental level, the restructuring of the system proposed in this book would change the incentives of physicians in ways that would guarantee they'd try to reduce costs. Since doctors order most healthcare, the rest of the medical neighborhood would have no choice but to follow suit.

Hospitals, for example, would have their prices administratively set after negotiations with the government. Naturally, they'd try to increase their volume to compensate—one reason some health policy experts favor global budgets for hospitals. But the specialists who work in hospitals would have an incentive to lower costs, as would the hospitalists hired by the primary care groups. And in markets where the groups had a choice of hospitals, they'd tend to refer to facilities that offered an optimal combination of high quality and low cost. Thus, hospitals that tried to game the payment system would lose out in the long run.

In this environment, when a doctor or a case manager decided where to send patients after hospital discharge, they'd probably choose the most cost-effective care setting that could help the patient recover. They'd also be likely to refer patients to post-acute care providers that the primary care groups favored. Since nursing homes and home care agencies depend on these referrals, they'd also have incentives to provide appropriate, high-quality care.

It's also important to remember that the physicians who belong to ACOs today receive only a portion—and in many cases, a small portion—of their income from those ACOs. The bulk of their revenue comes from fee for service, much of it from private health plans that pay significantly more than Medicare does.

In contrast, the primary care groups in the reform model would receive all their income from a single payer that would pay Medicare rates. Only by cutting waste and saving money could they raise their incomes above that level. The same would be true for the specialists. The alignment of incentives across the board would have a significant impact on physician behavior.

The competition among primary care groups in each region would also force the groups to reduce costs and provide high-quality care. While the provider report cards for consumers would not show details on specialty care and surgical outcomes, the specialist quality measures would be incorporated into the PCP group scores. Those published ratings would show how successful the groups had been in guiding care and selecting the best local specialists.

For all these reasons, it can be expected that the physician-led reform model would cut costs by an order of magnitude more than the Medicare Shared Savings Program.

BARRIERS TO WASTE REDUCTION

Even in a healthcare system dedicated to value-based care, there would be a few major barriers to the kinds of waste reduction described above. First, there's the ethical challenge: Physicians might be tempted to skimp on care when they have financial incentives to cut costs. Second, there's a practical obstacle: As explained in Chapter 5, clinical guidelines are not infallible, and large parts of medicine have never been subjected to rigorous trials. Third, because of the many gaps in clinical knowledge, it can be difficult for physicians to distinguish between beneficial and non-beneficial care before they provide it.

Regarding the ethical dimension, insurance companies often are criticized when they deny coverage for what doctors and patients view as financial reasons. Physicians encounter this every day when they request prior authorization for a test, a drug, or a procedure that they believe could benefit their patient. But in groups that take financial risk, physicians themselves have incentives to limit the amount and types of care to what they think is necessary. In other words, they must balance their duty to the patient against their role as stewards of scarce healthcare resources.

On the other hand, fee-for-service payment motivates physicians to do more for patients, regardless whether it's necessary or not. In some cases, doctors may order tests or do procedures of questionable value to protect themselves against malpractice suits; but studies of defensive medicine have shown that it actually raises health costs by a fairly small percentage.[13] More often, physicians overtreat patients because of individual practice patterns or because they practice in areas where that's the standard of care.[14-15] As long as doctors believe there's a chance that the patient will benefit from low-value care, they can justify their decision to provide that care.

The Institute of Medicine, in its book *Crossing the Quality Chasm*, neatly encapsulated the contrasting incentives of fee for service and prepaid or budgeted care.

> Under fee for service, there is a potential for overuse of services by increasing the intensity of care and treating more patients. Also, since the method is based on individual units of care or service, it can be difficult to coordinate payment across the many members of a care team. . . .
>
> The advantages of a budgeted approach are that it provides an incentive to control costs and produce care efficiently, and can encourage innovation in cost-reducing technologies, use of lower-cost settings of care, and investment in health promotion and disease prevention. . . . Disadvantages include the potential for risk selection to avoid patients who might be high-cost users of care, and the potential to provide insufficient or reduced quality of services to minimize costs and stay within budget.[16]

Risk adjustment can eliminate the temptation to shun higher-risk patients, and the use of data analytics—which hardly existed when the IOM book was written—can help at-risk groups stay within their budgets without skimping on care. To be successful, the primary care groups in the physician-led reform model would have to incentivize their doctors to provide high-quality care, first and foremost. Kaiser Permanente's physicians, for example, receive salaries and are not directly incentivized to cut costs. Instead, the group culture has internalized efficiency. "Separating clinical decision making from actual payment is what drives quality," Isaacs says. "That's patient-centered care, where you're doing what's best for the patient."

Wasteful vs. Beneficial Care

One reason waste is hard to eliminate is that it's often difficult to detect. In the book *The Hippocratic Myth*, M. Gregg Bloche, MD, a professor of law at Georgetown University, says that while up to 30% of healthcare might be wasted, "we don't know, until after the fact, which care is pointless under what conditions."[17]

While one might expect that experienced physicians know how to distinguish between beneficial and non-beneficial care, that assumption presupposes that they've been able to keep up with the latest studies, Bloche told me in an interview. Moreover, he noted, "the majority of clinical scenarios are not situations that have been studied and analyzed in a randomized controlled fashion. Even when there have been randomized controlled trials, the inclusion criteria required to make such studies effective statistically are pretty narrow. That's great from the perspective of doing a good study. But the more you narrow the inclusion criteria, the less relevant your study is to patients in the wild."

Nevertheless, there are many common scenarios where doctors know perfectly well whether care is being wasted. That's why three of four U.S. physicians said in a 2017 survey that the frequency with which doctors order unnecessary medical tests and procedures is a serious problem for the health system (see Chapter 5).[18]

Meanwhile, busy doctors can't keep up with the flood of new evidence, and many of them prescribe drugs pushed by sales reps brandishing biased studies. Even when physicians follow guidelines based on rigorous trials, some of their patients don't respond well to what those guidelines recommend. Hence, if a group requires its doctors to follow agreed-upon protocols, they must be given the freedom to deviate from them.

Despite all these caveats, however, it's physicians who provide, order, or supervise most of the care that patients receive. Consequently, they are the only healthcare players who can significantly reduce the waste in the system. But they're not going to do it under external pressure. Rather than being buffaloed by insurance companies, as many doctors are today, they should take the buffalo by the horns and manage care themselves. Because physicians have a trust relationship with their patients, they also have a unique ability to persuade patients that more care isn't always better care. If our country is going to make a real effort to cut waste enough to make healthcare affordable, physicians are the ones to do it.

THE PAYOFF

To understand how all of this might affect physician income in our reform model, let's start with the fact that primary care physicians would be prepaid for their own services. If their risk-adjusted capitation rate were equivalent to Medicare fee-for-service payments, they'd be losing a substantial chunk of the higher-paid health plan income they'd received before the transition to single payer. So, for the purpose of calculating lost income, let's assume that both primary care doctors and specialists are continuing to be paid fee for service.

According to one study, private insurers pay physicians other than surgeons roughly 130% of Medicare rates.[19] But only 43% of their patients, on average, are privately insured.[20] Medicaid, which accounts for nearly 17% of patients in the average practice, pays between 66% and 72% of Medicare rates.[21-22]

The Urban Institute estimates that the revenue of the average physician would drop by 13% under Medicare for All.[23] The PERI researchers at UMass Amherst, in contrast, estimate that average physician fees would fall by 7%–9%.[24] As I did earlier in estimating how much waste could be safely eliminated, I'll take the middle ground between these two estimates, which is about 10%.

To calculate how much the primary care groups would have to save to make up for this loss, we first need to know what the average cost of care is. According to the 2019 CMS actuarial report, spending on personal healthcare in 2018 was nearly $10,000 per person.[25] If Medicare for All had saved 10% of that in reduced administrative costs, the remaining cost per person at the current spending level would have been $9,000 in 2019.

Let's say that a PCP group could save 1% of that amount the first year, or $90 per patient. If a doctor had 2,000 patients, he or she would save $180,000 on his or her patient panel.

Now, let's further assume that the government and the group split the savings 50/50. In that case, the group would receive $90,000 on behalf of the physician.

However, there would be others to pay before getting to the bottom line. Infrastructure vendors like Aledade now take around 40% of their ACO clients' portion of shared savings. But they could probably be paid a lot less if they had the volume of business the reform model would give them. For the sake of argument, let's assume that they would receive 25% of the group's share of the savings.

Specialists would also have to be compensated above the Medicare rates they'd receive from the government. Since they wouldn't be taking financial risk, they'd get smaller bonuses than would the primary care doctors. In this example, I'll assume they get 25% of the savings that flow back to the primary care groups.

After subtracting the amounts going to the infrastructure vendor and the specialists, the primary care doctor would be left with $45,000. In 2019, the average primary care physician in the U.S. earned $237,000, according to the 2019 Medscape Physician Compensation Report.[26] If PCPs' average income were 10% lower than that under Medicare for All, they would garner a bonus nearly twice as big as their lost income of $23,700.

Effects on Specialists

Specialists would not fare as well. In 2019, consultants' average income was $341,000. Because doctors in various specialties earn very different amounts, it's impossible to estimate how much Medicare for All would lower any particular physician's income. We can safely assume, however, that the bonuses specialists would get from the primary care groups would not make up for it in most cases, if they received only a quarter of 50% of the total cost savings.

Nevertheless, specialists now make considerably more money than primary care doctors do. They'd still be earning more than PCPs at Medicare rates, and the bonuses they'd receive would help raise their income closer to what they used to earn. If a PCP group did so well that it generated larger bonuses for specialists, they might be able to recover or exceed their former level of income.

It might be objected that the shared savings going to the primary care groups would be gross income, not net income. But most of a group's overhead would be covered by primary care capitation and the payments to infrastructure vendors, which are already accounted for. The additional expense for ancillary staff such as care managers and social workers would be distributed across the physicians in the group; therefore, it wouldn't have too much of an effect on any single doctor's net income.

Setting Benchmarks

How well could a primary care group do in this scheme? That would depend partly on how the government set their benchmark and how often it was rebased. As discussed in Chapter 9, the benchmark would have to be risk-adjusted. It would probably follow the MSSP's hybrid model, mixing the group's historical cost experience with regional costs so as not to disadvantage the more efficient groups. Rebasing could be done at set intervals, as the MSSP does now at the end of contract terms. The MSSP's current five-year interval might work best.

With these parameters, a group starting out at average efficiency in a region with average costs might be able to achieve 5% savings within five years, adding 1% more each year. At that point, they'd enjoy a bonus of 5% of total costs in relation to their benchmark. Calculating this amount as we did earlier (again with 2019 numbers), the group would save $450 per patient. If a doctor had 2,000 patients, the annual savings would equal $900,000. The group would get half of that, or $450,000, and would have to pay $225,000 to its infrastructure vendor and specialists, leaving $225,000 for each doctor's share of savings. In this scenario, the PCPs would be earning nearly twice as much as they do today! The next year, however, they'd earn much less because of the rebasing and would have to save more to build larger bonuses.

When a group saved 5%, it would not be halfway to the goal of eliminating the 10% of costs deemed to be avoidable waste. That's because the first 5% of savings would be based on the group's initial benchmark, which in this example would have been set five years earlier. In the interim, the national health expenditure (NHE) per capita would continue rising, perhaps at the current rate of 3%–4% a year. So, each year after the first, the additional 1% that the group saved would be less than 1% of contemporaneous spending, which would be higher than total costs in the benchmark year. Unless the group's incremental savings rate were considerably more than 1% per year, it might never eliminate 10% of costs at the higher level of health spending.

Nevertheless, there must be a limit to how much the physician-led reform model could reduce waste before it cut into necessary care. At some point, a PCP group would approach maximum efficiency in providing high-quality care. As a result, its ability to generate savings would drop off. At that point, annual payments to the group might be set somewhere between their maximum past bonus and their current payout, with some adjustment for inflation. From there on out, they'd be competing with other highly efficient groups on quality rather than cost.

Savings to the System

According to the latest report from the CMS actuaries, the NHE was expected to grow at an average annual rate of 5.5% from 2018 to 2027. On a per capita basis, it was projected to increase 3.9% in 2019 and 4.9% in 2027. By comparison, gross domestic product (GDP) per capita was expected to grow 4% in 2019 and 3.7% in 2027. If these projections are correct, NHE per capita will increase faster than GDP per capita in 2027.[27]

If the physician-led reform model could cut total health costs per capita by 2% in 2027, and the single-payer system kept half of those savings, the difference between GDP growth and health spending growth in that year would largely disappear. If the model could somehow reduce costs by 4% per capita, yielding a 2% net savings to the government, the percentage of GDP going to healthcare would actually decline.

To achieve that long-sought goal, however, the government must do something about soaring drug prices, which are not under physicians' control. In addition, our country must finally reach an agreement about how to approach the coverage of new medical technologies before they break the bank. The final chapter of this book addresses these important issues.

CHAPTER 12

Drugs and The Technology Challenge

Alec Smith of Minneapolis was just 26 when he died of diabetic ketoacidosis. His entirely preventable death was attributed to a lack of insulin, which he could no longer afford after he aged out of his parents' health insurance. The monthly cost of the insulin he needed to survive was $1,300. That was more than he could pay on his $35,000 annual salary as a restaurant manager. He earned too much to be on Medicaid, and a health plan on the state health insurance exchange would have cost him $450 a month. The plan's $7,600 deductible meant he still couldn't have paid for his insulin. So, he rationed what insulin he had left and he died.

In a heartbreaking statement to the press, Alec's mother, Nicole Smith-Holt, blamed the drug companies. "The price of insulin has gone up over 1,200 percent in 20 years," she said. "It's not affordable. You're price-gouging people who need this one product to live, to survive."[1]

U.S. insulin prices nearly doubled from just 2012 to 2016. Eli Lilly, for example, raised its insulin prices by 20.8% in 2014, 16.9% in 2015, and 7.6% in 2016. In 2007, Lilly's Humalog cost $74 a vial. In 2017, the same vial cost $269, although the drug's patent had expired. Mike Magee, MD, who used to work at Lilly, estimates that Americans with diabetes spend about $572 a month to treat their condition, most of it for insulin.[2]

The protests of people with diabetes who cannot afford their medications have had some effect. A class action lawsuit was filed in 2017 against Eli Lilly, Sanofi, and Novo Nordisk, alleging that they colluded to artificially inflate U.S. prices of their insulin products.[3] A similar civil action was filed against the three drug makers—which together account for 90% of insulin sales—and the three top pharmacy benefit managers in 2017.[4] Both actions are still in early stages.

Meanwhile, a bevy of bills to reduce prescription drug prices have been introduced in Congress.[5] One of these measures, described below, passed the House at the end of 2019;[6] however, at the time of this writing, none of the drug price bills had a strong chance of being adopted into law. One reason is that many lawmakers are protective of the pharmaceutical industry, which fiercely opposes any legislation that smacks of price controls.

U.S. drug prices are three to four times as high as those in other major countries.[7] The main reason is that, unlike other nations' governments, ours does not negotiate drug prices with pharmaceutical companies or set prices based on international norms. Because Medicare and private insurers cover most new FDA-approved drugs without consideration of cost or comparative effectiveness, drug makers can set their prices at whatever level the market will bear.[8] In many other countries, the value of new drugs is considered in coverage decisions or in the prices that drug companies are allowed to charge.[9-10]

Creating Demand

Even if Congress could somehow get its act together to lower drug prices, drug spending would keep rising because of new, patented medications, many of which are no more effective than similar products already on the market. Since insurers will cover these "me-too" drugs, pharmaceutical firms have a strong incentive to develop them. They can also promote these medications through direct-to-consumer TV ads that aren't allowed in any other country except New Zealand.[11]

With the help of this kind of marketing, drug makers can create demand for new medications used to treat conditions that weren't considered major health problems in the past. Take Peyronie's disease, for example. If you never heard about this condition before you saw the TV ads with curved penises, you're not alone. This rare disease was not on the radar screen of most people before Endo Pharmaceuticals started running ads for its Xiaflex therapy. In the fourth quarter of fiscal 2018, Endo's sales of Xiaflex popped 30% to $80 million.[12]

Other medications are marketed to people with more familiar but non-life-threatening conditions such as insomnia, dry eye disease, plaque psoriasis, and attention deficit hyperactivity disorder. Any condition that is long-lasting and will require people to take pills for years or for life is a natural target for profit-making drug companies. They're much less interested in producing acute-care drugs, such as antibiotics, that are taken for brief periods.

The development and promotion of all these new medications, not surprisingly, has greatly expanded the market for prescription drugs. According to one study, 59% of U.S. adults used prescription drugs in 2011–2012, a significant increase from the 51% who used them in 1999–2000. The prevalence of polypharmacy—multiple prescriptions to the same individual—also increased, to 15% in 2011–2012 from 8% 12 years earlier.[13]

Therefore, it's not just the prices, but also the increased volume of prescription drugs that contributes to the rise in health costs. While the percentage of U.S. health spending represented by prescription drugs hasn't grown—it has hovered around 9%–10% of national health expenditures for several years[14]—pharmaceuticals have kept pace with the increasing costs in other healthcare sectors.

The growth in the number of new drugs is part of the overall expansion of medical technology that has helped to drive up health costs. While this is happening around the world, the role of technology is accentuated in U.S. cost growth. In a 2017 *Health Affairs Blog* post, Gregg Bloche, Neel Sukhatme, and John L. Marshall said:

> Many factors influence health spending, including coverage expansion, the balance of bargaining power between payers and providers, and the aging of the United States' population. But the persistent driving force behind rising medical spending is technological advance, fueled by health insurance's promise of rich reward and unchecked by insistence that advances deliver clinical benefit worth their cost.[15]

Later in this chapter, I'll delve further into the impact of medical technology on costs and how it could undermine the cost-reduction effects of the physician-led reform model. But first let's turn our attention to the impact of high drug prices and what can be done to lower them without harming innovation.

WHY ARE DRUG PRICES SO HIGH?

U.S. drug prices are continuing to grow at a rapid rate. From Jan. 1, 2012 to Dec. 31, 2017, a recent study found, 49 top-selling, brand-name drugs had a median cost increase of 76%. (Cost was defined as the combination of insurer payments and consumer out-of-pocket costs.) Of the 36 medications available during the entire five-year period, 28 had a median price increase of over 50% and 16 more than doubled in price.[16]

Some drug price increases cannot be attributed to any improvement in the effectiveness of medications, according to the Institute for Clinical and Economic Review (ICER), a private, nonprofit organization that assesses the value of new drugs. In 2018, ICER found seven top-selling drugs had net price increases (after rebates and discounts) of 10% or more without any new evidence of improvement in health benefits. These medications included Humira (15.8% increase), Lyrica (22.2%), Truvada (23.1%), Rituxan (13.8%), Neulasta (13.4%), Cialis (32.5%), and Tecfidera (9.8%). The additional sales due to these net price changes ranged from $313 million for Tecfidera to $1.857 billion for Humira. Altogether, these seven medications alone pushed up drug costs by $5.1 billion from 2017 to 2018.[17]

These findings suggest that many brand-name drugs are overpriced in the United States relative to their clinical benefit to patients. Drug makers have no reason not to price their products aggressively, since neither the government nor private payers negotiate with them on price. What the payers do instead is contract with pharmacy benefit managers (PBMs). These middlemen, which include very large firms, negotiate with the drug makers on behalf of insurance companies and Medicare Part D drug plans.

PBMs Rake It in from All Sides

To simplify a very complex subject, the PBMs bargain with the pharmaceutical firms mainly on the prices of expensive brand-name medications that have competitors in a particular therapeutic area. In return for getting rebates that average about 20%, the PBMs ensure that a drug is covered by the health plan and gets placed in a preferred tier. (Health plans usually have two to four tiers of drug pricing, each with different patient copays.) Rather than passing on all of the rebates to the insurers, PBMs keep some of the money as part of their business model.[18]

How much they retain is a matter of debate. A recent GAO study found that most Part D drug plan agreements with PBMs require them to pass on all of the rebates they receive from drug makers. Under these contracts, the PBMs also earn little money from "spread pricing," in which they keep the difference between the amount they pay the pharmacy for a drug on behalf of an insurer and the amount the PBM charges the plan, the GAO said.[19]

However, the report added, PBMs earn more money from spread pricing and rebate retention in their transactions with commercial plans. One study found that the percentage of rebates that PBMs passed on to insurers and employers rose from 78% in 2012 to 91% in 2016. But many smaller health plans and self-insured employers said they hadn't seen that increase.[20]

During the same time period, it was reported elsewhere, total rebates to PBMs increased from $39.7 billion to $89.5 billion.[21] These growing rebates, drug makers complained, had forced them to raise list prices substantially. If so, this shows that the PBMs haven't had much impact on the overall increase in drug costs—the pharma firms have just raised their prices to absorb the rebates. The PBMs and their clients also haven't made drugs cheaper for consumers. Even if PBMs have increased the portion of rebates they pass on to insurers, there's no evidence that patients have received any relief in the form of lower copays or lower premiums.

The Commonwealth Fund points to another drawback of PBMs: They have an incentive to favor high-priced drugs over lower-priced ones. Because their rebates are often calculated as a percentage of a medication's list price, they get a larger rebate for more expensive drugs. To the extent that they keep part of those rebates, they make more money.[22]

GENERIC DRUGS

Under the Hatch-Waxman Act of 1984, generic drug manufacturers can get FDA approval for their products without having to prove they are "biologically equivalent" to the brand-name drugs they're based on. (Biosimilar drugs, however, need to be tested for equivalence to approved biological medicines under a 2009 statute.) When the Hatch-Waxman law was passed, fewer than 15% of prescriptions were for generic drugs.[23] By 2016, the percentage had mushroomed to 82%. Nevertheless, brand-name drugs still generated 78% of sales volume.[24]

This can be partly explained by the fact that generic drugs cost 30%–80% less than the related brand-name medications.[25] Moreover, drug makers can maintain those high prices for brand-name products even in the face of generic competition. One study about drug price increases showed that costs grew at about the same rate for the 17 products with generic equivalents and the 32 drugs still under patent. "This finding suggests that prices of brand-name drugs are not largely affected by the presence of generic drugs," the authors said.[26]

Much of the continuing success of brand-name drugs—whether or not they have generic competition—can also be attributed to the pharmaceutical companies' marketing to physicians and their direct-to-consumer TV ads. Currently, the drug makers spend nearly $5.5 billion a year on TV advertising.[27] It has also been calculated that drug firms spend an average of more than $20,000 per physician annually on marketing efforts that include detailing, gifts, samples, meals, travel, and consultancy fees.[28]

Even though drug makers can maintain their prices after a generic enters the market, the non-branded drug still reduces the demand for the brand-name product. So pharmaceutical companies do everything they can to forestall the emergence of generic competitors. Some firms extend their 20-year patent on a medicine by making minor changes in the drug's chemical structure, mode of action, or administration. In other cases, the manufacturers pay off generic producers to delay the market introduction of their products.[29]

Some pharmaceutical companies bring out their own generic medications. The most famous example of this is Nexium, "the purple pill," which Astra Zeneca introduced in 2001, just as its patent on the equivalent brand-name drug Prilosec was about to expire. Thanks to a big TV advertising campaign, Nexium racked up blockbuster sales.[30]

In May 2019, Eli Lilly introduced Lispro, the generic equivalent of its Humalog insulin product, at a price of $137 per vial or $265 for five KwikPens—about half of what Humalog costs. However, several months after Lispro became available, GoodRx data showed that only 8% of prescription fills for the drug at pharmacies were for Lispro; the rest were for Humalog. This raised the question of whether Lilly was really promoting Lispro or had just released it to head off Congressional moves to cut insulin prices.[31]

Generic Prices Rise

Meanwhile, generic drug companies have been busy raising their own prices. The best-known example is Turing Pharmaceuticals, helmed by the now-imprisoned "pharma bro" Martin Shkreli, which bought the rights to an old generic antiparasitic drug and immediately jacked up its price from $18 to $750. Other generic firms have raised the prices of older medications significantly, the *New York Times* reported.[32]

The prices of many other generic drugs have increased less dramatically over time. In fact, a GAO study found that the average price of 1,400 generic drugs that were available from 2010 to 2015 fell slightly during that period. But more than 300 of these medications had at least one price increase of 100% or more, the GAO said.[33]

In another study that analyzed data for over 6,000 generic products, the researchers found that in 2014, about half of the drugs had price increases in excess of the growth in the medical consumer price index. Twenty-eight percent of the drugs had price rises of greater than 15%, and 23% had price growth of more than 20%.[34]

In theory, the growing abundance of generics on the market should have reduced overall drug costs over time. However, that hasn't happened because of the growth in generic prices and because high prices for brand-name drugs have persisted despite generic competition. So, we can't look to generic medications to solve the problem of high drug costs.

LEGISLATIVE GRIDLOCK

A few bills to lower drug prices were pending in Congress in early 2020. Nevertheless, none of these measures was likely to become law. Like legislation on nearly every other issue, progress on these bills has been blocked by the rancorous split between Republicans and Democrats. In addition, opposition from pharmaceutical companies makes it difficult to wrangle enough votes for any bill that would harm this powerful special interest.

Late in 2019, for example, the Democratic-majority House passed legislation that would lower drug costs partly by allowing the government to negotiate prices directly with pharmaceutical companies. Because of that provision alone, it was predicted that the bill would go nowhere in the Republican-controlled Senate.[35]

The House Democrats' bill, H.R. 3, includes two other elements. First, it would limit the out-of-pocket drug costs of Medicare beneficiaries to $2,000 annually. Second, the bill aims to decrease prices for drugs sold to Medicare patients immediately and retroactively. All manufacturers that, since 2016, have raised the prices of their products more rapidly than the inflation rate would either have to lower the price of the drug or pay the above-inflation amount to the Treasury as a rebate.

H.R. 3 also would give the Secretary of Health and Human Services the authority to negotiate a portion of drug prices for both Medicare and the private market. The HHS secretary could bargain on prices for between 50 and 250 branded drugs with very high costs. An international reference price index derived from a drug's average price in six other countries would be used as a target price ceiling.

The Congressional Budget Office (CBO) estimated that allowing HHS to negotiate drug prices would lower government healthcare spending by $456 billion over a decade and that the inflationary rebates would save another $36 billion.[36]

Meanwhile, a bipartisan drug price bill passed the Senate Finance Committee in July 2019. The most important feature of that legislation would require drug makers to limit price increases to Medicare Part D plans or pay rebates to the government, starting in 2022. Seniors' out-of-pocket costs would be capped at $3,100 per year. According to the CBO, the rebates in the Senate plan would save Medicare beneficiaries $21 billion and the government $34.6 billion over a decade.[37]

Drug companies oppose even that legislation, claiming that it would limit funds for research and would force up prices to commercial insurers. Predictably, Senate Majority Leader Mitch McConnell (R-KY) has refused to bring the bill to the floor for a vote.[38]

BIG PHARMA'S POSITION

Every time the issue of government price negotiations has been raised, the pharmaceutical companies have argued that they need high prices to cover their R&D costs and that if prices were lowered, there would be fewer life-saving cures.

A 2016 study by a drug industry-funded institute found it costs $2.5 billion–$3 billion to develop and bring a new drug to market.[39] But that's the price tag for a new molecular therapy created from scratch. In 2018, only 32% of FDA approvals were for novel, first-in-class therapies.[40] A GAO study found that from 2008 to 2014, new molecular therapies that served previously unmet medical needs or advanced patient care accounted for an average of 13% of FDA approvals.[41]

In a 2004 book, Marcia Angell, MD, a former editor of the *New England Journal of Medicine*, cited two other reasons pharmaceutical industry estimates of R&D costs are flawed. Only a small fraction of novel drugs are developed by the drug companies themselves, she noted; the rest mostly are licensed or acquired from university or government laboratories or biotechnology companies. In addition, she pointed out, nearly half of the average cost to create a new drug—which was then said to be $802 million—represented the "opportunity" cost of drug development. In other words, this was how much the drug company could have made if it had invested the R&D funds elsewhere.[42]

Growing Drug Profits

Whatever the costs of developing new drugs, it's incontestable that drug makers' U.S. sales have soared. From 2006 to 2015, the GAO report found, pharmaceutical and biotech sales in the U.S. increased from $534 billion to $775 billion in 2015 dollars.

Two-thirds of drug companies saw increases in their average profit margins from 2006 to 2015, the GAO noted. Among the 25 largest pharmaceutical firms, the average profit margin was 15%–20%, far above the 4%–9% range for the leading companies in other industries.

Pharmaceutical R&D spending worldwide rose modestly from $82 billion in 2008 to $89 billion in 2014. In contrast, drug companies' marketing outlays in the United States alone ballooned from $17.7 billion in 1997 to almost $30 billion in 2016. While it's not clear how much global marketing costs have increased, it's very clear where the drug makers' priorities are.

One of those priorities is to maintain the status quo on U.S. drug prices. With just 4% of the world's population, our country represents 45% of the global pharmaceutical market. In 2016, the U.S. market share was valued at $446 billion.[43] And the sky-high drug prices in the United States fund the bulk of pharmaceutical research; therefore, any attempt to lower U.S. drug prices significantly would reduce research funds as well as drug makers' profits.

Under Medicare for All, the government theoretically would be able to negotiate drug prices or set them at a level close to what other countries pay. According to one study, if negotiated prices were 26% above the international reference price level, that would be sufficient to fund current R&D spending by U.S. drug companies.[44]

Nevertheless, the pharmaceutical companies would be certain to howl that placing any limit on their prices would strangle research. They'd have an appreciative audience among many politicians as well as physicians, researchers, and patient advocates. So, despite the power of a government-run single-payer system, regulators would encounter stiff political headwinds if they tried to cut drug prices to anywhere near international levels.

A better strategy for the government might be to combine international reference pricing with a value-based approach to drug pricing. This method would be more acceptable to the drug companies and more politically palatable than simply cutting prices across the board. Moreover, the United States also needs to take cost-effectiveness into account to cope with the explosion of new medical technologies. To understand how value-based pricing might work for both new and existing drugs, we must look at how countries around the world are trying to address the rising costs of new technologies.

TECHNOLOGY VS. PRICES

Medical technologies include drugs, devices, tests, and procedures. Considered as a whole, these technologies are the key driver of growth in health costs, according to Georgetown University professor Gregg Bloche and his associates.

Bloche, *et al.*, view insurance coverage as the chief enabler of these technological innovations. In their earlier-cited *Health Affairs Blog* post, they said, "Drug and device developers, clinical researchers, and their financial backers anticipate coverage for new tests and treatments with little concern for whether they add substantial therapeutic value, and they make research and development decisions accordingly."[45]

In an interview, Bloche further explained, "If you're a technology developer, you can reasonably anticipate that if your product achieves a low but significant health gain, insurers are going to be under pressure to pay for it."

Insurers *do* cover most new drugs, although they may make it difficult for patients to access the ones that they deem to be low-value, notes Peter Neumann, director of the Center for the Evaluation of Value and Risk in Health at the Institute for Clinical Research and Health Policy Studies at Tufts Medical Center in Boston.

"It's hard to find a payer who says we're not paying for that thing because it's not cost-effective," he says. "Instead, they put restrictions on products based on the strength of the evidence, probably influenced by the cost-effectiveness and certainly by the clinical effectiveness. You can get that expensive new drug for multiple sclerosis or rheumatoid arthritis, but you have to fail all the cheap drugs first."

Despite these cost control efforts, the proliferation of new technologies is a bigger cost driver than all the waste and fraud in the system, says Amitabh Chandra, a professor of public policy and business administration at the Harvard Kennedy School. "The number one reason why insurance premiums increase is these medical technologies that have dubious or small medical effectiveness," he says.

Technology and Prices

Health policy experts assign different weights to the role of prices and technology in cost growth. In the famous article "It's the Prices, Stupid," by the late health economist Uwe Reinhardt and his colleagues,[46] and a 2019 follow-up piece by the surviving coauthors,[47] the health economists argued that high U.S. prices explain most of why our health costs are so much higher than those in other advanced countries.

The other major contributor to cost growth, they acknowledged, is "service intensity," which includes technology. However, they said, it's hard to define service intensity or separate it from price.

Bloche agreed that other countries have lower health costs than the U.S. does principally because their national health systems can negotiate lower prices with providers. But, even if the U.S. had a single-payer system, he noted, it would only be able to get a one-time cost-reduction by bargaining with providers. After that, he said, cost growth would resume at about the same rate as in other advanced countries because of new technology.

However, it's difficult to distinguish the impact of technological advances from price growth. As the availability of technology increases, so do the prices charged for care. In 2015, for example, the United States had 39 MRI units per one million people, compared to the Organisation for Economic Co-operation and Development (OECD) median of 12.6. Similarly, the United States had 41 CT scanners per million in 2015, compared to the OECD median of 17.8.[48] American providers use those machines routinely, ordering expensive imaging tests far more often than do their peers in other OECD countries.[49] And as it happens, our overall health costs are much higher than in those other nations.

New procedures also increase costs, partly because they don't always replace older procedures. After angioplasties and stents came along, for example, millions of people had those procedures, but there was no decrease in the number of coronary artery bypass graft procedures.[50] Other minimally invasive procedures have replaced open surgeries, but have resulted in more people getting the laparoscopic operations.[51]

Changing practice patterns have also increased spending on some drugs. For example, statin drugs have benefited many people at risk for heart disease, but over time, changes in clinical guidelines have expanded the eligibility of patients for these cholesterol-lowering drugs. A recent analysis suggested that statin use in low-risk patients has little value and wastes healthcare resources.[52]

It has also been suggested—usually by drug companies—that some new technologies save money because they prevent hospitalization or detect disease at an early stage, when it can be treated more cheaply. This is frequently true in individual cases. But when experts analyze the impact of technology on population health costs over time, they find that it increases costs more often than it saves money.

"New technologies tend to increase overall costs," says Neumann. For example, he notes, genomic tests are being developed to determine which medications a particular patient will respond to best. Such tests might reduce the amount of wasteful drug spending, but any savings that accrued from the use of this technology, Neumann says, would be overwhelmed by the number of people having their genomes sequenced and getting those tests.

COST-EFFECTIVENESS ANALYSIS

The ability of a country to afford new technology is directly proportional to the increase in its wealth. But as every nation except the United States has learned, there are limits to what people can afford to spend on healthcare. Hence there is an increasing recognition—mostly abroad, but also in certain quarters here—of the importance of cost-effectiveness analysis (CEA).

CEA is one branch of health technology assessment (HTA), which also includes comparative effectiveness research (CER). CEA depends on CER, but health technology assessment doesn't always include CEA. For example, the Patient-Centered Outcomes Research Institute (PCORI), which was established by the Affordable Care Act, compares the effectiveness of tests and treatments but is prohibited from doing CEA. Nevertheless, as we'll see, PCORI does sometimes determine that a particular technology is low-value.

At the other end of the HTA spectrum is the U.K.'s National Institute for Health and Care Excellence (NICE). NICE is a governmental organization that tells the National Health Service (NHS) which new drugs and other technologies to cover. Its recommendations, based on a combination of CEA and CER, are legally binding.

Many countries with national insurance have adopted CEA because it helps them select the new technologies that will provide the greatest health benefit within a budget. CEA is rarely applied to coverage decisions in the U.S., however. During the runup to Obamacare, the debate over whether to consider CEA in coverage decisions "raised the specter of rationing and government interference in patient care," noted Alan Garber and Harold Sox in a 2010 article.[53] This explains the limitation on PCORI's activities. Moreover, any consideration of cost is forbidden in Medicare coverage determinations. Medicare's "coverage with evidence development" process seeks to get around that prohibition by limiting coverage until additional evidence of effectiveness is provided for expensive new interventions.

Recently, a private, not-for-profit organization that uses CEA to evaluate drug pricing has begun to gain traction among U.S. payers and pharmaceutical companies. The Institute for Clinical and Economic Review (ICER), whose report on unjustified price increases was mentioned earlier, has built credibility in recent years with a series of health technology assessments funded mainly by private foundations. ICER will be discussed at length later.

The Basics of CEA

According to Garber and Sox, cost-effectiveness analysis "is a method designed to assess the comparative impacts of expenditures on different health interventions.... It is based on the premise that for any given level of resources available, society ... wishes to maximize the total aggregate health benefits conferred.... Cost-effectiveness compares the health effects that result from alternative uses of a given amount of health resources."[54]

NICE goes further than that by estimating the "opportunity costs" created by the adoption of a new technology. These opportunity costs result when the technology absorbs resources that might otherwise be devoted to other healthcare services or even to the non-healthcare needs of a country, such as education or defense. Because the United Kingdom has a fixed healthcare budget, NICE has repeatedly stated that it considers an appropriate threshold for product approval to be the "opportunity cost of programs displaced by new, more costly technologies."[55]

The United States, which doesn't have an overall budget for healthcare, has never looked at technological advances in this way. Nevertheless, some ICER reports refer to a "budget impact threshold" above which a drug or product would likely contribute significantly to excessive growth in health costs.[56]

The cost-effectiveness thresholds used in CEA are customarily expressed in "quality-adjusted life years" (QALYs). A QALY combines the additional years of life that can be gained through the use of the technology with the expected quality of those years. The QALY scale is based on such health states as "completely healthy," "blind," "immobilized," and "dead." There are multiple health states for each condition, adding up to thousands of these categories.

Large numbers of patients have filled out surveys in which they rated different health states on a scale from 0 (death) to 1 (full health). In CEA studies, the numerical results of these quality-of-life ratings are applied to the number of years that patients can expect to live as the result of a particular treatment. If the quality-of-life value for an operation that leaves a patient incontinent is 0.5, for instance, and that person's added life expectancy is 12 years, the treatment would provide 6 QALYs. QALYs apply equally to everyone in a population, whether they're young or old, male or female, rich or poor.[57]

Joe Selby, MD, the former director of PCORI, views the quality-of-life aspect as the Achilles' heel of CEA. (Selby says he is speaking for himself, not PCORI.) A healthy person and a sick person, for example, might have different evaluations of what their quality of life would be if they were on dialysis, he points out.

Neumann, in contrast, says it's wrong to look at CEA from the perspective of individual patients who have a disease. "We should think about what the insurance would cover before we know we have the disease. Through insurance, you're buying a package of benefits that would be covered in case you have the illness. So how much would you be willing to pay to add some new technology to that package on the very small chance you'll need it? It's a hard calculation to do. But that's how we should think about it."

Defining CE Thresholds

The span of cost-effectiveness thresholds in various countries is huge, ranging from about $25,000 to $200,000 per QALY gained. Moreover, HTA bodies build flexibility into their thresholds. Even NICE, which has not increased its threshold range of 20,000–30,000 British pounds ($25,800–$38,700) since 2001, has made exceptions in recent years for treatments of "very rare diseases" and the later stages of terminal disease.[58]

ICER uses a threshold range of $100,000–$150,000 per QALY gained—a gamut that some experts consider fairly reasonable for the United States. The lower end of this range comes mainly from what the World Health Organization has calculated that our country can afford to pay, based on its GDP per capita, says David Whitrap, vice president of communications and outreach for ICER.

Cost-effectiveness thresholds also can be based on the amount that patients would be willing to pay for an additional year of life, he notes. Many surveyed patients say that they'd give about two years of their income to live an extra year.

NICE uses a third CEA approach tied to opportunity costs, as mentioned earlier. Its experts compare "the incremental cost-effectiveness of a new technology with the cost-effectiveness threshold. This indicates whether or not the health expected to be gained from its use exceeds the health expected to be lost elsewhere as other health-care activities are displaced."[59]

There is no evidentiary basis for the cost-effectiveness threshold used by NICE, the authors noted.[60] The same is true for HTA bodies in other nations. One systematic review published in 2018 found that 17 countries had formal cost-effectiveness thresholds, of which 13 were based on willingness to pay. Most of the thresholds fell within the WHO range of one to three times GDP per capita. But the authors concluded, "Presently, there is no commonly agreed-upon value or method for determining C/E thresholds."[61]

Nevertheless, Chandra says, CEA is important for two reasons: First, in the absence of CEA, we end up paying for a raft of new technologies that cost more in insurance premiums and taxes than their incremental benefit to patients. Second, he says, not subjecting new products to CEA sends a signal to manufacturers that they should create more of these "dubious new technologies," because we'll pay for them. "So, the lack of cost-effectiveness analysis creates strong incentives to bring less cost-effective drugs and devices to markets."

INTERNATIONAL EXPERIENCE

The U.K. single-payer system entails more rigorous government control than any other healthcare system in the world. So, it's not surprising that NICE also takes a more rigorous approach to CEA than other countries do. While NICE recommends that the NHS cover most things that it deems to be clinically effective, it draws the line at some expensive, low-value technologies.

This approach sometimes leads to clashes with public opinion. One recent example involved NICE's rejection of coverage for five drugs because their cost far exceeded its C/E threshold. According to one report, "this decision resulted in patients suffering from chronic lymphocytic leukaemia and mantle cell lymphoma not having access to medication that could improve their quality of life."[62]

In another case, NICE declined to approve Pfizer's crizotinib for advanced lung cancer. While this drug targeted only a small subset of lung cancer patients with a specific genetic mutation, Pfizer priced at it at 7,800 pounds ($10,000) per month, which translated to 195,000 pounds ($250,000) per QALY. After the company offered to reduce the price, the drug still would have cost over 100,000 pounds ($129,000) per QALY, and NICE decided it was not cost-effective.[63]

Chandra takes a dim view of NICE's low C/E threshold range. "British taxpayers routinely forgo medical treatments that are cost-effective but are deemed cost ineffective by NICE," he says. "Folks in the U.K. might love that and say, 'look how little we spend on healthcare.' But if you were to ask a sick child or the parents of a child who has cystic fibrosis in the U.K., 'where would you rather live, in America or the U.K.,' the answer would be America. So the U.K. has erred too much on one side of the tradeoff. I don't think what they've done is responsible. It's an irresponsible country in the way they treat the sick."

As noted earlier, however, NICE has become more flexible during the past decade. In 2009, the agency began assigning greater weight to QALYs achieved in terminal diseases. In practice, it now uses a threshold of 50,000 pounds ($64,500) per QALY for these end-of-life technologies.

Since 2016, NICE experts have been able to recommend that cancer drugs be funded even if they have high incremental cost-effectiveness ratios. And in 2017, NICE adopted a threshold of 100,000-300,000 pounds ($129,000–$387,000) for treatments of "very rare diseases."[64]

Canadian Approach

Canada has national health insurance, but it doesn't cover outpatient drugs. Hence, Canadians have to pay for medications out of pocket or buy private drug insurance. The government sets drug prices using an international reference price system; however, while costs are far below those of the United States, Canada has the second-highest drug prices in the world.[65]

In response to public protests, the Trudeau government in 2019 announced new policies to reduce drug prices and allow the government to consider cost-effectiveness in coverage decisions.[66]

The Canadian Agency for Drugs and Technologies in Health (CADTH), an independent, not-for-profit organization created by the government, already does this on an advisory basis.[67] CADTH performs health technology assessments, including CER and CEA. It uses a cost-effectiveness threshold of just under $100,000 per QALY gained for new drugs.[68] When a new medication exceeds that threshold, CADTH sometimes recommends it only for particular types of patients or in particular situations.

For example, the agency has recommended that lanadelumab be reimbursed for routine prevention of attacks of hereditary angioedema (HAE) only if the patient is at least 12 years old, the diagnosis is made by a specialist in the condition, and the patient has experienced at least three HAE attacks within any four-week period before initiating lanadelumab therapy. It also has recommended that the drug's price, currently $534,000 a year, be reduced by at least 59%. At the lower price, CADTH concluded, the incremental cost-effectiveness ratio of lanadelumab would be $50,000 per QALY compared with Cinryze, another therapy for HAE.[69]

The German Solution

Germany doesn't use an explicit C/E threshold to determine the value of new drugs. Instead, the government allows a new drug approved by the European Medicines Agency (EMA) to go on the market at whatever list price its manufacturer sets for the first year. During that year, the country's Institute for Quality and Efficiency in Health Care (IQWiG) evaluates the drug's comparative effectiveness based on clinical evidence, including the studies that the manufacturer submitted to the EMA. The IQWiG sends its report to a government committee, which, after public hearings, decides whether the medication offers major, moderate, minor, or no incremental benefit compared to existing treatments.[70]

If a drug offers more benefit than its comparators do, the German "sickness funds" association negotiates a price with the drug company based on comparative effectiveness and other factors. If the medicine offers no added benefit, the insurers will pay no more for it than they pay for the alternatives in its therapeutic class. If the sickness funds and the drug maker can't reach an agreement, an arbitration panel sets the price or the company withdraws the drug.

Prior to 2011, when this system was established, drug prices in Germany were 26% higher than the average across Europe. Now they're substantially lower, according to a McKinsey & Co. report.[71] Moreover, it doesn't appear that innovation has been harmed. From 2011 to 2017, the German system conducted assessments of pricing for 186 drugs. Of these, only 35 went to arbitration and just 30 were withdrawn from the market.[72]

ICER'S IMPACT IN THE UNITED STATES

Founded in 2005 by David Pearson, MD, the Institute for Clinical and Economic Review (ICER) is an "independent and nonpartisan research organization that objectively evaluates the clinical and economic value of prescription drugs, medical tests, and other health care and health care delivery innovations," according to its website. Best-known as an independent watchdog on drug pricing, ICER assesses the efficacy and cost-effectiveness of new drugs and some other new technologies. Its reports establish "value-based benchmarks" that indicate how drugs should be priced in relation to their value in improving outcomes. All of ICER's funding, the organization says, comes from nonprofit foundations and other "conflict-free" sources.[73]

To a greater extent than health technology assessment (HTA) bodies in other countries, ICER involves patients in its research from the start. When ICER begins reviewing a new drug—usually about eight months before the FDA is expected to approve it—the organization reaches out to patient communities, including patient advocacy groups, and starts getting their input on the burden of the disease and what outcomes matter most to them, Whitrap says. This dialog continues throughout the assessment process and public hearings that also involve experts and manufacturers.

As mentioned earlier, ICER uses a C/E threshold range of $100,000–$150,000 per QALY gained. If a new drug or other technology exceeds that range, ICER will recommend that its price be reduced. ICER evaluated 90 drugs from 2015 through December 2019, Whitrap says. Of those products, only 30 were priced below ICER's upper boundary of cost-effectiveness—that is, $150,000 per QALY gained.

For most of its comparative effectiveness research, ICER, like other HTA organizations, does meta-analyses of existing studies. ICER is forced to do this because drug companies rarely perform head-to-head trials that compare their new products with other medications in the same therapeutic class.

Cost-Effective, High-Cost Drugs

Because the QALY represents the degree to which a treatment extends and improves patients' lives, some breakthrough treatments for people with serious disabilities or illnesses can generate more QALYs than lower-priced drugs and can therefore justify a higher price. Among the very expensive drugs that ICER has found to be cost-effective are:

- CAR-T therapy for childhood leukemia at $475,000 per treatment.
- Emicizumab for hemophilia at $450,000 per year.
- Personalized lung cancer drugs at $90,000 per year.[74]

Another drug that turned out to be surprisingly cost-effective, Whitrap says, is Zolgensma, a gene therapy for spinal muscular atrophy. Novartis, Zolgensma's manufacturer, captured headlines when it priced the drug—which only has to be administered once—at $2.1 million. ICER considers Zolgensma to be cost-effective because it provides a potential cure for an always fatal childhood disease.

ICER set the drug's value-based price benchmark at $1.1 million–$1.9 million to fall below the threshold of $150,000 per QALY gained. ICER also assigned Zolgensma a price benchmark of $1.2 million–$2.1 million, based purely on the number of years it added.[75] Novartis then cut the price to $2.1 million from the $4 million–$5 million it had planned to ask, according to Whitrap.

New Drugs for Common Conditions

Despite its stratospheric price, Zolgensma is not likely to have a major impact on health costs because it treats a rare condition. Other lower-priced, cost-effective drugs could have a much bigger effect on overall costs because they could be taken by millions of people.

One example is oral semaglutide, which ICER says has long-term cost-effectiveness for people with type 2 diabetes. This condition affects approximately 28 million people in the United States. Because of the large number of people who might be eligible for the drug, ICER's report on the drug includes a budget impact threshold of $819 million over five years. At oral semaglutide's net price, the report notes, only 7% to 14%

of eligible U.S. patients could be treated before the drug's cost to the nation crossed this threshold.[76]

ICER raises this flag, Whitrap says, to alert healthcare decision makers that the short-term impact of an expensive drug for a big population could affect health costs significantly. Such an effect was felt in 2014 when two new drugs for hepatitis C caused drug costs to skyrocket and jolted national health spending upward.[77]

The same phenomenon is expected to occur on a much bigger scale when the first Alzheimer's disease drug is developed, notes Neumann. "Everybody will want it if it works. But we can't possibly provide Alzheimer's treatments to all eligible patients. We'll probably restrict it and negotiate the price of it and fight a lot about it."

ICER and Price Negotiations

Whitrap says that ICER's reports have begun to affect price negotiations between U.S. payers and drug companies, and outside observers agree. "Perhaps the greatest impact of these reports thus far has been to exert pressure on manufacturers when drug prices exceed ICER's threshold of value and societal affordability," wrote Laura Pizzi, a professor at Rutgers University, in a 2016 article.[78]

"Payers are really taking to heart ICER's analyses," Matt Sussman, head of modeling and evidence at Boston Health Economics, a healthcare analytics and consulting company, said in an interview. "They're considering the cost-effectiveness of the prices derived from those analyses."

According to Sussman, ICER reports are increasingly being discussed in price negotiations. A white paper from ICON, another consulting firm, supports his observation. In an ICON survey, more than three-quarters of payer executives—including those from pharmacy benefit managers, managed care organizations, and integrated delivery networks—said they were familiar with ICER. Fifty-five percent of respondents said they used the ICER findings in rebate/pricing discussions with drug makers. Sixty-four percent of the respondents said they used the reports as part of their research on the effectiveness of new medications.[79]

DEVICES AND PROCEDURES

New devices, tests, and procedures can also be evaluated for cost-effectiveness. However, as mentioned at the outset, cost-effectiveness can't be determined without first establishing how effective a technology is compared with the alternatives. This is a major obstacle to doing CEA for medical devices because of the shortage of data on their effectiveness. While both the FDA and the EMA require proof of a drug's safety and efficacy, a study points out, "the evidence hurdle for licensing of medical devices has traditionally been much lower than for pharmaceutical products."[80]

Government regulators usually require only small clinical trials of medical devices, and the FDA doesn't require collection of long-term efficacy data. Regulators also apply the concept of "substantial equivalence" to medical devices. In the United States, if a new device has the same or similar mechanism of action and intended use and is at least as safe or effective as an earlier model or a model from another manufacturer, it is considered to be substantially equivalent to the earlier model.[81]

A review of 96,000 U.S. clinical trials found that fewer than a third of procedure and device studies were randomized controlled trials (RCTs) and just 14% were blinded. Thus, most clinical evidence for devices is from observational studies and registries.[82]

There are good reasons RCTs are less-common for devices and procedures than for drugs. Some experts question the ethics of sham procedures and random allocation in medical device trials, and doctors and patients tend to agree with them.

Robotic surgery offers a perfect example, notes Selby, the former PCORI director. "Some people just believed robotic surgery was better, and some doctors had been trained in robotic surgery. So, they and their patients didn't want to be in a randomized trial, even if that was the best way to answer the question."

NICE deals with some new devices and procedures by ruling that there isn't enough evidence to recommend them. Where sufficient evidence exists for a particular device, NICE experts evaluate its cost-effectiveness. In some cases, the agency allows a new technology to be covered only in the context of research. Examples include the use of stent-graft placement in abdominal aortic aneurysm and percutaneous mitral valve annuloplasty.[83]

Coverage with Evidence Determination

That approach is nearly identical to Medicare's coverage with evidence determination (CED). Under this program, CMS conditionally covers a new technology while collecting additional evidence on the technology's effectiveness. The patients who receive the drug, device, or procedure must be in a clinical trial.[84] Current examples of these technologies include the artificial heart, cochlear implantation, transcatheter aortic valve replacement, and vagus nerve stimulation for treatment-resistant depression. About two dozen technologies currently are covered under CED, although others have been covered, as well, in the 15 years since CMS launched the program.[85]

In some cases, CMS's efforts to control the introduction of these technologies have failed. In February 2019, for example, CMS announced it would provide CED for CAR T-cell cancer therapies.[86] These personalized biologic drugs cost $373,000–$475,000, and the supportive care they require can double those prices.[87] According to Neumann, CMS tried to negotiate an agreement to cover the drugs only if short-term outcomes were positive, but the deal fell apart. In late 2019, CMS announced a national coverage determination for CAR-T therapies.[88]

PCORI AND EXISTING TECHNOLOGY

In contrast to most HTA bodies, the Patient-Centered Outcomes Research Institute (PCORI) evaluates existing, rather than new technologies. The agency funds comparative effectiveness research (CER) and studies on how to improve the effectiveness of healthcare delivery. For example, PCORI has underwritten studies comparing online vs. in-person care for managing skin conditions, the effect of shared decision-making on patients with congestive heart failure, and antibiotics for children. The latter study supported the use of narrow-spectrum rather than broad-spectrum antibiotics for most children with earaches or strep throat.[89]

A current PCORI trial seeks to determine the proper dosage of aspirin prescribed to patients for secondary prevention after a heart attack or a stroke. Two-thirds of doctors, Selby notes, prescribe an adult dose of aspirin and one-third of them advise taking baby aspirin. While the larger doses might be more protective, he says, people who take adult aspirin have more side effects, including GI bleeding.

A major strength of PCORI's approach is that, unlike other HTA entities, which depend mostly on existing studies, PCORI funds new trials designed to answer particular questions. These are "pragmatic" trials that test hypotheses in real-world settings rather than with carefully selected participants, as in drug trials.

About 70% of PCORI's pragmatic CER trials are randomized controlled trials, which provide more reliable data than do observational studies, Selby says. Going forward, however, PCORI may fund more observational studies, which provide faster results and are easier to do than RCTs.

"The challenge with an RCT is that it's based on people willing to be in the trial and be randomized," Selby notes. "That's usually a small fraction of the eligible people. So, an observational study gives you a broader view of everybody who's getting the treatment."

PCORI has also widened and accelerated its research by funding PCORnet, a nation-wide clinical trial network that analyzes EHR data on various interventions.[90] The big challenge here, Selby says, is that the data from different EHRs need to be standardized and cleaned up—tasks that eat up nearly half of PCORnet's budget.

How PCORI Studies Are Used

Many PCORI-funded studies have been published in peer-reviewed journals, and some of the results have been incorporated into clinical practice guidelines, Selby says. UptoDate, an online research source many physicians use in their daily work, has also built a couple of dozen PCORI-funded studies into its evidence base, he adds.

Some PCORI trials have identified low-value interventions. For example, a large randomized trial looked at people with type 2 diabetes who take oral medications but not insulin. It compared patients who self-monitored their glucose daily with fingerstick strips to patients who didn't do it and to those who did it with nurse coaching. After one year, it found there were no differences among the three groups in their blood sugar levels, hypoglycemia, hospital visits, need to start using insulin, or quality of life.

What this means, Selby says, is that the United States is spending about $2 billion a year on fingerstick strips that patients of this type don't need. In other words, the spending is wasted. New clinical guidelines include the evidence from this trial, and PCORI is now looking at how best to implement it with doctors and patients.

In some cases, this kind of research can eliminate the need to do cost-effectiveness analysis, Selby asserts. For example, CER alone can show that the lower-cost option (such as no fingerstick tests) is better than or at least as good as the higher-cost option.

"In that case, you don't need to do CEA, because you know the lower-cost option is more cost-effective," he says. "You do CER to show that the drug is better and has fewer side effects than the other drug, and you know what patients are paying for it. So if they're paying more for treatment A than treatment B, but B has better outcomes, you know which is the appropriate treatment to choose."

Selby objects to CEA in principle, not only because of the challenges in defining quality of life, but also because most of these analyses use questionable assumptions to model cost-effectiveness, in his view. But he supports programs like ICER to the extent that they can help payers negotiate lower prices with drug companies.

"I'd support having this country think about its healthcare budget and how much it had to spend, and being more proactive in negotiation. And if CEA was a more effective tool, that would be great. But you have to get the cost-effectiveness right, and it's very difficult to get it to a point where American patients will accept it as fair."

NEW DIRECTIONS

The introduction of new technologies must be controlled in some manner to constrain the growth in health spending. In addition, the comparative effectiveness of existing technologies must be studied to find out which ones really contribute to health and which ones don't.

The federal government will have to negotiate with pharmaceutical companies as part of any effective program to reduce drug prices. Some kind of international reference pricing could help the United States in that endeavor, as it has helped other countries. But instead of drug prices being whacked across the board, cost-effectiveness analysis should be applied, where appropriate, to determine how best to allocate healthcare resources.

This will become even more important under Medicare for All, which must have a budget to control costs. And it is critical to the physician-led reform model: Even if that model can reduce as much waste as predicted in this book, all those gains could eventually be swept away by new technologies if they're given free rein.

Chandra agrees. If a public option plan or a single-payer system covers everything, he predicts, "it's going to be an all-you-can-eat buffet for manufacturers of these dubious drugs."

Possible Solutions

A German-style system of assigning comparative values to new drugs, based on evidence, could possibly lower drug prices in the United States. If the goal were to reduce prices to a justifiable level without eliminating incentives for innovation, some drug companies might get behind it.

Unlike Germany, ICER uses cost-effectiveness analysis to determine fair prices for drugs. While this approach raises questions about methodology, it has a growing number of supporters in the U.S. Among them is Chandra, who thinks ICER is going in the right direction but still lacks sufficient evidence for many of its decisions. He especially likes the way that ICER involves patients and patient advocacy groups in its determinations.

"When the U.S. goes to CEA, the way to do it is to have multiple ICERs evaluating the cost-effectiveness of technologies," he says. "If any one of them got it wrong, over time the others would have an incentive to get it right. That's a uniquely American solution to the problem, rather than giving it to the government. Government won't have the patience to talk to patients [about what matters to them]."

Currently, ICER lacks the resources to undertake a project of this magnitude. Chandra envisions that, under his scheme, ICER-like entities might be funded by government grants, private payers, and drug and device manufacturers.

He stresses the need to foster competition among these entities. "It's a hard problem for a single organization to solve. So we don't want to rely too much on an organization that does it imperfectly. We want to have more comparisons and more information."

Public Attitudes

It's unclear whether the public will accept the results of studies showing that some life-saving treatments are not cost-effective. For example, there are many drugs on the market for colorectal cancer, but they deliver a minimal therapeutic benefit, Bloche and Sukhatme point out in a law review article. In most cases, these medications extend life for no more than three months, yet cost between $50,000 and $250,000. The most expensive drug provides just a month and a half of extra life. Yet, because of what has been called the "rule of rescue," hospitals and doctors cannot withhold beneficial care in such cases.

"Once a test or treatment becomes state of the art, ethical practice bars withholding it based on cost," the coauthors note.[91]

Therefore, they propose to rein in the development of new low-value technologies before they're approved and come into common use. They'd tie payment rates and the length of patent protection for future tests and treatments to emerging evidence of therapeutic value. In their view, this would channel R&D away from me-too and marginal advances and reward real innovations. It's a clever idea, but drug and device companies probably would depict this approach as an enemy of innovation.

Rationing by Price

Except in situations governed by the rule of rescue, the United States rations care by price. If you don't have money or insurance, you receive care only when you're so sick that hospitals can't turn you away. But if you're well-off and well-insured, you can receive as much care as your money will buy. There's no national healthcare budget, so providers and technology companies can take an increasingly large percentage of the national wealth.

Under Medicare for All, in contrast, everyone would have access to all necessary care, regardless of income, but we'd need a system to determine which care was necessary. And the public would have to accept that system, as people do in other countries.

The conundrum is how to balance the good of society against the welfare of the individual in healthcare. Today, mainly because of politics, national efforts to reach such a consensus have reached an impasse. "If progressives come up with a scheme that limits healthcare spending in the Medicare program or other public programs in an administrative fashion, Republicans are going to call that rationing," Bloche notes. "And if Republicans come up with schemes that limit healthcare spending by voucherizing the Medicare program, Democrats will call that rationing. And being accused of rationing healthcare is about the worst thing that can happen politically."

Ultimately, the fate of health technology assessment, like that of Medicare for All, depends on whether Americans develop the sense of social solidarity that we see in other advanced countries. Currently, the chances of that happening in the United States are slim. But perhaps when enough people have lost access to the healthcare they need to survive or live decent lives, the public will see the light and support the changes needed to make first-class, comprehensive healthcare available to all.

Final Thoughts

Controlling health costs isn't easy. If it were, millions of Americans wouldn't be struggling to pay their healthcare bills. It isn't easy for other countries, either; that's why their health costs are rising along with ours, although from lower levels. They have the same challenges with technology that we do, but their systems are better positioned to control costs because they operate within a budget.

If we want to do the same, we'll have to move to national health insurance, as other advanced nations have done. Our system won't look like that of any other country, because we have our own unique culture and way of doing things; however, because our multi-payer system has failed so miserably, it's likely we'll move to a single-payer system at some point.

During the transition period, which could last 10 years or more, we'd have to restructure the healthcare delivery system. Applying Medicare for All to the current system would guarantee that costs would continue to rise faster than our ability to pay, partly because the need to budget resources runs counter to the incentive of fee for service to do more. Physicians can be incentivized to greatly reduce the waste in the system if they can share in the savings to a sufficient degree. And, because physicians order most care, they can bring hospitals and post-acute-providers along with them.

While all of this is going on, the government must also take steps to address the costs of new technologies and cut the cost of current ones to a level that society can afford. This is going to be a tall order, but as Chapter 12 shows, similar efforts are already well underway in various countries. Even in the U.S., we're seeing the birth of cost-consciousness in health technologies.

There are no guarantees that any of this will work. Nevertheless, the reform proposal described in this book stands a better chance of success than trying to graft Medicare for All onto a dysfunctional delivery system while giving carte blanche to drug and device companies.

All the entrenched interests in the industry oppose Medicare for All, which threatens each of them in different ways. How much more they'd dislike physician-led healthcare reform is open to debate. In either scenario, insurance companies would be phased out, and hospitals would lose income and market power. Drug and device companies would have to adjust to lower prices. Many physicians are open to Medicare for All, and primary care doctors would do well under the model described in this book. But the majority of doctors would probably resist having to change their practice arrangements and, more important, how they practice.

If the public supported the transition to a new healthcare system, the healthcare industry might eventually accept Medicare for All. However, a large chunk of the population depends on healthcare or health insurance for their livelihoods. The question is how many of those people might be laid off as a result of healthcare reform, and how they would react politically.

Healthcare Drives the Economy

In the fourth quarter of 2018, healthcare surpassed manufacturing and retail to become the largest source of jobs in the United States. While millions of people were getting laid off during the Great Recession, healthcare added jobs every month—even before Obamacare took hold.[1] From the start of the recession in 2008 through the end of 2014, the sector gained 2.5 million positions.[2] In 2015, as the uninsured rate dropped, healthcare added nearly 475,000 jobs.[3] And the growth continued unabated until the start of the COVID-19 pandemic. In September 2019 alone, 38,800 new healthcare jobs were created, representing nearly 30% of overall U.S. hiring.[4] Even in the midst of the pandemic, the industry added an estimated 312,400 jobs in May 2020, after losing 1.4 million jobs in April, according to the Bureau of Labor Statistics (BLS).[5]

As of May 2019, 12% of Americans worked in healthcare. This included ambulatory healthcare services, hospitals, and nursing and residential care facilities.[6] However, it didn't encompass health insurance companies, which employed more than 500,000 people in 2018.[7] In addition, the U.S. pharmaceutical industry had 854,000 employees in 2014, not counting drug distribution workers and retail pharmacists.[8]

While these statistics show how important healthcare is to the national economy, they don't fully capture the role healthcare plays in local economies. In many cities and regions, healthcare is the largest employer. In some rural areas, local hospitals are the only employers paying decent wages. When rural hospitals go under—as many have in recent years—it's financially devastating to the surrounding areas.

Big Job Losses

So, what would be the impact of Medicare for All—even without a restructuring of the system—on national employment?

In 2016, when Bernie Sanders unveiled his first Medicare for All plan, UMass Amherst economist Gerald Friedman estimated that it would result in the loss of about 2 million jobs for people who worked in insurance and medical billing.[9] According to a recent study by the PERI Institute, 1.06 million jobs would be lost in healthcare administration alone.[10] But it's unclear how many additional positions healthcare providers would shed as a result of lower payments.

In Chapter 1, I cited a study of what might happen if hospital payments were suddenly reduced to Medicare levels across the board. In that scenario, the study estimated, up to 1.5 million hospital jobs would disappear if healthcare systems reduced labor costs enough to compensate for the lower payment levels.

Fewer people would forfeit their jobs under the restructuring I've proposed, because provider payments wouldn't be reduced as much as they would under the current MFA proposals. Moreover, the pain of this major economic change would be spread out over many more years. So fewer people would be turned loose on the job market in any particular year, cushioning the impact of healthcare reform.

Still, the economy would have difficulty absorbing the loss of this many jobs, and the ripple effect would extend far beyond that in local economies. The dislocation produced by these changes would also occur during a period when it would become increasingly difficult to provide well-paying jobs for Americans displaced by technology and outsourcing—not to mention COVID-19.

The solution to this problem goes far beyond the scope of this book. Politicians will eventually have to grapple with the giant challenge that technological change poses to our economy. Retraining and green jobs won't cut it. Even infrastructure-related jobs will provide only a temporary boost. But this country can't continue to depend on healthcare as a job-creating machine, because we can't afford it anymore.

There are those who argue that healthcare reform is impossible and/or undesirable because of its negative economic impact.[11] Others maintain that Medicare for All would actually increase the number of jobs in the larger economy.[12] But, even if reform causes some job losses, that must be weighed against the need of all Americans for affordable, comprehensive healthcare. There will inevitably be a tradeoff. But giving up and saying that nothing can be done is not a solution.

Eventually, the current healthcare system will be swept away when it becomes unaffordable to enough people. The question is whether we'll end up with something much better or something much worse.

COVID-19's Impact

As the press date for this book approaches, the COVID-19 pandemic has already claimed more than 100,000 lives in the U.S. and is continuing to surge in many areas of the country. The Trump Administration has predicted that up to 240,000 Americans might die in this pandemic[13]—a number some regard as conservative, given the uncoordinated national response to the emergency.[14]

Already in these early days, the COVID-19 crisis has changed U.S. healthcare. Hospitals and health systems are expected to start running out of cash within a few months,[15] and independent physician practices will hit that wall sooner as their patient volume drops. A survey in early April 2020 by the Medical Group Management Association (MGMA) found that on average, 55% of practices had seen a decrease in revenue and 60% had experienced a decline in patient volume since the start of the pandemic.[16]

While a Congressional rescue package authorized CMS to advance up to three months' worth of Medicare payments to physicians as loans,[16] the agency later cut off this lifeline. Meanwhile, restrictions on the forgiveness of Small Business Administration loans are said to limit their value to physician practices.[18]

Some independent practices, already stressed by the tough market before COVID-19, are reportedly throwing in the towel and seeking to affiliate with health systems. Joshua Halvorson, a principal with ECG Management Consultants, says that the prospect of financial ruin will drive many practices into hospitals' arms, leading to a further consolidation of the industry.

However, Halee Fischer-Wright, MD, president and CEO of MGMA, takes the opposite position. She predicts that, as the COVID-19 crisis cuts into health systems' bottom lines, they will start shedding employed practices that are no longer bringing in income or generating admissions.

While it's impossible to foretell which way this will go, hospitals are expecting hard times because of COVID-19 losses and the ban on elective procedures in many states. Some hospitals have already begun to furlough staff, including physicians.[19-20]

Medicare for All: Sooner Rather Than Later?

Besides showing us the value of single-payer healthcare, as noted in Chapter 1, the COVID-19 crisis may even bring it on. Health insurance premiums are forecast to rise by 40% or more in 2021 because of the costs of coronavirus testing and treatment.[21] If premiums jump by only 20%, that could break the back of private insurance, which is already unaffordable for many employers and workers. The best alternative, in that scenario, would be Medicare for All.

Most major health insurers, including United, Anthem, Cigna, Humana, Aetna, and locally owned Blue Cross Blue Shield plans,[22-23] have waived COVID-19 cost-sharing, including copayments and deductibles, for a limited period of time. But they'll eventually pass that on to customers in the form of higher premiums.

Meanwhile, the huge layoffs precipitated by the crisis have driven up the number of uninsured.[24] According to one estimate, 3.5 million people lost their coverage through March 2020.[25] Unemployed people without insurance are certainly in no condition to foot the bill for COVID-19 treatment, which could bankrupt them after a single day in the hospital.

What all of this shows is that our hybrid system of private and public healthcare financing is spectacularly unsuited for emergencies like this one. Moreover, because of the pandemic, the glaring inadequacy of the system is becoming apparent to many people who never had a major health problem before. Coupled with the anticipated skyrocketing of insurance premiums, this new public realization might be enough to usher in single-payer health care.

The timing of this epochal shift depends not only on the perception of average Americans, but also on the financial calculus of the major industry players. When they finally recognize that Medicare for All will benefit both them and their patients, and that the only alternative is a systemic collapse, they will make it happen.

Endnotes

CHAPTER 1

1. Starr P. *The Social Transformation of American Medicine: The Rise of a Sovereign Profession and the Making of a Vast Industry*. New York: Basic Books;1982:404-405.

2. Stein J. What Rep. John Conyers's sweeping single-payer health care bill would actually do. *Vox*. Aug. 28, 2017. https://www.vox.com/policy-and-politics/2017/8/28/16114436/john-conyers-single-payer-insurance.

3. Krugman P. Health reform realities. *New York Times*. Jan. 18, 2016. https://www.nytimes.com/2016/01/18/opinion/health-reform-realities.html?action=click&pgtype=Homepage&clickSource=story-heading&module=opinion-c-col-left-region&region=opinion-c-col-left-region&WT.nav=opinion-c-col-left-region&_r=0.

4. Megerian C, Levey NN. Tightening Democratic race revives party's old debate over healthcare. *The Los Angeles Times*. Jan. 15, 2016. https://www.latimes.com/politics/la-na-democrats-universal-healthcare-20160115-story.html.

5. Blumberg Y. 70% of Americans now support Medicare-for-all—here's how single-payer could affect you. *CNBC Money*. Aug. 28, 2018. https://www.cnbc.com/2018/08/28/most-americans-now-support-medicare-for-all-and-free-college-tuition.html.

6. McCarthy J. Seven in 10 maintain negative view of U.S. healthcare system. Gallup news release. Jan. 14, 2019. https://news.gallup.com/poll/245873/seven-maintain-negative-view-healthcare-system.aspx.

7. Fried J, Shakir M, Herzog M. Another look at the midterms: public not ready for Medicare for All. *Health Affairs* (blog). Dec. 19. 2018. https://www.healthaffairs.org/do/10.1377/hblog20181217.603723/full.

8. Foran C, Barrett T. Trump signs coronavirus relief legislation into law. CNN. March 19, 2020. https://www.cnn.com/2020/03/18/politics/coronavirus-congress-relief-senate-house/index.html

9. Gaffney A. America's extreme neoliberal healthcare system is putting the country at risk. The Guardian. March 21, 2020. https://www.theguardian.com/commentisfree/2020/mar/21/medicare-for-all-coronavirus-covid-19-single-payer

10. Tolbert J, Orgera K, Singer N, Damico A. Key facts about the uninsured population. *Kaiser Family Foundation Issue Brief*. Dec. 13, 2019. https://www.kff.org/uninsured/issue-brief/key-facts-about-the-uninsured-population.

11. Benchmark Employer Survey Finds Average Family Premiums Now Top $20,000. Kaiser Family Foundation press release, Sept. 25, 2019. https://www.kff.org/health-costs/press-release/benchmark-employer-survey-finds-average-family-premiums-now-top-20000.

12. Altman D. Employer-based coverage is unaffordable for low-wage workers. *Axios*. Sept. 26, 2019. https://www.axios.com/employer-based-coverage-is-unaffordable-for-low-wage-workers-f6855a5e-83ed-452e-825a-7ed966dd0f3b.html.

13. Benchmark Employer Survey Finds Average Family Premiums Now Top $20,000 . . .

14. Commonwealth Fund health care affordability index finds costs unaffordable for a quarter of working-Age adults with private health insurance. Commonwealth Fund press release. Nov. 20, 2015. http://www.commonwealthfund.org/publications/press-releases/2015/nov/commonwealth-fund-health-care-affordability-index.

15. Luthra S. Do 160 million Americans really like their health plans? *MedCity News*. Nov. 22, 2019. https://medcitynews.com/2019/11/do-160-million-americans-really-like-their-health-plans/?utm_

campaign=MCN%20Daily%20Top%20Stories&utm_source=hs_email&utm_medium=email&utm_content=79859455&_hsenc=p2ANqtz--w3Sqflkw9GAo_-IKx_Wircw_pCBl9IUFjsJc8ywIrHATQTR953TQ3X2Hv3atYZYFnDU1jHdBm8D5u6Vly4d4-0-SSlw&_hsmi=79859455.

16. Frist B, Hamburg M. Understanding the burning platform of health care spending growth. *Health Affairs* (blog), March 21, 2019. https://www.healthaffairs.org/do/10.1377/hblog20190320.106452/full.

17. Warren E. Ending the stranglehold of health care costs on American families. *Medium.com*. Nov. 1, 2019. https://medium.com/@teamwarren/ending-the-stranglehold-of-health-care-costs-on-american-families-bf8286b13086.

18. Yglesias M. Joe Biden's health care plan, explained. *Vox*, July 16, 2019, https://www.vox.com/2019/7/16/20694598/joe-biden-health-care-plan-public-option

19. Klein E. It's time to move past employer-based health insurance. Vox. April 9, 2020. https://www.vox.com/2020/4/9/21210353/coronavirus-health-insurance-biden-sanders-medicare-for-all

20. Health Care. Joe Biden 2020 website. https://joebiden.com/healthcare.

21. Sullivan S. Biden moves closer to Sanders on health care and student debt. Washington Post. April 9, 2020. https://www.washingtonpost.com/politics/biden-moves-closer-to-sanders-on-health-care-and-student-debt/2020/04/09/7ca45ce2-7a70-11ea-9bee-c5bf9d2e3288_story.html

22. Medicare for All Act of 2019. Sen. Bernie Sanders website. https://www.sanders.senate.gov/download/medicare-for-all-act-of-2019?id=0DD31317-EF09-4349-A0D4-0510991EF748&download=1&inline=file.

23. Weissert W. Warren says getting to "Medicare for All" will take 3 years. *Associated Press*. Nov. 15, 2019. https://www.yahoo.com/lifestyle/warren-says-she-won-t-172213168.html.

24. Ending the stranglehold of health care costs on American families . . .

25. Kaplan T, Goodnough A, Sanger Katz M. Elizabeth Warren proposes $20.5 trillion health care plan. *New York Times*. Nov. 1, 2019. https://www.nytimes.com/2019/11/01/us/politics/elizabeth-warren-medicare-for-all.html?action=click&module=Top%20Stories&pgtype=Homepage.

26. Kliff S, Scott D. We read Democrats' 9 plans for expanding health care. Here's how they work. *Vox*, March 20, 2019. https://www.vox.com/2018/12/13/18103087/medicare-for-all-explained-single-payer-health-care-sanders-jayapal.

27. Kocher R, Berwick DM. Policies for making health care in the United States better. *Health Affairs* (blog). June 6, 2019. https://www.healthaffairs.org/do/10.1377/hblog20190530.216896/full/?utm_source=Newsletter&utm_medium=email&utm_content=Kocher+and+Berwick%3A+What+To+Do+While+Considering+Medicare+for+All%3B+Wisconsin+Medicaid+Expansion%3B+The+Specialty+Palliative+Care+Workforce&utm_campaign=HAT.

28. Ault A. Many doctors feel angry, undervalued by Warren's health plan. *Medscape Medical News*. Nov. 11, 2019. https://www.medscape.com/viewarticle/921060

29. Medicare for America summary. https://delauro.house.gov/sites/delauro.house.gov/files/Medicare_for_America_Summary.pdf.

30. Medicare for America Act of 2018. https://delauro.house.gov/sites/delauro.house.gov/files/Medicare_for_America_Act_.pdf.

31. *Ibid.*

32. We read Democrats' 9 plans for expanding health care . . .

33. Altman A. The detail that could make Medicare for all generous—and expensive. *Axios*. Jan. 9, 2019. https://www.axios.com/medicare-for-all-out-of-pocket-costs-7aa80feb-ea06-4f35-a43a-9cfc719ab897.html.

34. Holahan J, Buettgens M, Clemans-Cope L, Favreault MM, Blumberg LJ, Ndwandwe S. The Sanders single-payer health care plan: the effect on national health expenditures and federal and private spending. Urban Institute. May 2016. https://www.urban.org/research/publication/sanders-single-payer-health-care-plan-effect-national-health-expenditures-and-federal-and-private-spending.

35. Blumberg LJ, Holahan J, Buettgens M, Gangopadhyaya A, Garrett B, *et al.* From incremental to comprehensive health insurance reform: how various reform options compare on coverage and costs. Urban Institute. Oct. 2019. https://www.urban.org/sites/default/files/2019/10/15/from_incremental_to_comprehensive_health_insurance_reform-how_various_reform_options_compare_on_coverage_and_costs.pdf.

36. Katz J, Quealy K, Sanger-Katz M. Would "Medicare for All" save billions or cost billions? *New York Times.* April 10, 2019. https://www.nytimes.com/interactive/2019/04/10/upshot/medicare-for-all-bernie-sanders-cost-estimates.html.

37. The Sanders single-payer health care plan . . .

38. Friedman G. Yes, we can have improved Medicare for All. White paper. Dec. 11, 2018. https://businessinitiative.org/wp-content/uploads/2019/01/We-Can-Have-Improved-M4A-Friedman-ilovepdf-compressed.pdf.

39. Pollin R, Heintz J, Arno P, Wicks-Lim J, Ash M. Economic analysis of Medicare for All. Political Economic Research Institute. Nov. 30, 2018. https://www.peri.umass.edu/publication/item/1127-economic-analysis-of-medicare-for-all

40. Yes, we can have improved Medicare for All . . .

41. Blahous C. The costs of a national single-payer healthcare system. Mercatus Center. July 30, 2018. https://www.mercatus.org/publications/federal-fiscal-policy/costs-national-single-payer-healthcare-system.

42. From incremental to comprehensive health insurance reform . . .

43. Would "Medicare for All" save billions or cost billions?

44. Medicare Payment Advisory Commission. National health care and Medicare spending. http://www.medpac.gov/docs/default-source/data-book/jun17_databooksec1_sec.pdf?sfvrsn=0.

45. Zuckerman S, Skopec L, Epstein M. Medicaid physician fees after the ACA primary care fee bump. Urban Institute. March 2017. https://www.urban.org/sites/default/files/publication/88836/2001180-medicaid-physician-fees-after-the-aca-primary-care-fee-bump_0.pdf.

46. Livingston S. Employer health plans pay hospitals 241% of Medicare. *Modern Healthcare.* May 9, 2019. https://www.modernhealthcare.com/payment/employer-health-plans-pay-hospitals-241-medicare?utm_source=modern-healthcare-alert&utm_medium=email&utm_campaign=20190509&utm_content=hero-headline.

47. Medicaid physician fees after the ACA primary care bump . . .

48. Luthi S. Medicaid buy-in proposals prompt similar worries as "Medicare for all." Modern Healthcare. Oct. 17, 2018. https://www.modernhealthcare.com/article/20181017/NEWS/181019897/medicaid-buy-in-proposals-prompt-similar-worries-as-medicare-for-all.

49. Schulman KA, Milstein A. The implications of "Medicare for All" for US hospitals. *JAMA.* 2019;321(17):1661–1662. doi:10.1001/jama.2019.3134. https://jamanetwork.com/journals/jama/fullarticle.

50. The costs of a national single-payer healthcare system . . .

51. The Sanders single-payer health care plan . . .

52. Ault A. Majority of healthcare professionals support single payer system, poll says. *Medscape Medical News.* Dec. 18, 2018, https://www.medscape.com/viewarticle/906703#vp_1.

53. Kliff S. Obama just approved a $214 billion plan to fix Medicare. That's a big deal. *Vox.* April 16, 2015. https://www.vox.com/2015/3/17/8232071/medicare-doc-fix-sgr.

54. Many Doctors Feel Angry, Undervalued by Warren's Health Plan . . .

55. Firth S. AMA president: it's still "no" to single payer. *MedPage Today*. Oct. 17, 2018. https://www.medpagetoday.com/publichealthpolicy/healthpolicy/75775.

56. Doherty R, Cooney TG, Mire RD, *et al*; Health and Public Policy Committee and Medical Practice and Quality Committee of the American College of Physicians. Envisioning a better U.S. health care system for all: a call to action by the American College of Physicians. *Ann Intern Med*. 2020;172:S3–S6. doi: https://doi.org/10.7326/M19-2411.

57. American Association of Medical Colleges (AAMC). New research shows increasing physician shortages in both primary and specialty care. AAMC news release. April 11, 2018. https://news.aamc.org/press-releases/article/workforce_report_shortage_04112018.

58. Frakt A. A sense of alarm as rural hospitals keep closing. *New York Times*, Oct. 29. 2018. https://www.nytimes.com/2018/10/29/upshot/a-sense-of-alarm-as-rural-hospitals-keep-closing.html.

59. Rojas-Burke J. What happens when hospitals abandon inner cities. *Covering Health*. July 9, 2014. https://healthjournalism.org/blog/2014/07/what-happens-when-hospitals-abandon-inner-cities.

60. Congressional Budget Office (CBO). Key design components and considerations for establishing a single-payer health care system. CBO report. May 2019, 22. https://www.cbo.gov/system/files/2019-05/55150-singlepayer.pdf.

61. Would "Medicare for All" Save Billions or Cost Billions?

62. Berwick DM, Hackbarth AD. Eliminating waste in US health care. *JAMA*. 2012;307(14):1513-1516. doi:10.1001/jama.2012.362. https://jamanetwork.com/journals/jama/fullarticle/1148376

63. Institute of Medicine. The healthcare imperative: lowering costs and improving outcomes. Workshop series summary. 2010. https://www.ncbi.nlm.nih.gov/books/NBK53942.

64. Sanders, Medicare for All Act of 2019 . . .

65. Jayapal P, Dingell D. Medicare for All Act of 2019: summary. https://jayapal.house.gov/wp-content/uploads/2019/02/Medicare-for-All-Act-of-2019_Summary-002.pdf.

66. Economic analysis of Medicare for All . . .

67. *Ibid*.

68. Institute of Medicine, *Crossing the Quality Chasm: A New Health System for the 21st Century*. Washington, DC: National Academy Press; 2001:3.

69. International Profiles. The Commonwealth Fund. May 2017. https://www.commonwealthfund.org/sites/default/files/documents/___media_files_publications_fund_report_2017_may_mossialos_intl_profiles_v5.pdf.

CHAPTER 2

1. Summary of the Affordable Care Act. Kaiser Family Foundation. March 2017. http://files.kff.org/attachment/Summary-of-the-Affordable-Care-Act

2. Brill S. *America's Bitter Pill: Money, Politics, Backroom Deals, and The Fight to Fix Our Broken Healthcare System*. New York: Random House; 2015:36-37.

3. Orszag's health warning. *Wall Street Journal*. Dec. 29, 2008. https://www.wsj.com/articles/SB123051170671838473.

4. Health care reform tops Obama's priority list. *PBS News Hour*. June 8, 2009. https://www.pbs.org/newshour/health/health-jan-june09-healthpreview_06-08.

5. Fleming C. 2009 U.S. health spending estimated at $2.5 trillion. *Health Affairs* (blog). Feb. 4, 2010. 10.1377/hblog20100204.003786. https://www.healthaffairs.org/do/10.1377/hblog20100204.003786/full

6. Jones S. Obama: National debt problem "is very simple": "We use a lot of healthcare." *CNS News.com*. Feb. 23, 2016. https://www.cnsnews.com/news/article/susan-jones/obama-national-debt-problem-very-simple-we-use-lot-healthcare.

7. Health care reform tops Obama's priority list . . .

8. Tolbert J, Orgera K, Singer N, Damico A. Key facts about the uninsured population. *Kaiser Family Foundation Issue Brief*. Dec. 13, 2019. https://www.kff.org/uninsured/issue-brief/key-facts-about-the-uninsured-population

9. Cohn J. Here's what's really going on with Obamacare premiums. *Huffington Post*. April 12, 2016. https://www.huffingtonpost.com/entry/obamacare-premiums_us_570d94a8e4b0ffa5937d7963.

10. Kennelly R. What are the 2019 federal poverty levels? iHealth Agents. https://help.ihealthagents.com/hc/en-us/articles/225377107-What-are-the-2019-Federal-Poverty-Levels-.

11. Washington Post Staff. *Landmark: The Inside Story of America's New Health-Care Law and What It Means for Us All*. Washington, D.C.: Washington Post;2010:86.

12. Scott D. A requiem for the individual mandate. *Vox*. April 13, 2018. https://www.vox.com/policy-and-politics/2018/4/13/17226566/obamacare-penalty-2018-individual-mandate-still-in-effect.

13. Geisel J. Health insurance exchange signups surging. *Business Insurance*. Jan. 6, 2016. http://www.businessinsurance.com/article/20160106/NEWS03/160109918/u-s-centers-for-medicare-and-medicaid-services-reports-health?tags=%7C62%7C63%7C67%7C74%7C307%7C329%7C278.

14. Pozen RC. How Obamacare inadvertently threatens the financial health of small businesses,and what states should do about it. *Forbes*. Nov. 12, 2015. https://www.forbes.com/sites/forbesleadershipforum/2015/11/12/how-obamacare-inadvertently-threatens-the-financial-health-of-small-businesses-and-what-to-do-about-it/#3a4fb5f61bb6.

15. Holan AD. Lie of the year: "If you like your health care plan, you can keep it." *Politifact*. Dec. 12, 2013. https://www.politifact.com/truth-o-meter/article/2013/dec/12/lie-year-if-you-like-your-health-care-plan-keep-it.

16. Carnevale ML. Obama: "If you like your doctor, you can keep your doctor." *Wall Street Journal*. June 15, 2009. https://blogs.wsj.com/washwire/2009/06/15/obama-if-you-like-your-doctor-you-can-keep-your-doctor.

17. Polsky D, Weiner J. The skinny on narrow networks in health insurance marketplace plans. Data brief. Penn Leonard Davis Institute of Health Economics and Robert Wood Johnson Foundation. June 2015. https://www.rwjf.org/content/dam/farm/reports/issue_briefs/2015/rwjf421027.

18. State Health Insurance Marketplace Types. Kaiser Family Foundation. 2020. https://www.kff.org/health-reform/state-indicator/state-health-insurance-marketplace-types/?currentTimeframe=0&selectedRows=%7B%22states%22:%7B%22all%22:%7B%7D%7D,%22wrapups%22:%7B%22united-states%22:%7B%7D%7D%7D&sortModel=%7B%22colId%22:%22Location%22,%22sort%22:%22asc%22%7D.

19. 58% favor repeal of health care law. *Rasmussen Reports*. June 7, 2010. http://www.rasmussenreports.com/public_content/politics/current_events/healthcare/june_2010/58_favor_repeal_of_health_care_law.

20. Tanden N. A short history of Republican attempts to repeal Obamacare. *Politico*. Jan. 30, 2014. https://www.politico.com/magazine/story/2014/01/house-republicans-obamacare-repeal-votes-102911.

21. Efforts to repeal the Patient Protection and Affordable Care Act. *Wikipedia*. https://en.m.wikipedia.org/wiki/Efforts_to_repeal_the_Patient_Protection_and_Affordable_Care_Act.

22. Liptak A. Supreme Court upholds health care law, 5-4, in victory for Obama. *New York Times*. June 28, 2012. https://www.nytimes.com/2012/06/29/us/supreme-court-lets-health-law-largely-stand.html.

23. Young J. These were the most important Obamacare stories of 2015. *Huffington Post*. Dec. 31, 2015. http://www.huffingtonpost.com/entry/most-important-obamacare-stories-2015_56859b80e4b014efe0da7822.

24. Goodnough A, Pear R. Texas judge strikes down Obama's Affordable Care Act as unconstitutional. *New York Times*. Dec. 14, 2018. https://www.nytimes.com/2018/12/14/health/obamacare-unconstitutional-texas-judge.html?action=click&module=Top%20Stories&pgtype=Homepage.

25. Keith K. Fifth Circuit strikes mandate, remands on rest of ACA. *Health Affairs* (blog). Dec. 19, 2019. 10.1377/hblog20191219.863104.

26. Keith K. Supreme Court denies expedited review of Texas. *Health Affairs* (blog). Jan. 21, 2020. https://www.healthaffairs.org/do/10.1377/hblog20200121.699161/full/?utm_source=Newsletter&utm_medium=email&utm_content=Vaccine+Infrastructure+And+Education%3B+Supreme+Court+Denies+Expedited+Review+Of+Texas%3B+Medicare+s+Voluntary+Bundled+Payment+For+Joint+Replacement+Surgery&utm_campaign=HAT.

27. Liptak A, Goodnough A. Supreme Court to Hear Obamacare Appeal. New York Times. March 2, 2020. https://www.nytimes.com/2020/03/02/us/supreme-court-obamacare-appeal.html

28. Pear R. Trump officials broaden attack on health law, arguing courts should reject all of it. March 25, 2019. https://www.nytimes.com/2019/03/25/us/politics/obamacare-unconstitutional-trump-aca.html?action=click&module=Top%20Stories&pgtype=Homepage.

29. Hiltzik M. No, Marco Rubio didn't score a blow against Obamacare—he merely hurt patients. *Los Angeles Times*. Dec. 10, 2015. http://www.latimes.com/business/hiltzik/la-fi-mh-no-marco-rubio-didn-t-score-20151210-column.html?ref=yfp.

30. Corlette S, Miskell S, Lerche J, Giovannelli J. Why are many co-ops failing? *Commonwealth Fund* report. Dec. 2015. https://www.commonwealthfund.org/sites/default/files/documents/___media_files_publications_fund_report_2015_dec_1847_corlette_why_are_many_coops_failing.pdf.

31. Cohn J. Trump threatens coverage of millions if Democrats won't negotiate on ACA repeal. *Huffington Post*. April 12, 2017. https://www.huffingtonpost.com/entry/trump-threatens-coverage_us_58eebb13e4b0bb9638e13674.

32. Pear P, Haberman M, Abelson R. Trump to scrap critical health care subsidies, hitting Obamacare again. *New York Times*. Oct. 12, 2017. https://www.nytimes.com/2017/10/12/us/politics/trump-obamacare-executive-order-health-insurance.html.

33. Livingston S. Several health insurers win lawsuits over unpaid federal subsidies. *Modern Healthcare*. Feb. 15, 2019. https://www.modernhealthcare.com/article/20190215/NEWS/190219945.

34. Carolyn Y. Johnson, UnitedHealth Group to exit Obamacare exchanges in all but a handful of states. *Washington Post*. April 19, 2016. https://www.washingtonpost.com/news/wonk/wp/2016/04/19/unitedhealth-group-to-exit-obamacare-exchanges-in-all-but-a-handful-of-states/?utm_term=.03b8c0ec6806.

35. Bryan B. America's 3rd largest health insurers is losing $300 million on Obamacare. *Yahoo Finance*. Aug. 2, 2016. https://finance.yahoo.com/news/americas-third-largest-health-insurer-152157576.html.

36. Aetna drops Obamacare in most states. *Reuters*. Aug. 15, 2016. https://www.huffingtonpost.com/entry/aetna-obamacare_us_57b262cbe4b0c75f49d7eb27.

37. Lucia K, Giovannelli J, Curran E, Corlette S. Beyond UnitedHealthcare: how are other publicly traded insurers faring on the marketplaces? *To the Point*. The Commonwealth Fund. June 1, 2016. https://www.commonwealthfund.org/blog/2016/beyond-unitedhealthcare-how-are-other-publicly-traded-insurers-faring-marketplaces?redirect_source=/publications/blog/2016/jun/beyond-unitedhealthcare-how-insurers-faring-on-marketplaces.

38. Hiltzik M. Healthcare shocker: these insurers are making money on Obamacare. *Los Angeles Times.* April 27, 2016. https://www.latimes.com/business/hiltzik/la-fi-hiltzik-obamacare-profits-20160427-snap-htmlstory.html.

39. Cohn J. Here's what's really going on with Obamacare premiums. *Huffington Post.* April 12, 2016. https://www.huffingtonpost.com/entry/obamacare-premiums_us_570d94a8e4b0ffa5937d7963.

40. Hiltzik M. Dirty little secret: insurers actually are making a mint from Obamacare. *Los Angeles Times.* Feb. 16, 2016. https://www.latimes.com/business/hiltzik/la-fi-mh-insurers-are-making-a-mint-from-obamacare-20160216-column.html.

41. Jost T. House passes AHCA: how it happened, what it would do, and its uncertain Senate future. *Health Affairs* (blog). May 4, 2017. https://www.healthaffairs.org/do/10.1377/hblog20170504.059967/full.

42. *Ibid.*

43. Andrews M. Limited outreach, shorter sign-up time may cause insurance headaches in 2018. *NPR News.* Oct. 24, 2017. https://www.npr.org/sections/health-shots/2017/10/24/559565543/limited-outreach-shorter-sign-up-time-may-cause-insurance-headaches-in-2018.

44. Pollitz K, Tolbert J, Diaz M. Further reductions in navigator funding for federal marketplace states. *Kaiser Family Foundation Data Note.* Sept. 24, 2018. https://www.kff.org/health-reform/issue-brief/data-note-further-reductions-in-navigator-funding-for-federal-marketplace-states.

45. Limited outreach, shorter sign-up time . . .

46. Armour S, Burton TM. Cheaper health plans with less coverage move forward. *Wall Street Journal.* Aug. 1, 2018. https://www.wsj.com/articles/cheaper-health-plans-with-less-coverage-move-forward-1533121200.

47. Faux Z, Mosendz P, Tozzi J. Health insurance that doesn't cover the bills has flooded the market under Trump. *Bloomberg Businessweek.* Sept. 17, 2019. https://www.bloomberg.com/news/features/2019-09-17/under-trump-health-insurance-with-less-coverage-floods-market.

48. Tavernise S, Gebeloff R. Immigrants, the poor and minorities gain sharply under affordable care act. *New York Times.* April 17, 2016. https://www.nytimes.com/2016/04/18/health/immigrants-the-poor-and-minorities-gain-sharply-under-health-act.html?hp&action=click&pgtype=Homepage&clickSource=story-heading&module=second-column-region&region=top-news&WT.nav=top-news&_r=0.

49. Medicaid enrollment changes following the ACA. Medicaid and CHIP Payment and Access Commission. https://www.macpac.gov/subtopic/medicaid-enrollment-changes-following-the-aca.

50. Health Insurance Exchanges 2019 Open Enrollment Report. CMS news release. March 25, 2019. https://www.cms.gov/newsroom/fact-sheets/health-insurance-exchanges-2019-open-enrollment-report.

51. Marketplace Enrollment 2014-2019. Kaiser Family Foundation. https://www.kff.org/health-reform/state-indicator/marketplace-enrollment/?currentTimeframe=0&sortModel=%7B%22colId%22:%22Location%22,%22sort%22:%22asc%22%7D.

52. Berchick ER, Barnett JC, Upton RD. Health insurance coverage in the United States: 2018. U.S. Census Bureau. Nov. 2019. https://www.census.gov/content/dam/Census/library/publications/2019/demo/p60-267.pdf.

53. Keith K. Uninsured rate rose in 2018, says Census Bureau report. *Health Affairs* (blog). Sept. 11, 2019. https://www.healthaffairs.org/do/10.1377/hblog20190911.805983/full/?utm_source=Newsletter&utm_medium=email&utm_content=Event%3A+Military+Health+Systems%3B+Census+Bureau%3A+Uninsured+Rate+Rose+In+2018%3B+ACO+Participation+Numbers+Worth+Watching%3B+Health+Spending+And+Social+Spending+In+High-Income+Countries&utm_campaign=HAT+9-11-19.

54. Cohn J. Democrats finally see a chance to make Obamacare better. *Huffington Post*. March 23, 2018. https://www.huffingtonpost.com/entry/obamacare-elizabeth-warren-bernie-sanders-democrats_us_5ab42b66e4b0decad048532e.

55. Sanger-Katz M. Even insured can face crushing medical debt, study finds. *New York Times*. Jan. 5, 2016. http://www.nytimes.com/2016/01/06/upshot/lost-jobs-houses-savings-even-insured-often-face-crushing-medical-debt.html?hp&action=click&pgtype=Homepage&clickSource=story-heading&module=first-column-region&region=top-news&WT.nav=top-news&_r=1.

56. Pear R. Many say high deductibles make their health law insurance all but useless. *New York Times*. Nov. 14, 2015. http://www.nytimes.com/2015/11/15/us/politics/many-say-high-deductibles-make-their-health-law-insurance-all-but-useless.html?hp&action=click&pgtype=Homepage&clickSource=story-heading&module=first-column-region&region=top-news&WT.nav=top-news.

57. Fehr R, Cox C, Levitt L. Insurer participation in ACA marketplaces. *Kaiser Family Foundation Issue Brief*. Nov. 14, 2018. https://www.kff.org/health-reform/issue-brief/insurer-participation-on-aca-marketplaces-2014-2019.

58. McCarthy N. The number of uninsured Americans is rising again—and young adults are most likely to lack coverage. *Forbes*. Sept. 18, 2019. https://www.forbes.com/sites/niallmccarthy/2019/09/18/the-number-of-uninsured-americans-is-rising-again--and-young-adults-who-are-most-likely-to-lack-coverage/#26e775455b62.

59. The Affordable Care Act under the Trump Administration . . .

60. Antonisse L, Garfield R, Rudowitz R, Guth M. The effects of Medicaid expansion under the ACA: updated findings from a literature review. *Kaiser Family Foundation Issue Brief*. Aug. 15, 2019. https://www.kff.org/medicaid/issue-brief/the-effects-of-medicaid-expansion-under-the-aca-updated-findings-from-a-literature-review-august-2019.

61. The public's views on the ACA. Kaiser Family Foundation. Jan. 23, 2019. https://www.kff.org/interactive/kff-health-tracking-poll-the-publics-views-on-the-aca/#?response=Favorable--Unfavorable&aRange=twoYear.

62. Fiedler M, Aaron HJ, Adler L, Ginsburg PB, Young CL. Building on the ACA to achieve universal coverage. *N Engl J Med*. 2019;380:1685-88. doi: 10.1056/NEJMp1901532. https://www.nejm.org/doi/full/10.1056/NEJMp1901532?query=TOC.

63. CMS. About the CMS Innovation Center. https://innovation.cms.gov/About.

64. CMS, Innovation Models. https://innovation.cms.gov/initiatives/#views=models.

65. Berwick DM, Nolan TW, Whittington J. The Triple Aim: care, health and cost. *Health Affairs*. May/June 2008, 759-769. https://www.healthaffairs.org/doi/full/10.1377/hlthaff.27.3.759.

66. Characteristics of office-based physician visits. National Center for Health Statistics. 2016. https://www.cdc.gov/nchs/products/databriefs/db331.htm.

67. Institute of Medicine. *Crossing the Quality Chasm: A New Health System for the 21st Century*. Washington, D.C.: National Academies Press;2001:3.

68. Shortell, SM, Schmittdiel J. Prepaid groups and organized delivery systems. *Toward a 21st Century Health System: The Contributions and Promise of Prepaid Group Practice*. Enthoven AC and Tollen J, eds. San Francisco: John Wiley & Sons;2004:7-11.

69. Terry K. *Rx for Health Care Reform*. Nashville: Vanderbilt University Press;2007:177.

70. Sisko AM, Keehan SP, *et al*. National health expenditure projections, 2018-27: economic and demographic trends drive spending and enrollment growth. *Health Affairs*. 38(3):491-501. https://www.healthaffairs.org/doi/abs/10.1377/hlthaff.2018.05499.

71. Davis K, Guterman S, Bandeali F. The Affordable Care Act and Medicare. *Commonwealth Fund Issues Brief.* June 9, 2015. https://www.commonwealthfund.org/publications/fund-reports/2015/jun/affordable-care-act-and-medicare.

72. Fontana E, Hawes K. Map: See the 2,599 hospitals that will face readmissions penalties this year. *Advisory Board Co. Daily Briefing.* Sept. 27, 2018. https://www.advisory.com/daily-briefing/2018/09/27/readmissions.

73. The Affordable Care Act and Medicare . . .

74. Boccuti C, Casillas G. Aiming for fewer hospital U-turns: the Medicare hospital readmissions reduction. *Kaiser Family Foundation Issue Brief.* March 10, 2017. https://www.kff.org/report-section/aiming-for-fewer-hospital-u-turns-the-medicare-hospital-readmission-reduction-program-issue-brief.

75. CMS. Hospital-Acquired Condition Reduction Program. https://www.cms.gov/medicare/medicare-fee-for-service-payment/acuteinpatientpps/hac-reduction-program.html.

76. Castellucci M. Drop in hospital-acquired conditions saves $7.7 billion. *Modern Healthcare.* Jan. 29, 2019. https://www.modernhealthcare.com/article/20190129/NEWS/190129927?utm_source=modernhealthcare&utm_medium=email&utm_content=20190129-NEWS-190129927&utm_campaign=dose.

77. CMS. The hospital value-based purchasing (VBP) program. https://www.cms.gov/Medicare/Quality-Initiatives-Patient-Assessment-Instruments/Value-Based-Programs/HVBP/Hospital-Value-Based-Purchasing.html.

78. CMS. CMS hospital value-based purchasing program results for fiscal year 2019. Dec. 3, 2018. https://www.cms.gov/newsroom/fact-sheets/cms-hospital-value-based-purchasing-program-results-fiscal-year-2019.

79. CMS. Bundled payments for care improvement initiative. Jan. 30, 2014. http://www.cms.gov/Newsroom/MediaReleaseDatabase/Fact-sheets/2014-Fact-sheets-items/2014-01-30-2.html.

80. Seldman J. Some providers leave government's bundled payment program; those remaining expand participation. Avalere Health. Dec. 14, 2015. http://avalere.com/expertise/managed-care/insights/some-providers-leave-governments-bundled-payment-program-those-remaining-ex.

81. Terry K. CMS finalizes mandatory hip and knee bundled payment program. *Medscape Medical News.* Nov. 18, 2015. https://www.medscape.com/viewarticle/854714.

82. Terry K. CMS proposes to cut mandatory bundling programs. *Medscape Medical News.* Aug. 16, 2017. https://www.medscape.com/viewarticle/884371.

83. O'Brien J. CMS cancels bundled payment programs, continuing shift toward voluntary models. Health Leaders. Dec. 1, 2017. https://www.healthleadersmedia.com/finance/cms-cancels-bundled-payment-programs-continuing-shift-toward-voluntary-models.

84. Liao JM, Emanuel EJ, Polsky DE, *et al.* National representativeness of hospitals and markets in Medicare's mandatory bundled payment program. *Health Aff.* 38(1):44-53. https://www.healthaffairs.org/doi/pdf/10.1377/hlthaff.2018.05177.

85. CMS. MIPS overview. https://qpp.cms.gov/mips/overview.

86. Page L. MIPS: Will you earn more or less money? *Medscape Business of Medicine.* June 22, 2016. https://www.medscape.com/viewarticle/864936_5.

87. Verma S. 2018 quality payment program (QPP) performance results. CMS (blog). Jan. 6, 2020. https://www.cms.gov/blog/2018-quality-payment-program-qpp-performance-results.

88. CMS. Advanced alternative payment models. https://qpp.cms.gov/apms/advanced-apms.

89. Verma S. Quality payment program (QPP) year 1 performance results. CMS (blog). Nov. 8, 2018. https://www.cms.gov/blog/quality-payment-program-qpp-year-1-performance-results.

90. 2018 quality payment program (QPP) performance results . . .

91. Kaiser Family Foundation. Summary of new health reform law. 2010. https://kaiserfamily foundation.files.wordpress.com/2013/01/8061.pdf.

92. National Committee on Quality Assurance (NCQA). Patient-centered medical home (PCMH). https://www.ncqa.org/programs/health-care-providers-practices/patient-centered-medical-home-pcmh.

93. CMS. Comprehensive primary care initiative. https://innovation.cms.gov/initiatives/comprehensive-primary-care-initiative/.

94. *Ibid.*

95. CMS. Comprehensive primary care: 2016 fast facts. https://innovation.cms.gov/files/x/cpci-fastfacts2016.pdf

96. CMS. Comprehensive primary care plus. https://innovation.cms.gov/initiatives/comprehensive-primary-care-plus

97. CMS. Primary care first: foster independence, reward outcomes. April 22, 2019. https://www.cms.gov/newsroom/fact-sheets/primary-care-first-foster-independence-reward-outcomes.

98. CMS. Primary care first options. https://innovation.cms.gov/initiatives/primary-care-first-model-options.

99. Peikes D, Dale S, Ghosh A, *et al.* The comprehensive primary care initiative: effects on spending, quality, patients, and physicians. *Health Aff.* 37(6):890-99. https://www.healthaffairs.org/doi/pdf/10.1377/hlthaff.2017.1678.

100. Hodach R, Grundy P, Jain A, Weiner M. *Provider-Led Population. Health Management: Key Strategies for Healthcare in the Cognitive Era, 2d Ed.* Indianapolis: John Wiley & Sons;2016:26.

101. Castellucci M, Dickson V. Medicare ACOs saved CMS $314 million in 2017. *Modern Healthcare.* Aug. 30, 2018. https://www.modernhealthcare.com/article/20180830/NEWS/180839987/medicare-acos-saved-cms-314-million-in-2017.

102. Verma S. Interest in 'Pathways to Success' grows: 2018 ACO results show trends supporting program redesign continue. *Health Affairs* (blog). Sept. 30, 2019. https://www.healthaffairs.org/do/10.1377/hblog20190930.702342/full/?utm_source=Newsletter&utm_medium=email&utm_content=CMS+Administrator+Seema+Verma+On+The+Medicare+Shared+Savings+Program%3B+The+Demise+of+the+ACA+s+Multi-State+Plan+Program%3B+Coverage+Of+Children+With+Medical+Complexity&utm_campaign=HAT.

103. *Ibid.*

104. CMS. Medicare shared savings program fast facts. Jan. 2018. https://www.cms.gov/medicare/medicare-fee-for-service-payment/sharedsavingsprogram/downloads/ssp-2018-fast-facts.pdf.

105. Dawe C, Lewine C. Five simple charts show that risk-based ACOs are working. *Health Affairs* (blog). Dec. 13, 2017. https://www.healthaffairs.org/do/10.1377/hblog20171212.585293/full/.

106. Terry K. ACOs get some relief in Medicare shared savings program. *Medscape Medical News.* June 13, 2016. https://www.medscape.com/viewarticle/864707.

107. CMS. New accountable care organization model opportunity: Medicare ACO Track 1+ Model. https://www.cms.gov/Medicare/Medicare-Fee-for-Service-Payment/sharedsavingsprogram/Downloads/New-Accountable-Care-Organization-Model-Opportunity-Fact-Sheet.pdf.

108. MSSP fast facts . . .

109. Terry K. Redesigned MSSP imposes risk on ACOs more quickly. *Medscape Medical News.* Dec. 24, 2018. https://www.medscape.com/viewarticle/906934.

110. CMS. Medicare shared savings program. https://www.cms.gov/Medicare/Medicare-Fee-for-Service-Payment/sharedsavingsprogram/about.html.

111. Verma S. More ACOs taking accountability under MSSP through "Pathways to Success." https://www.healthaffairs.org/do/10.1377/hblog20190717.482997/full/?utm_source=Newsletter&utm_medium=email&utm_content=CMS+Administrator+Seema+Verma+On+ACO+Accountability%3B+Autistic+Perspectives+Needed%3B+Disparities+Among+Elderly+Dual+Eligibles&utm_campaign=HAT+7-17-19.

112. National Association of Accountable Care Organizations. Survey shows ACOs' concerns about the effect of COVID-19. April 2020. https://www.naacos.com/assets/docs/pdf/2020/SurveyReportACO-EffectsCOVID19-04132020.pdf.

113. Bleser WK, Singletary E, Crook HL, Gonzalez-Smith J, Saunders RS, McClellan MB. Maintaining progress toward accountable care and payment reform during a pandemic, part I: utilization and financial impact. April 14, 2020. https://www.healthaffairs.org/do/10.1377/hblog20200410.281882/full/.

114. Joszt L. HHS sets goals to move Medicare payments from volume to value. *American Journal of Managed Care* Newsroom. Jan. 26, 2015. https://www.ajmc.com/newsroom/hhs-sets-goals-to-move-medicare-payments-from-volume-to-value.

115. *Ibid.*

116. Miliard M. HHS gets to value-based reimbursement goal ahead of schedule. *Healthcare IT News.* March 3, 2016. https://www.healthcareitnews.com/news/hhs-gets-value-based-reimbursement-goal-ahead-schedule?mkt_tok=3RkMMJWWfF9wsRonuarLde%2FhmjTEU5z16u4uXaG1gYkz2EFye%2BLIHETpodcMTcFqMrrYDBceEJhqyQJxPr3MLtINwNlqRhPrCg%3D%3D.

117. Adoption of alternative payment models continues to increase with 34% of payments tied to value-based care. Health Care Payment Learning & Action Network news release. Oct. 22, 2018. https://www.prnewswire.com/news-releases/adoption-of-alternative-payment-models-continues-to-increase-with-34-of-payments-tied-to-value-based-care-300734881.html.

118. APM Framework. Health Care Payment Learning & Action Network. 2017. http://hcp-lan.org/workproducts/apm-refresh-whitepaper-final.pdf.

119. Payment reform has grown significantly, though not across methods likely to transform health care. Catalyst for Payment Reform press release. Dec. 4, 2019. https://www.catalyze.org/about-us/cpr-in-he-news/new-national-scorecards/.

120. Five simple charts show that risk-based ACOs are working . . .

121. Sisko AM, Keehan SP, *et al.* National health expenditure projections, 2018-27: Economic and demographic trends drive spending and enrollment growth. *Health Aff.* 38(3):491-501. https://www.healthaffairs.org/doi/pdf/10.1377/hlthaff.2018.05499.

122. The Affordable Care Act and Medicare . . .

123. National health expenditure projections, 2018-27 . . .

124. Blumenthal D, Abrams A. The Affordable Care Act at 10 Years—Payment and Delivery System Reforms. New England Journal of Medicine. February 26, 2020. DOI: 10.1056/NEJMhpr1916092. https://www.nejm.org/doi/full/10.1056/NEJMhpr1916092?query=TOC

CHAPTER 3

1. Abdela A, Steinbaum M. The United States has a market concentration problem. *FTC Issue Brief.* Sept. 2018. https://www.ftc.gov/system/files/documents/public_comments/2018/09/ftc-2018-0074-d-0042-155544.pdf.

2. Merritt Hawkins. 2019 survey: final-year medical residents. https://www.merritthawkins.com/uploadedFiles/merritthawkins_2019_resident_survey_release.pdf.

3. Schoen C, Collins SR. The big five health insurers' membership and revenue trends: implications for public policy. *Commonwealth Fund Policy Brief.* Dec. 4, 2017. https://www.commonwealthfund.org/publications/journal-article/2017/dec/big-five-health-insurers-membership-and-revenue-trends.

4. Firth S. Healthcare mergers: good, bad, or both? *MedPage Today.* Nov. 23, 2015. http://www.medpagetoday.com/PublicHealthPolicy/HealthPolicy/54856.

5. American Medical Association. Competition in health insurance: 2018 update. https://www.ama-assn.org/system/files/2018-11/competition-health-insurance-us-markets_1.pdf.

6. Morse S. PwC: Hospital mergers not yielding IT, clinical or operational efficiencies. *Healthcare IT News.* March 29, 2016. https://www.healthcareitnews.com/news/pwc-hospital-mergers-not-yielding-operational-efficiencies?mkt_tok=3RkMMJWWfF9wsRonuKzJc%2B%2FhmjTEU5z16u4uXaG1gYkz2EFye%2BLIHETpodcMTcZnMrrYDBceEJhqyQJxPr3MLtINwNlqRhPrCg%3D%3D.

7. Gaynor M, Mostashari F, Ginsburg P. Health care's crushing lack of competition. *Forbes.* June 28, 2017. https://www.forbes.com/sites/realspin/2017/06/28/health-cares-crushing-lack-of-competition/#2943fcee14ff.

8. Bealieu ND, Dafney LS, Landon BE, *et al.* Changes in quality of care after hospital mergers and acquisitions. *N Engl J Med.* 2020; 382:51-59. doi: 10.1056/NEJMsa1901383. Jan. 2, 2020. https://www.nejm.org/doi/full/10.1056/NEJMsa1901383.

9. Kacik A. Beth Israel Deaconess and Lahey Health complete merger. *Modern Healthcare.* March 1, 2019. https://www.modernhealthcare.com/mergers-acquisitions/beth-israel-deaconess-and-lahey-health-complete-merger?utm_source=modern-healthcare-daily-dose-friday&utm_medium=email&utm_campaign=20190301&utm_content=article2-headline.

10. Kacik A. Catholic Health Initiatives, Dignity Health combine to form CommonSpirit Health. *Modern Healthcare.* Feb. 1, 2019. https://www.modernhealthcare.com/article/20190201/NEWS/190209994?utm_source=modernhealthcare&utm_medium=email&utm_content=20190201-NEWS-190209994&utm_campaign=mh-alert.

11. Schencker L. Advocate Health Care finalizes merger with Wisconsin hospital system. *Chicago Tribune.* April 2, 2018. https://www.chicagotribune.com/business/ct-biz-advocate-aurora-merger-done-20180403-story.html.

12. Kacik A. Atrium Health, Wake Forest Baptist Health and Wake Forest University to merge. *Modern Healthcare.* April 10, 2019. https://www.modernhealthcare.com/finance/atrium-health-wake-forest-baptist-health-and-wake-forest-university-merge?utm_source=modern-healthcare-alert&utm_medium=email&utm_campaign=20190410&utm_content=hero-headline.

13. Dietsche D. Why some health system merger plans work out but others are nixed—and why you should care. *MedCity News.* April 11, 2019. https://medcitynews.com/2019/04/health-system-merger/?utm_campaign=MCN%20Daily%20Top%20Stories&utm_source=hs_email&utm_medium=email&utm_content=71700257&_hsenc=p2ANqtz--o7h798t2iwMfTYALBvEdEvngaXLoY-TWvGuZca-JZME6bfoFYH-99GjU44X3oboprneH5mRnC9osjzEf0z636brqxDkw&_hsmi=71700257.

14. Abelson R. Small, piecemeal mergers in health care fly under regulators' radars. *New York Times.* April 8, 2016. https://www.nytimes.com/2016/04/09/business/small-piecemeal-mergers-in-health-care-fly-under-regulators-radars.html?hpw&rref=business&action=click&pgtype=Homepage&module=well-region&region=bottom-well&WT.nav=bottom-well.

15. Schencker S. FTC challenges NorthShore, Advocate mega-merger in Illinois. *Modern Healthcare.* Dec. 18, 2015. http://www.modernhealthcare.com/article/20151218/NEWS/151219865.

16. Melnick GA, Fonkych K. Hospital prices increase in California, especially among hospitals in the largest multi-hospital systems. *Inquiry.* June 9, 2016. https://journals.sagepub.com/doi/full/10.1177/0046958016651555.

17. Health care's crushing lack of competition . . .

18. Cooper Z, Craig S, Gaynor M, Harish NJ, Krumholz HM, Reenen JV. Hospital prices grew substantially faster than physician prices for hospital-based care in 2007-14. *Health Aff.* 39(2):184-89. https://healthcarepricingproject.org/sites/default/files/hlthaff.2018.05424.pdf.

19. White C, Whaley C. Prices paid to hospitals by private health plans are high relative to Medicare and vary widely. *RAND Health Research report.* 2019. https://www.rand.org/pubs/research_reports/RR3033.html.

20. Health care's crushing lack of competition . . .

21. Scheffler RM, Glied SA. Differing impacts of market concentration on affordable care act marketplace premiums. *Commonwealth Fund* (blog). May 2, 2016. https://www.common-wealthfund.org/publications/journal-article/2016/may/differing-impacts-market-concen-tration-affordable-care-act?redirect_source=/publications/in-the-literature/2016/may/differing-impacts-market-concentration-aca-marketplace-premiums.

22. Health care's crushing lack of competition . . .

23. *Ibid.*

24. Landman J, Moore K, Muhlestein DB, Smith NJ, Winfield LD. What is driving total cost of care? An analysis of factors influencing total cost of care in U.S. healthcare markets. June 2018. Healthcare Financial Management Association report. https://leavittpartners.com/wp-content/uploads/2018/06/Total-Cost-of-Care-Executive-Summary-2018.pdf.

25. Ault A. For first time, more doctors employed than self-employed: AMA. *Medscape Medical News.* May 9, 2019. https://www.medscape.com/viewarticle/912791#vp_1.

26. Terry K. Hospitals continue to acquire more physician practices. *Medscape Medical News.* Feb. 22, 2019. https://www.medscape.com/viewarticle/909411.

27. Kane CK and Emmons DW. New Data on Physician Practice Arrangements: Private Practice Remains Strong Despite Shifts Toward Hospital Employment. AMA Policy Research Perspectives. 2013. https://www.ama-assn.org/sites/ama-assn.org/files/corp/media-browser/premium/health-policy/prp-physician-practice-arrangements_0.pdf.

28. The engagement gap. Jackson Healthcare white paper. https://indd.adobe.com/view/2a8b5500-6f78-42a5-8a57-638305e1c8b1.

29. Kane CF. Updated data on physician practice arrangements: For the first time, fewer physicians are owners than employees. *AMA Policy Research Perspectives.* https://www.ama-assn.org/system/files/2019-05/prp-fewer-owners-benchmark-survey-2018.pdf.

30. Singleton T, Miller P. The physician employment trend: What you need to know. *Fam Pract Manag.* 2015 Jul-Aug;22(4):11-15. https://www.aafp.org/fpm/2015/0700/p11.html.

31. Terry K. One in 5 residents doubt career choice, despite ample job offers. *Medscape Medical News.* May 16, 2019. https://www.medscape.com/viewarticle/913082.

32. Hancock J. When the hospital is boss, that's where doctors' patients go. *Kaiser Health News.* Sept. 9, 2015. http://khn.org/news/when-the-hospital-is-boss-thats-where-doctors-patients-go.

33. Terry K. Site-neutral payments are less than meets the eye, experts say. *Medscape Medical News.* Dec. 6, 2018. https://www.medscape.com/viewarticle/906146.

34. *Ibid.*

35. Terry K. Court overturns CMS' site-neutral payment policy; doc groups upset. *Medscape Medical News.* Sept. 19, 2019. https://www.medscape.com/viewarticle/918744.

36. LaPointe J. CMS to repay site-neutral payments to hospitals, appeal case. *RevCycle Intelligence.* Dec. 16, 2019. https://revcycleintelligence.com/news/cms-to-repay-site-neutral-payments-to-hospitals-appeal-case.

37. Haelle T. Physician-hospital integration tied to higher prices. *Medscape Medical News*. Oct. 20, 2015. http://www.medscape.com/viewarticle/852900.

38. Evans M. Hospitals hire more doctors, outpatient prices increase. *Modern Healthcare* (blog). Oct. 19, 2015. http://www.modernhealthcare.com/article/20151019/BLOG/151019915

39. Kacik A. Rapid rise in hospital-employed physicians increases costs. *Modern Healthcare*. March 16, 2018. https://www.modernhealthcare.com/article/20180316/TRANSFORMATION02/180319913.

40. Jones Sanborn B. Hospitals are losing money on employed physicians: Here's how to save the bottom line and your staff. *Healthcare Finance News*. May 31, 2018. https://www.healthcarefinancenews.com/news/hospitals-are-losing-money-employed-physicians-heres-how-save-bottom-line-and-your-staff

41. Sullivan L, McCaw C. Evaluating reasons for physician practice losses. Healthcare Financial Management Association. Dec. 2014. No longer available online.

42. Physicians Foundation. 2018 survey of America's physicians: Practice patterns & perspectives. Sept. 2018. https://physiciansfoundation.org/wp-content/uploads/2018/09/physicians-survey-results-final-2018.pdf.

43. 2019 physician inpatient/outpatient revenue survey . . .

44. One in 5 residents doubt career choice, despite ample job offers . . .

45. 2018 survey of America's physicians: practice patterns & perspectives . . .

46. Small, piecemeal mergers in health care fly under regulators' radars . . .

47. The engagement gap . . .

48. Kane CK. Updated data on physician practice arrangements: For the first time, fewer physicians are owners than employees. *AMA Policy Research Perspectives*. https://www.ama-assn.org/system/files/2019-05/prp-fewer-owners-benchmark-survey-2018.pdf.

49. *Ibid.*

50. Casalino LP, Devers KJ, Lake TK. Benefits of and barriers to large medical group practice in the United States. *Arch Intern Med.* 2003;163(16):1958-64. doi:10.1001/archinte.163.16.19. https://jamanetwork.com/journals/jamainternalmedicine/fullarticle/215993.

51. Enthoven AC, Tollen J (eds.) *Toward a 21st Century Health System: The Contributions and Promise of Prepaid Group Practice.* San Francisco: John Wiley & Sons;2004:xxvii-xlix.

52. Benefits of and barriers to large medical group practice in the United States . . .

53. Casalino LP, Pesko MF, Ryan AM, Mendelsohn JL, Copeland KR, *et al.* Small primary care physician practices have low rates of preventable hospital admissions. *Health Aff* 33(9):1680-88. https://www.healthaffairs.org/doi/pdf/10.1377/hlthaff.2014.0434.

54. Haefner M. With 8K more physicians than Kaiser, Optum is "scaring the crap out of hospitals." *Becker's Hospital Review*. April 9, 2018. https://www.beckershospitalreview.com/payer-issues/with-8k-more-physicians-than-kaiser-optum-is-scaring-the-crap-out-of-hospitals.html.

55. Bannow T. FTC approves UnitedHealth-DaVita deal with conditions. *Modern Healthcare*. June 19, 2019. https://www.modernhealthcare.com/mergers-acquisitions/ftc-approves-unitedhealth-davita-deal-conditions?utm_source=modern-healthcare-alert&utm_medium=email&utm_campaign=20190619&utm_content=hero-headline.

56. With 8K more physicians than Kaiser, Optum is "scaring the crap out of hospitals" . . .

57. Finnegan J. How many VA doctors are there? No one really knows, GAO report says. *Fierce Healthcare*. Oct. 20, 2017. https://www.fiercehealthcare.com/practices/va-doctors-number-unknown-gao-report.

58. Tracer Z. 30,000 strong and counting, UnitedHealth gathers a doctor army, *Bloomberg News*. April 9, 2018. https://www.bloomberg.com/news/articles/2018-04-09/30-000-strong-and-counting-unitedhealth-gathers-a-doctor-army.

59. Galewitz P. Insurance titan drops doctors, needy patients 'caught in the middle.' Kaiser Health News. Feb. 26, 2020. https://www.medscape.com/viewarticle/925778.

60. The OptumCare footprint. OptumCare website. http://campaign.optum.com/content/optumcare/en/about-optumcare/health-care-providers/practice-models-locations.html.

61. Livingston S. Texas Blues insurer to open primary-care clinics. *Modern Healthcare.* April 8, 2019. https://www.modernhealthcare.com/care-delivery/texas-blues-insurer-open-primary-care-clinics?utm_source=modern-healthcare-daily-dose&utm_medium=email&utm_campaign=20190408&utm_content=article4-headline.

62. Partners in primary care to open five new senior-focused primary care centers in Houston. Humana press release. May 8, 2019. https://www.linkedin.com/jobs/view/1236840570/?refId=870ceac6-7aa8-4833-946c-08de5f82a08f&trk=eml-vjr-similar-job-title&midToken=AQEdQ4kQWRA91g&trkEmail=eml-email_jobs_viewed_job_reminder_01-null-26-null-null-8gti9%7Ejw27gyee%7E2f-null-jobs%7Eview.

63. Anthem Inc. to acquire Beacon Health Options. Anthem press release. June 6, 2019. https://ir.antheminc.com/news-releases/news-release-details/anthem-inc-acquire-beacon-health-options?field_nir_news_date_value%5Bmin%5D=2019.

64. Kacik A. Private equity infuses healthcare with $63B investment. *Modern Healthcare.* April 18, 2019. https://www.modernhealthcare.com/finance/private-equity-infuses-healthcare-63b-investment?utm_source=modern-healthcare-daily-dose-thursday&utm_medium=email&utm_campaign=20190418&utm_content=article3-headline.

65. Gondi S, Song Z. Potential implications of private equity investments in health care delivery. *JAMA.* 2019;321(11):1047-48. doi:10.1001/jama.2019.1077. https://jamanetwork.com/journals/jama/fullarticle/2727259?guestAccessKey=58f92bb3-01c7-4e7d-a5c3-ced30a11642c&utm_source=silverchair&utm_medium=email&utm_campaign=article_alert-jama&utm_content=etoc&utm_term=031519.

66. Monegain B. 5 ways retail clinics are poised to upend healthcare. *Healthcare Finance News.* April 21, 2017. https://www.healthcarefinancenews.com/news/5-ways-retail-clinics-are-poised-upend-healthcare.

67. Truong K. Walgreens to launch in-store primary care clinics in partnership with VillageMD. *Medcity News.* April 10, 2019. https://medcitynews.com/2019/04/walgreens-to-launch-in-store-primary-care-clinics-in-partnership-with-villagemd/?utm_campaign=MCN%20Daily%20Top%20Stories&utm_source=hs_email&utm_medium=email&utm_content=71661012&_hsenc=p2ANqtz-94canA5cFQquOtMLJRFLZQwkuxbsjV_RLaRyLRnFIl5tscpmst1u33PtjJifYn-b6sokiy8gO77Trw2VfKRu4oenOk5jA&_hsmi=71661012

68. Bannow T. CVS to aggressively expand healthcare services in stores. *Modern Healthcare.* June 4, 2019. https://www.modernhealthcare.com/patient-care/cvs-aggressively-expand-healthcare-services-stores?utm_source=modern-healthcare-daily-dose-tuesday&utm_medium=email&utm_campaign=20190604&utm_content=article1-headline.

69. Meyer M. Walmart tests leap into healthcare business by opening second clinic. *Modern Healthcare.* Jan. 31, 2020. https://www.modernhealthcare.com/providers/walmart-tests-leap-healthcare-business-opening-second-clinic?utm_source=modern-healthcare-daily-dose-friday&utm_medium=email&utm_campaign=20200131&utm_content=article4-headline.

70. Ginsburg P. Health care market consolidations: impacts on cost, quality and access. Testimony to California Senate Committee on Health. March 16, 2016. https://www.brookings.edu/testimonies/health-care-market-consolidations-impacts-on-costs-quality-and-access.

CHAPTER 4

1. Starfield B, Shi L, Grover A, Macinko J. The effects of specialist supply on populations' health: Assessing the evidence. *Health Aff.* 2005 Jan-Jun; Suppl Web Exclusives: W5-97-107. https://doi.org/10.1377/hlthaff.w5.97.

2. Baicker K, Chandra A. Medicare spending, the physician workforce, and beneficiaries' quality of care. *Health Aff.* 2004 Jan-Jun;Suppl Web Exclusives: W4-184.97. https://doi.org/10.1377/hlthaff.w4.184.

3. Fine MD. Presentation, Society of Primary Care Policy Fellows. March 26, 2009. Archived by Robert Graham Center. https://www.graham-center.org/content/dam/rgc/documents/publications-reports/presentations/universal-primary-care.pdf.

4. Lazris A, Roth A, Brownlee S. No more lip service; It's time we fixed primary care (part one). *Health Affairs* (blog). Nov. 20, 2018. https://www.healthaffairs.org/do/10.1377/hblog20181115.750150/full/.

5. Goroll AH. Does primary care add sufficient value to deserve better funding? *JAMA Intern Med.* 2019;179(3):372-73. doi:10.1001/jamainternmed.2018.6707. https://jamanetwork.com/journals/jamainternalmedicine/article-abstract/2721034.

6. Nash D. Pondering the primary care predicament. *MedPage Today.* May 16, 2019. https://www.medpagetoday.com/columns/focusonpolicy/79883?xid=nl_mpt_DHE_2019-05-17&eun=g1342670d0r&utm_source=Sailthru&utm_medium=email&utm_campaign=Daily%20Headlines%2014%20day%202019-05-17&utm_term=NL_Daily_DHE_14signups.

7. Agency for Healthcare Research and Quality (AHRQ). The number of practicing primary care physicians in the United States. AHRQ. https://www.ahrq.gov/research/findings/factsheets/primary/pcwork1/index.html.

8. Barbet C, Sahni N, Kocher R, Chernew M. Physician workforce trends and their implications for spending growth. *Health Affairs* (blog). July 28, 2017. https://www.healthaffairs.org/do/10.1377/hblog20170728.061252/full.

9. *Ibid.*

10. No more lip service; It's time we fixed primary care (part one) . . .

11. Physicians Foundation. 2018 survey of America's physicians: Practice patterns & perspectives. https://physiciansfoundation.org/wp-content/uploads/2018/09/physicians-survey-results-final-2018.pdf.

12. AAMC. New research shows increasing physician shortages in both primary and specialty care. American Association of Medical Colleges press release. April 11, 2018. https://news.aamc.org/press-releases/article/workforce_report_shortage_04112018.

13. Verma S. Putting our rethinking rural health strategy into action. CMS (blog). May 8, 2019. https://www.cms.gov/blog/putting-our-rethinking-rural-health-strategy-action.

14. American Association of Nurse Practitioners. NP Fact Sheet. https://www.aanp.org/about/all-about-nps/np-fact-sheet.

15. American Association of Physician Assistants. About the AAPA. https://www.aapa.org/news-central/press-room.

16. AHRQ. The number of nurse practitioners and physician assistants practicing primary care in the U.S. Agency for Healthcare Research and Quality. Sept. 2012. https://www.ahrq.gov/research/findings/factsheets/primary/pcwork2/index.html.

17. Vleet AV, Paradise J. Tapping nurse practitioners to meet rising demand for primary care. *Kaiser Family Foundation Issue Brief.* Jan. 20, 2015. https://www.kff.org/medicaid/issue-brief/tapping-nurse-practitioners-to-meet-rising-demand-for-primary-care.

18. Terry K. Telehealth, urgent care, retail clinics getting more popular. *Medscape Medical News.* April 2, 2019. https://www.medscape.com/viewarticle/911252.

19. Monegain M. 5 ways retail clinics are poised to upend healthcare. *Healthcare Finance*. April 21, 2017. https://www.healthcarefinancenews.com/news/5-ways-retail-clinics-are-poised-upend-healthcare.

20. Personal communication with Urgent Care Association spokesman.

21. Dickson V. MedPAC votes to cut payments for free-standing ERs. *Modern Healthcare*. April 5, 2018. https://www.modernhealthcare.com/article/20180405/NEWS/180409947/medpac-votes-to-cut-payments-for-free-standing-ers.

22. Stoimenoff L, Newman N. The essential role of the urgent care center in population health. Urgent Care Association of America white paper. 2018.

23. Johnson DW, Richie W. Getting urgent about urgent care: Health systems go big on retail. *4Sight Health Market Corner Commentary*. May 21, 2019. https://gallery.mailchimp.com/8a4b f5d1617f86a90e5a909f0/files/20ac8d84-9835-4e33-93b1-eeb79a25d03f/4sightHealth. UrgentAboutUrgentCare.CB.MCC.5_21_19.01.pdf?utm_source=4sight+Health+Readers& utm_campaign=d05b8fc5a8-CMS+Misdirection_COPY_01&utm_medium=email&utm_ term=0_96b6d85309-d05b8fc5a8-147472109.

24. Livingston S. Humana announces virtual primary-care plan. *Modern Healthcare*, April 24. 2019. https://www.modernhealthcare.com/insurance/humana-announces-virtual-primary-care-plan?utm_source=modern-healthcare-daily-dose-wednesday&utm_medium=email&utm_ campaign=20190424&utm_content=article4-headline.

25. Pupillo J. Study: retail clinics contribute to higher health care costs. March 24, 2016. American Academy of Family Physicians website. https://www.aafp.org/news/practice-professional-issues/20160324retailclinics.html.

26. Hargraves J, Frost A. Trends in primary care visits. Health Care Cost Institute. Nov. 15, 2018. https://www.healthcostinstitute.org/research/publications/hcci-research/entry/trends-in-primary-care-visits.

27. Thousands of resident applicants celebrate NRMP match results. National Resident Matching Program press release. March 15, 2019. http://www.nrmp.org/one-nine-press-release-thousands-resident-physician-applicants-celebrate-nrmp-match-results.

28. Terry K. One in 5 residents doubt career choice despite ample job offers. *Medscape Medical News*. May 16, 2019. https://www.medscape.com/viewarticle/913082.

29. Medscape Physician Compensation Report 2019. https://www.medscape.com/slideshow/2019-compensation-overview-6011286?src=ban_comp2019_desk_mscpmrk_hp#2.

30. One in 5 residents doubt career choice . . .

31. Bodenheimer T, Berenson RA, Paul Rudolf. The primary care-specialty income gap: why it matters. *Ann Intern Med*. 2007;146;301-06. doi: https://doi.org/10.7326/0003-4819-146-4-200702200-00011.

32. Sinsky C, Colligan L, Li L, Prgomet M, Reynolds S, *et al*. Allocation of physician time in ambulatory practice: a time and motion study in 4 specialties. *Ann Intern Med*. 165(11):753-60. doi:10.7326/M16-0961. https://adfm.org/media/1476/ann-2016-time-study.pdf.

33. Hoff TJ. *Next in Line: Lowered Care Expectations in the Age of Retail and Value-Based Health*. Oxford: Oxford University Press;2017:98.

34. Peckham C. Physician burnout: it just keeps getting worse. *Medscape Family Medicine*. Jan. 26, 2015, https://www.medscape.com/viewarticle/838437_3

35. Direct Primary Care. AAFP website. https://www.aafp.org/practice-management/payment/dpc.html.

36. Haefner M. 7 things to know about the rise of fee-based direct primary care. *Becker's Hospital Review*. March 19, 2018. https://www.beckershospitalreview.com/hospital-physician-relationships/7-things-to-know-about-the-rise-of-fee-based-direct-primary-care.html.

37. Corba KL, Watson M. Direct primary care may be the link to the 'fourth aim' of healthcare. *Medical Economics*. July 10, 2018. https://www.medicaleconomics.com/business/direct-primary-care-may-be-link-fourth-aim-healthcare.

38. Jabbarpour Y, Coffman M, Habib A, Chung Y, Liaw W, *et al*. Executive summary: Advanced primary care: A key contributor to successful ACOs. PCPCC and Robert Graham Center. https://www.pcpcc.org/sites/default/files/resources/PCPCC%202018%20Executive%20Summary.pdf.

39. NCQA, MACRA and NCQA Recognition Programs. https://www.ncqa.org/programs/health-care-providers-practices/patient-centered-medical-home-pcmh/benefits-support/macra.

40. Nash D. Healthcare reform's Rx for primary care. *MedPage Today*. Aug. 18, 2010. www.medpagetoday.com/Columns/21750.

41. American Academy of Family Physicians, American Academy of Pediatrics, American College of Physicians, and American Osteopathic Association. Joint principles of the patient-centered medical home. March 2007. www.aafp.org/dam/AAFP/documents/practice_management/pcmh/initiatives/PCMHJoint.pdf.

42. Nutting P, Miller WL, Crabtree, BF, Jaen CR, Stewart E, Stange KC. Initial lessons from the first national demonstration project on practice transformation to a patient-centered medical home. *Ann Fam Med* 2009;7:254-60. doi: 10.1370/afm.1002. https://www.ncbi.nlm.nih.gov/pmc/articles/PMC2682981.

43. Executive Summary: Advanced primary care: a key contributor to successful ACOs . . .

44. Jabbarpour Y, DeMarchis E, Bazemore A, Grundy P. Executive Summary: The impact of primary care practice transformation on cost, quality, and utilization. Patient-Centered Primary Care Collaborative (PCPCC) and Robert Graham Center. https://www.pcpcc.org/sites/default/files/resources/pcmh_evidence_es_071417%20FINAL.pdf.

45. *Next in Line: Lowered Care Expectations in the Age of Retail and Value-based Health.* 30-31.

46. Executive Summary: Advanced primary care: a key contributor to successful ACOs . . .

47. Bodenheimer T, Ghorob A, Willard-Grace R, Grumbach K. The 10 building blocks of high-performing primary care. *Ann Fam Med*. 12(2):166-71. doi: 10.1370/afm.1616. Accessed at http://www.annfammed.org/content/12/2/166.full.pdf.

48. Bodenheimer T. Anatomy and physiology of primary care teams. *JAMA Intern Med*. 179(1):61-2. doi:10.1001/jamainternmed.2018.5550. https://jamanetwork.com/journals/jamainternalmedicine/article-abstract/2716182.

49. Bodenheimer T. Building powerful primary care teams. Unpublished manuscript for Mayo Clinical Proceedings provided by the author.

50. Aledade Medicare ACOs Improve Quality of Care and Health Outcomes, Save Medicare Over $69 Million in 2018. Aledade press release. Sept. 30, 2019. https://www.aledade.com/aledade-medicare-acos-improve-quality-care-and-health-outcomes-save-medicare-over-69-million-2018.

51. Leventhal R. Aledade expands ACO scope to California healthcare market. *Healthcare Innovation*. May 31, 2019. https://www.hcinnovationgroup.com/policy-value-based-care/accountable-care-organizations-acos/news/21082863/aledade-expands-aco-scope-to-california-healthcare-market.

52. Terry K. EHRs: 5 ways to put data into action: Physicians share strategies to improve quality metrics, chronic care. *Medical Economics*. June 10, 2014. http://www.modernmedicine.com/sites/default/files/legacy/mm/digital/ME/me061014_ezine_FIN.pdf

53. Rama A. Payment and delivery in 2018: participation in medical homes and accountable care organizations on the rise while fee-for-service revenues remain stable. *AMA Policy Research Perspectives*. https://www.ama-assn.org/system/files/2019-09/prp-care-delivery-payment-models-2018.pdf.

CHAPTER 5

1. Kallmes DF, Comstock BA, *et al.* A randomized controlled trial of vertebroplasty for osteoporotic spine fractures. *N Engl J Med.* 361(6):569-79. doi: 10.1056/NEJMoa0900563.

2. Buchbinder R, Osborne RH, *et al.* A randomized trial of vertebroplasty for painful osteoporotic vertebral fractures. *N Engl J Med.* 361(6):557-68. doi: 10.1056/NEJMoa0900429.

3. Firanescu CE, de Vries J, Lodder P, Venmans A, *et al.* Vertebroplasty versus sham procedure for painful acute osteoporotic vertebral compression fractures (VERTOS IV): randomised sham controlled clinical trial. *BMJ.* 361:k1551. https://doi.org/10.1136/bmj.k1551.

4. Buchbinder R, Johnston RV, *et al.* Vertebroplasty for treating spinal fractures due to osteo-porosis. *Cochrane Collaborative.* Nov. 6, 2018. https://www.cochrane.org/CD006349/MUSKEL_vertebroplasty-treating-spinal-fractures-due-osteoporosis.

5. Institute of Medicine. *Crossing the Quality Chasm: A New Health System for the 21st Century.* Washington, D.C.: National Academies Press; 2001:3.

6. Fineberg HV. A successful and sustainable health system—how to get there from here. *N Engl J Med.* 366:1020-1027 doi: 10.1056/NEJMsa1114777. https://www.nejm.org/doi/full/10.1056/NEJMsa1114777

7. Berwick DM, Hackbarth AD. Eliminating waste in US health care. *JAMA.* 2012;307(14):1513-16.

8. Institute of Medicine. The healthcare imperative: lowering costs and improving outcomes: workshop series summary. 2010. https://www.ncbi.nlm.nih.gov/books/NBK53942.

9. Gee E, Spiro T. Excess administrative costs burden the U.S. healthcare system. Center for American Progress (blog). April 8, 2019. https://www.americanprogress.org/issues/healthcare/reports/2019/04/08/468302/excess-administrative-costs-burden-u-s-health-care-system.

10. Emanuel EJ. Democrats are having the wrong health care debate. *New York Times.* Aug. 2, 2019. https://www.nytimes.com/2019/08/02/opinion/democrats-health-care.html?action=click&module=Opinion&pgtype=Homepage.

11. Fisher ES, Wennberg DE, Stukel TA, Gottlieb DJ, Lucas FL, Pinder EL. The implications of regional variations in Medicare spending: Part I, the content, quality, and accessibility of Care. *Ann Intern Med.* 138(4):273-87. doi: https://doi.org/10.7326/0003-4819-138-4-200302180-00006.

12. Fisher ES, Wennberg DE, T. Stukel TA, Gottlieb DJ, Lucas FL, Pinder EL. The implications of regional variations in Medicare spending: Part 2, health outcomes and satisfaction with care. *Ann Intern Med.* 138(4):288-98. doi: https://doi.org/10.7326/0003-4819-138-4-200302180-00007

13. The implications of regional variations in Medicare spending: Part I, the content, quality, and accessibility of care . . .

14. Chassin M, Kosecoff J, Park RE, *et al.* Does inappropriate use explain geographic variations in the use of health care services: a study of three procedures. *JAMA.* 258(18):2533-37. doi:10.1001/jama.1987.03400180067028. https://jamanetwork.com/journals/jama/article-abstract/369138.

15. Gawande A. The cost conundrum: what a Texas town can teach us about health care. *The New Yorker.* June 1, 2009. https://www.newyorker.com/magazine/2009/06/01/the-cost-conundrum.

16. Molitor D. The evolution of physician practice styles: evidence from cardiologist migration. *Am Econ J Econ Policy.* 10(1):326-56. doi: 10.1257/pol.20160319. https://www.ncbi.nlm.nih.gov/pmc/articles/PMC5876705.

17. Gawande A. Overkill. *The New Yorker.* May 11, 2015. https://www.newyorker.com/magazine/2015/05/11/overkill-atul-gawande

18. Farias V. No secret sauce: a proven, no-nonsense approach to MSSP. *Group Practice Journal.* April 2019. http://www.amga.org/wcm/SM/2019/04/680422.pdf.

19. Chassin MR. Quality of care: time to act. *JAMA*. 266(24):3472-73. doi: 10.1001/jama.1991. 03470240094040. https://jamanetwork.com/journals/jama/article-abstract/394108.

20. McGlynn Asch SM, Adams J, Keesey J, Hicks J, DeCristofaro A, Kerr EA. The quality of health care delivered to adults in the United States. *N Engl J Med*. 348:2635-45 doi: 10.1056/NEJMsa022615. https://www.nejm.org/doi/full/10.1056/NEJMsa022615.

21. Institute of Medicine. *To Err Is Human: Building a Safer Health System*. Washington, DC: National Academies Press;2000:1.

22. Rutherford PA, Provost LP, Kotagal. UR, Luther K, Anderson A. Achieving hospital-wide patient flow. Institute for Healthcare Improvement white paper. Cambridge, Mass.: Institute for Healthcare Improvement; 2017.

23. *Crossing the Quality Chasm: A New Health System for the 21st Century*, 3.

24. Louden K. Creating a better discharge summary. *ACP Hospitalist*. March 2009. https://acphospitalist. org/archives/2009/03/discharge.htm.

25. O'Malley AS, Reschovsky JD. Referral and consultation communication between primary care and specialist physicians: finding common ground. *Arch Intern Med*. 171(1):56-65. doi:10. 1001/archinternmed.2010.480. https://jamanetwork.com/journals/jamainternalmedicine/ fullarticle/226367.

26. Eliminating waste in US health care . . .

27. *Ibid*.

28. Shekelle P. Overview of clinical practice guidelines. *UpToDate*. https://www.uptodate.com/contents/ overview-of-clinical-practice-guidelines.

29. Steinberg EP, Luce BR. Evidence-based? Caveat emptor. *Health Affairs*, Jan./Feb. 2005, 80-92. https://doi.org/10.1377/hlthaff.24.1.80.

30. *Ibid*.

31. Guggenheim R. Putting EBM to work (easier said than done). *Managed Care*. Dec. 2005. https:// www.managedcaremag.com/archives/2005/12/putting-ebm-work-easier-said-done.

32. Terry K. *Rx for Health Care Reform*. Nashville: Vanderbilt University Press;2007:103.

33. *Ibid*., 100.

34. National Quality Forum. NQF's work in quality measurement. http://www.qualityforum.org/ about_nqf/work_in_quality_measurement.

35. Rosenthal MB, Frank RG, Li Z, *et al*. Early experience with pay-for-performance. *JAMA*. 294(14):1788-93. doi:10.1001/jama.294.14.1788. https://jamanetwork.com/journals/jama/ fullarticle/201673.

36. Pearson SD. Schneider EC, Kleinman KP, Coltin KL, Singer JA. The impact of pay-for-performance on health care quality in Massachusetts, 2001-2003. *Health Affairs*, 27:4 (July/Aug. 2008). https:// www.healthaffairs.org/doi/full/10.1377/hlthaff.27.4.1167.

37. Centers for Medicare and Medicaid Services. Medicare Shared Savings Program Fast Facts. Jan. 2018. https://www.cms.gov/medicare/medicare-fee-for-service-payment/sharedsavingsprogram/ downloads/ssp-2018-fast-facts.pdf.

38. Sorondo BM, Allen A, Bayleran J, Doore S. Using a patient portal to transmit patient report health information into the electronic record: workflow implications and user experience. EGEMS. 4(3):7. doi: http://doi.org/10.13063/2327-9214.1237.

39. American Medical Association. Regulatory nightmare threatens care for America's seniors. Oct. 14, 2014. www.ama-assn.org/ama/pub/news/2014/2014-10-21-regulatory-nightmare-threatens-seniors.page

40. Choosing Wisely. Choosing Wisely: a report on the first five years. http://www.choosingwisely. org/wp-content/uploads/2017/10/Choosing-Wisely-at-Five.pdf.

41. Choosing Wisely. Facts and figures. http://www.choosingwisely.org/our-mission/facts-and-figures.

42. Choosing Wisely. Patient resources. http://www.choosingwisely.org/patient-resources.

43. Choosing Wisely: a report on the first five years . . .

44. Castellucci M. Low-value care persists five years into Choosing Wisely campaign. *Modern Health-care*. Oct. 24, 2017. https://www.modernhealthcare.com/article/20171024/NEWS/171029941/ low-value-care-persists-five-years-into-choosing-wisely-campaign.

45. Kerr EA, Kullgren JT, Saini SD. Choosing Wisely: how to fulfill the promise in the next 5 years. *Health Affairs*. 36(11): 2012-18. doi:10.1377/hlthaff.2017.0953. https://www.healthaffairs.org/doi/ pdf/10.1377/hlthaff.2017.0953.

46. Castellucci M. Spending on low-value services slowed from 2014 to 2016. *Modern Healthcare*. June 21, 2019. https://www.modernhealthcare.com/payment/spending-low-value-services-slowed-2014-2016?utm_source=modern-healthcare-daily-dose-friday&utm_medium=email&utm_campaign=20190621&utm_content=article2-headline.

47. Choosing Wisely: a report on the first five years . . .

48. Choosing Wisely: how to fulfill the promise in the next 5 years . . .

49. Cohen K. New West Physicians' journey to becoming a high-performing health system. *Group Practice Journal*. March 2016. http://www.amga.org/wcm/PI/Acclaim/2015/newWest.pdf.

50. Cohen K. Eliminating low-value care: a new model. *Journal of America's Physician Groups*. Spring 2019: 52-54. https://2h24dy2ehwvl3j7p7q1hih8t-wpengine.netdna-ssl.com/wp-content/ uploads/2019/04/JAPG_ConferenceEdition2019_finallores-1.pdf

51. Spending on low-value services slowed from 2014 to 2016 . . .

52. Daubs M. Lower back pain: best left unimaged. OptumCare website. https://professionals.optumcare. com/insights/outpatient-based/back-pain-unimaged.html?o=optum:EM:OC_9.1_2019:em:OC: lrn:Clinician_Insights_June:19f303306jr10&elq_mid=398&elq_cid=18457.

53. Cohen K. Designing evidence-based spine care. OptumCare website. https://professionals. optumcare.com/insights/outpatient-based/spine-care-team.html?o=optum:EM:OC_9.1_2019: em:OC:lrn:Clinician_Insights_June:19bvdyt06jr10&elq_mid=398&elq_cid=18457.

CHAPTER 6

1. Farias V. No secret sauce: a proven, no-nonsense approach to MSSP. *Group Practice Journal*. April 2019. http://www.amga.org/wcm/SM/2019/04/680422.pdf.

2. Centers for Medicare and Medicaid Services. Final rule creates pathways to success for the Medicare Shared Savings Program. Fact sheet. Dec. 21, 2018. https://www.cms.gov/newsroom/fact-sheets/ final-rule-creates-pathways-success-medicare-shared-savings-program

3. Berwick DM, Nolan TW, Whittington J. The Triple Aim: care, health and cost. *Health Affairs*, May/ June 2008, 759-69. https://www.healthaffairs.org/doi/full/10.1377/hlthaff.27.3.759.

4. Hodach R, Grundy P, Jain J, Weiner M. *Provider-Led Population. Health Management: Key Strate-gies for Healthcare in the Cognitive Era, 2d ed.* Indianapolis: John Wiley & Sons;2016:14-15.

5. Jabbarpour Y, Coffman M, Habib A, Chung Y, Liaw W, *et al.* Executive summary: Advanced primary care: a key contributor to successful ACOs. Patient-Centered Primary Care Collabora-tive (PCPCC) and Robert Graham Center. https://www.pcpcc.org/sites/default/files/resources/ PCPCC%202018%20Executive%20Summary.pdf.

6. Payment reform has grown significantly, though not across methods likely to transform health care. Catalyst for Payment Reform press release. Dec. 4, 2019. https://www.catalyze.org/about-us/cpr-in-the-news/new-national-scorecards/.

7. *Provider-Led Population Health Management*, 20.

8. Kaiser Family Foundation. Health care costs: a primer. May 1, 2012. https://www.kff.org/report-section/health-care-costs-a-primer-2012-report.

9. *Provider-Led Population Health Management*, 105.

10. *Ibid.*, 104.

11. Green DE, Hamory BH, Terrell GE, O'Connell J. A case report: cornerstone health care reduced the total cost of care through population segmentation and care model redesign. *Popul Health Manag.* 2017 Aug;20(4):309-17. doi: 10.1089/pop.2016.0105. Epub 2017 Jan 20. https://www.ncbi.nlm.nih.gov/pubmed/2810651

12. *Provider-Led Population Health Management*, 92-3.

13. Regenbogen SE, Cain-Nielsen AH, Syrjamaki JD, *et al.* Spending on postacute care after hospitalization in commercial insurance and Medicare around age sixty-five. *Health Affairs.* 38(9):1505-13. doi:10.1377/hlthaff.2018.05455. https://www.healthaffairs.org/doi/abs/10.1377/hlthaff.2018.05445.

14. Miliard M. In push to population health and value-based payments, health systems look to post-acute-care networks. *Healthcare IT News.* April 15, 2016. https://www.healthcareitnews.com/news/push-population-health-and-value-based-payments-health-systems-look-post-acute-care-networks.

15. Castellucci M. Home health saves Medicare money despite higher readmissions. *Modern Healthcare.* March 13, 2019. https://www.modernhealthcare.com/care-delivery/home-health-saves-medicare-money-despite-higher-readmissions?utm_source=modern-healthcare-daily-dose-wednesday&utm_medium=email&utm_campaign=20190313&utm_content=article1-headline.

16. *Ibid.*

17. Medicare patients are using fewer skilled nursing services. Avalere Health report. March 15, 2018. https://avalere.com/press-releases/medicare-patients-are-using-fewer-skilled-nursing-services.

18. Redesigned MSSP imposes risk on ACOs more quickly . . .

19. Terry K. Site-neutral payments are less than meets the eye, experts say. *Medscape Medical News.* Dec. 6, 2018. https://www.medscape.com/viewarticle/906146.

20. Terry K. CMS must pay hospitals what it withheld under site-neutral rule. *Medscape Medical News.* Oct. 22, 2019. https://www.medscape.com/viewarticle/920276.

21. *Provider-Led Population Health Management*, 198.

CHAPTER 7

1. Foden-Vencil K. How Oregon is getting 'frequent flyers' out of hospital ERs. *Kaiser Health News.* July 10, 2013. https://khn.org/news/emergency-room-frequent-flyers.

2. The world health report 2002 – reducing risks, promoting healthy life. World Health Organization. https://www.who.int/whr/2002/en.

3. Health care's blind side: the overlooked connection between social needs and good health. Robert Wood Johnson Foundation. http://www.rwjf.org/content/dam/farm/reports/surveys_and_polls/2011/rwjf71795.

4. Insights from McKinsey's consumer social determinants of health survey. McKinsey & Company. April 2019. https://www.mckinsey.com/industries/healthcare-systems-and-services/our-insights/insights-from-the-mckinsey-2019-consumer-social-determinants-of-health-survey.

5. Thomas-Henkel C, Schulman M. Screening for determinants of health in populations with complex needs: implementation considerations. Center for Health Care Strategies report. Oct. 2017. https://www.chcs.org/media/SDOH-Complex-Care-Screening-Brief-102617.pdf.

6. Khullar D, Chokshi DA. Health, income & poverty: where we are & what could help. *Health Aff.* 38(9):1505-13. doi: 10.1377/hpb20180817.901935. https://www.healthaffairs.org/do/10.1377/hpb20180817.901935/full.

7. McGinnis JM, Williams-Russo P, Knickman JR. The case for more active policy attention to health promotion. *Health Aff.* 21(2):78-93. https://doi.org/10.1377/hlthaff.21.2.78.

8. National Academies of Sciences, Engineering and Medicine. Integrating Social Care into the Delivery of Health Care: Moving Upstream to Improve the Nation's Health. Washington, DC: National Academies of Sciences, Engineering and Medicine;2019. https://www.nap.edu/catalog/25467/integrating-social-care-into-the-delivery-of-health-care-moving.

9. Horwitz LI, Chang C, et al. Quantifying Health Systems' Investment in Social Determinants of Health, By Sector, 2017-19. *Health Affairs* 39, No. 2(2020): 192-198. doi: 10.1377/hlthaff.2019.01246. https://www.healthaffairs.org/doi/10.1377/hlthaff.2019.01246.

10. Abir M, Hammond S, Iovan S, Lantz PM. Why more evidence Is needed on the effectiveness of screening for social needs among high-use patients in acute care settings. *Health Affairs* (blog). May 23, 2019. https://www.healthaffairs.org/do/10.1377/hblog20190520.243444/full/?utm_source=Newsletter&utm_medium=email&utm_content=Surprise+Billing%3B+Social+Needs+Among+High-Use+Patients%3B+Alice+Rivlin%3A+A+Consequential+Life%3B+ACA+Litigation+Round-Up%3B+GrantWatch&utm_campaign=HAT.

11. Castellucci M. Fee-for-service limits long-term work on social determinants, execs warn. *Modern Healthcare.* June 15, 2019. https://www.modernhealthcare.com/providers/fee-service-limits-long-term-work-social-determinants-execs-warn?utm_source=modern-healthcare-hits-wednesday&utm_medium=email&utm_campaign=20190619&utm_content=article3-headline.

12. Johnson SR. Kaiser to launch social care network. *Modern Healthcare.* May 6, 2019. https://www.modernhealthcare.com/care-delivery/kaiser-launch-social-care-network?utm_source=modern-healthcare-hits&utm_medium=email&utm_campaign=20190506&utm_content=article2-headline.

13. Johnson SR. CVS and Aetna to launch social care network. *Modern Healthcare.* July 24, 2019. https://www.modernhealthcare.com/providers/cvs-and-aetna-launch-social-care-network?utm_source=modern-healthcare-daily-dose-wednesday&utm_medium=email&utm_campaign=20190724&utm_content=article6-headline.

14. Minemyer P. Why UnitedHealthcare wants to expand diagnostic codes to the social determinants of health. *FierceHealthcare.* Feb. 11, 2019. https://www.fiercehealthcare.com/payer/why-united-healthcare-wants-to-expand-diagnostic-codes-to-social-determinants-health?mkt_tok=eyJpIjoiWmpRelpqVmhNemt6TjJRNCIsInQiOiI4SWdzc3dCRWtYeU1hK1RtRUlvbFNWbjAxYm5sUHZcL3drWkYxTjVhSDVSdnhFY1FQNDlMbkNFK2lUV3VTZU1mRXlzMFRXXajl6QUdJN1ZvazZSTXRNcWMwWTZ0ZDRSUThXM2J6RWFNZHExcmJ2TUJabkh6b095dFBVZnpupuRzRxek0ifQ%3D%3D&mrkid=629433&utm_medium=nl&utm_source=internal.

15. Miliard M. New BCBS Institute working with Lyft, CVS, Walgreens to tackle social determinants. *Healthcare IT News.* March 16, 2018. https://www.healthcareitnews.com/news/new-bcbs-institute-working-lyft-cvs-walgreens-tackle-social-determinants?mkt_tok=eyJpIjoiTkRabU5Ea3hNelpsTkRCSIsInQiOiJTZ3hLK1lKWTkwNW9uQjN2ZW1GRHlUNHNpDTG80R3JidnlFVGV4aENwdHFMZWxBU1ZEQVl6aG5wNWdaY1wvYk1OckttGOWREdjMwTjJaMm1cL2hQcHBSZ0RyXC84VEhkMElxSkhBUmxWR0NVZkN3MGZKWVNnRjVaZ0xjODdUdUY2YyOXozMyJ.

16. Minemyer P. Why New Jersey's top insurer wants to expand its work on the social determinants of health in 2019. *Fierce Healthcare.* Feb. 25, 2019. https://www.fiercehealthcare.com/payer/

why-horizon-bcbsnj-wants-to-expand-its-work-social-determinants-health-2019?mkt_tok=eyJpIjo
iTVdGaU16ZzBOR0l5TldRMiIsInQiOiJ5aWVlMEp4dE11MGlpeVN2eThzVlNHdlwvakNmX
C9tc3FVZ1VQbWtrRjVXeEo5dWVqczM3d2xlQUkzTG54eU9yXC9xelZTaVwvNHNqNkZPTFFi
SUlUVVNub1VnUW4wQTcxeUE5RllqS1dYQ2FCRTE0a3Y4ZEtXMGhYeEFBJaGcyYWp6Skwif
Q%3D%3D&mrkid=629433&utm_medium=nl&utm_source=internal.

17. The importance of social determinants of health data. eHealth Initiative report. March 25, 2019. https://www.ehidc.org/sites/default/files/resources/files/Importance%20of%20SDOH%20Data%20 March%202019.pdf.

18. Centers for Medicare and Medicaid Services (CMS). Accountable health communities model. https://innovation.cms.gov/initiatives/ahcm.

19. Trump administration drives down Medicare Advantage and Part D premiums for seniors. CMS press release. Sept. 24, 2019. https://www.cms.gov/newsroom/press-releases/trump-administration-drives-down-medicare-advantage-and-part-d-premiums-seniors.

20. Morse S. Few Medicare Advantage insurers use new benefit flexibility to address the social determinants of health. *Healthcare Finance News*. Sept. 23, 2019. https://www.healthcarefinancenews.com/ news/few-medicare-advantage-insurers-use-new-benefit-flexibility-address-social-determinants-health?mkt_tok=eyJpIjoiTUdZeVlqZGtaVFJrWkdReiIsInQiOiJ2b1VoWXVUNnBtVzhVRElqYU crQjhSM0VjQ3ltWm1XSFhNcFR6Rk1OZmx2NDNZZ3BMSVdWWWNweVQxREpEdnIwZW ZxWm1Bbkpmb2JtZTRlTno0Zm1QMGZ4aG0rYVBJOWhicEFLTUYyYlVvYnRWWK3NqZ0tW WlU0UVFtSkFIXC9yXC9BIn0%3D.

21. Bachrach D, Bernstein W, Augenstein J, Lipson M, Ellis R. Implementing New York's DSRIP program: implications for Medicaid payment and delivery system reform. Commonwealth Fund. April 2016. https://www.commonwealthfund.org/sites/default/files/documents/___media_files_ publications_fund_report_2016_apr_1871_bachrach_implementing_new_york_dsrip_v4.pdf

22. New York State Department of Health. DSRIP Overview. https://www.health.ny.gov/health_care/ medicaid/redesign/dsrip/overview.htm.

23. Implementing New York's DSRIP program . . .

24. *Ibid.*

25. Foden-Vencil K. Oregon's $2 billion Medicaid bet. *Kaiser Health News*. May 30, 2012. https://khn. org/news/oregon-cco.

26. Aney K. Former Oregon governor believes new approach needed on health care. *Blue Mountain Eagle*. Sept. 23, 2019. https://www.bluemountaineagle.com/news/former-oregon-governor-believes-new-approach-needed-on-health-care/article_b026a73a-f7ea-5cd1-a769-17734367cae2.html.

27. Terry K. Why physicians must step up, address social determinants of health. *Medical Economics*. Feb. 25, 2017. https://www.medicaleconomics.com/health-law-and-policy/why-physicians-must-step-address-social-determinants-health.

28. Community Care of North Carolina. Statewide "boots on the ground" and demonstrated ROI. https://www.communitycarenc.org/what-we-do/care-management.

29. Livingston S. Social determinants are core of North Carolina's Medicaid overhaul. *Modern Healthcare*. Aug. 3, 2018. https://www.modernhealthcare.com/article/20180803/TRANSFORMATION01/180809944/ social-determinants-are-core-of-north-carolina-s-medicaid-overhaul.

30. Why physicians must step up, address social determinants of health . . .

31. Klein S, Hostetter M. In Focus: Integrating behavioral health and primary care. Commonwealth Fund Quality Matters Archive. Aug./Sept. 2014. http://www.commonwealthfund.org/publications/ newsletters/quality-matters/2014/august-september/in-focus.

32. Nash D, Reifsnyder J, Fabius R, Pracilio V. *Population Health: Creating a Culture of Wellness*. Burlington, Mass.: Jones & Bartlett Learning;2011:126.

33. Johnson SR, Meyer H. Behavioral health: fixing a system in crisis. *Modern Healthcare Special Report*. https://www.modernhealthcare.com/reports/behavioral-health/#!.

34. Mental health by the numbers. National Alliance on Mental Illness. https://www.nami.org/learn-more/mental-health-by-the-numbers.

35. deGruy F. Mental health in the primary care setting. In *Primary Care: America's Health in a New Era*. Washington, D.C.: National Academies Press;1996.

36. Hodach R, Grundy P, Jain A, Weiner M. *Provider-Led Population. Health Management: Key Strategies for Healthcare in the Cognitive Era, 2nd ed*. Indianapolis: John Wiley & Sons;2016:209.

37. Integrating behavioral health into primary care. SAMHSA-HRSA Center for Integrated Health Systems. http://www.integration.samhsa.gov/integrated-care-models/behavioral-health-in-primary-care.

38. New NCQA patient-centered medical home standards raise the bar. March 24, 2014. National Committee for Quality Assurance (NCQA) press release. http://www.ncqa.org/newsroom/news-archive/2014-news-archive/news-release-march-24-2014.

39. Why behavioral health needs to be integrated into the patient-centered medical home . . .

40. *Ibid*.

41. In Focus: Integrating behavioral health and primary care . . .

42. Fraze TK, Brewster AL, Valerie A. Lewis. Prevalence of screening for food insecurity, housing instability, utility needs, transportation needs, and interpersonal violence by US physician practices and hospitals. *JAMA Netw Open*. 2019;2(9):e1911514. doi:10.1001/jamanetworkopen.2019.11514. https://jamanetwork.com/journals/jamanetworkopen/fullarticle/2751390

43. Thomas-Henkel C, Schulman M. Screening for determinants of health in populations with complex needs: implementation considerations. Center for Health Care Strategies. Oct. 2017. https://www.chcs.org/media/SDOH-Complex-Care-Screening-Brief-102617.pdf.

44. Gold R, Cottrell E, Bunce A, Middendorf M, Hollombe C, *et al*. Developing electronic health record (EHR) strategies related to health center patients' social determinants of health. *J Am Board Fam Med*. 2017 Jul-Aug; 30(4): 428-47. doi: 10.3122/jabfm.2017.04.170046.

45. Siwicki B. What population health IT vendors are doing to support SDOH. *Healthcare IT News*. Sept. 5, 2019. https://www.healthcareitnews.com/news/what-population-health-it-vendors-are-doing-support-sdoh?mkt_tok=eyJpIjoiT1dNMFpXUTBORGRoT0RGbCIsInQiOiI4eGltNDR0cWtHcTlNaWxuaXd6aEtvNVwvQkhYaWpNeW9JcjRQQnd5aFBQREtvSFNNMZVNPTGd2NCtsMHFzajByV1F2Uk5Rd1dvM3dUQ216YWtWWVJkaTBZUFwvTVJPTGJhSWxqLTcVRXMW5tREhPU1dmK2wrWnhtdkVyUUlweTJtIn0%3D.

46. Unite US website. https://www.uniteus.com

47. Social care coordination platform, Unite Us, partners with Kaiser Permanente to launch thrive local. Unite US press release. May 20, 2019. https://blog.uniteus.com/kaiser-permanente.

48. Miliard M. Investments in social determinants will pay off, with better outcomes and value. *Healthcare IT News*. Sept. 1, 2019. https://www.healthcareitnews.com/news/investments-social-determinants-will-pay-better-outcomes-and-value?mkt_tok=eyJpIjoiWTJFM1lUQXlOek5oTkd aaSIsInQiOiJldDJjajahwU0VGNzlBNDBsY0thVzZoc0NzbVdrdlVoaVJkbWhWRXhFTGZFTE9WS jRvcDBxZW5FdEpvNWklRa1IrRm1MckxHeG5DanJNelB2Q0pqbGJWUGlxYUJUU1FBWXVSd1dVS3BXaGw5Y1VKOEhMMjBGUmxLMzllY2hvdmhVZSJ9

49. Karen Handmaker, personal communication.

50. Provider-led population health management, 211.

51. Models of care for high-need, high-cost patients: an evidence synthesis. Commonwealth Fund Brief. Oct. 29, 2015. http://www.commonwealthfund.org/publications/issue-briefs/2015/oct/care-high-need-high-cost-patients?omnicid=EALERT91443&mid=%25%25emailaddr%25%25

52. Miller E, Nath T, Line L. Working together toward better health outcomes. Nonprofit Finance Fund, Center for Health Care Strategies, and Alliance for Strong Families and Communities report. June 2017. https://www.chcs.org/media/Working-Together-Toward-Better-Health-Outcomes.pdf

53. Freda B, Kozick D, Spencer A. Partners for health: lessons for bridging community-based organizations and health care organizations. Center for Health Care Strategies. Jan. 2018. https://www.chcs.org/media/CBO-HCO_Partnership_update_032018.pdf.

54. Nonprofit hospitals' community benefit requirements. *Health Affairs Policy Brief*. Feb. 25, 2018. https://www.rwjf.org/content/dam/farm/reports/issue_briefs/2016/rwjf426962.

55. *Ibid*.

56. The case for more active policy attention to health promotion . . .

CHAPTER 8

1. Ginsburg P. Health care market consolidations: impacts on cost, quality and access. Testimony to California Senate Committee on Health. March 16, 2016. https://www.brookings.edu/testimonies/health-care-market-consolidations-impacts-on-costs-quality-and-access.

2. Murray R. Setting hospital rates to control costs and boost quality: The Maryland experience. *Health Aff.* 28(5):1395-405. https://www.healthaffairs.org/doi/full/10.1377/hlthaff.28.5.1395

3. Roberts ET, Hatfield LA, McWilliams JM, Chernew ME, Done N, *et al.* Changes in hospital utilization three years into Maryland's global budget program for rural hospitals. *Health Aff.* 37(4):644-53. https://morningconsult.com/wp-content/uploads/2018/04/Health-Affairs-Maryland-2018-0112_p2.pdf.

4. Galarraga J, Pines JM. The challenging transformation of health care under Maryland's global budgets, *Health Affairs* (blog). Dec. 19, 2017. https://www.healthaffairs.org/do/10.1377/hblog20171214.96251/full/.

5. McDonough JE. Tracking the demise of state hospital rate setting. *Health Aff.* 16(1):142-9. https://doi.org/10.1377/hlthaff.16.1.142.

6. Sanger-Katz M. Why the less disruptive health care option could be plenty disruptive. *New York Times*. Dec. 3, 2019. https://www.nytimes.com/2019/12/03/upshot/public-option-medicare-for-all.html?action=click&module=Top%20Stories&pgtype=Homepage.

7. Kocher R, Berwick DM. Policies For making health care in the United States better. *Health Affairs* (blog). June 6, 2019. https://www.healthaffairs.org/do/10.1377/hblog20190530.216896/full/?utm_source=Newsletter&utm_medium=email&utm_content=Kocher+and+Berwick%3A+What+To+Do+While+Considering+Medicare+for+All%3B+Wisconsin+Medicaid+Expansion%3B+The+Specialty+Palliative+Care+Workforce&utm_campaign=HAT.

8. Terry K. *Rx for Health Care Reform*. Nashville: Vanderbilt University Press;2007:177.

9. Hancock J. When the hospital is boss, that's where doctors' patients go. *Kaiser Health News*. Sept. 9, 2015. http://khn.org/news/when-the-hospital-is-boss-thats-where-doctors-patients-go.

10. Casalino LP, Pesko MF, Ryan AM, Mendelsohn JL, Copeland KR, *et al.* Small primary care physician practices have low rates of preventable hospital admissions. *Health Aff.* 33(9):1680-88. https://www.healthaffairs.org/doi/pdf/10.1377/hlthaff.2014.0434.

11. Yetter EJ. Understanding corporate practice of medicine laws by state. *Physicians First Healthcare Partners* (blog). Aug. 25, 2017. https://www.physiciansfirst.com/blog/corporate-practice-of-medicine-laws-by-state.

12. Finnegan J. Private equity companies' acquisition of physician practices likely to accelerate. Fierce Healthcare. Jan. 10, 2019. https://www.fiercehealthcare.com/practices/private-equity-companies-acquisition-physician-practices-likely-to-accelerate.

13. Cohen JK. Separate EHRs pose care-coordination challenge for ACOs, OIG finds. *Modern Healthcare*. May 22, 2019. https://www.modernhealthcare.com/operations/separate-ehrs-pose-care-coordination-challenge-acos-oig-finds?utm_source=modern-healthcare-hits-wednesday&utm_medium=email&utm_campaign=20190522&utm_content=article1-headline.

14. Sisko AM, Keehan SP, *et al*. National health expenditure projections, 2018-27: economic and demographic trends drive spending and enrollment growth. *Health Aff.* 38(3):491-501. doi: 10.1377/hlthaff.2018.05499. https://www.healthaffairs.org/doi/pdf/10.1377/hlthaff.2018.05499. This report shows that Medicare spending increased by $41.5 billion in 2018. New MSSP savings were $739 million and gross program savings were $1.7 billion. So the total amount that Medicare itself saved was only 2% of the increase in Medicare costs.

15. Van de Water PN. Medicare Advantage upcoding, overpayments require attention. Center on Budget and Policy Priorities. Oct. 30, 2018. https://www.cbpp.org/blog/medicare-advantage-upcoding-overpayments-require-attention.

16. Edwards K, Richards R, Muhlestein D. The 2018 ACO survey: unique paths to success. Leavitt Partners white paper. March 2019. https://cdn2.hubspot.net/hubfs/4795448/2018%20ACO%20Survey%20Report%20March%202019.pdf?utm_campaign=White%20Papers&utm_source=hs_automation&utm_medium=email&utm_content=71259667&_hsenc=p2ANqtz-9bSZvAZfdNG1gtrLgnUt-0hZ3QSZ5OVhxrF3xc9K6DtQti9ZPMSrUapg4lqeANI7yajy42OqwJtfgxAZUSay9_hwDQ3A&_hsmi=71259667.

17. Robert Richards, Leavitt Partners, personal communication.

18. Physicians Foundation. 2018 survey of America's physicians: practice patterns & perspectives. https://physiciansfoundation.org/wp-content/uploads/2018/09/physicians-survey-results-final-2018.pdf.

19. Sharon Grace, AMGA, personal communication.

20. A majority of physicians now take part in an ACO. American Medical Association news release. Sept. 12, 2019. https://www.ama-assn.org/practice-management/payment-delivery-models/majority-physicians-now-take-part-aco.

21. Centers for Medicare and Medicaid Services (CMS). Shared Savings Program Participation Options. https://www.cms.gov/Medicare/Medicare-Fee-for-Service-Payment/sharedsavingsprogram/Downloads/ssp-aco-participation-options.pdf.

22. Verma S. Interest in 'Pathways to Success' grows: 2018 ACO results show trends supporting program redesign continue. *Health Affairs* (blog). Sept. 30, 2019. https://www.healthaffairs.org/do/10.1377/hblog20190930.702342/full/?utm_source=Newsletter&utm_medium=email&utm_content=CMS+Administrator+Seema+Verma+On+The+Medicare+Shared+Savings+Program%3B+The+Demise+of+the+ACA+s+Multi-State+Plan+Program%3B+Coverage+Of+Children+With+Medical+Complexity&utm_campaign=HAT.

23. CMS. Medicare Shared Savings Program: Fast Facts. Jan. 2018. https://www.cms.gov/Medicare/Medicare-Fee-for-Service-Payment/sharedsavingsprogram/Downloads/SSP-2018-Fast-Facts.pdf.

24. Muhlestein D. Bleser WK. Saunders RS, Richards R, Singletary E, McClellan MB. Spread of ACOs and value-based payment models in 2019: gauging the impact of Pathways to Success. *Health Affairs* (blog). Oct. 21, 2019. 10.1377/hblog20191020.962600. https://www.healthaffairs.org/do/10.1377/hblog20191020.962600/full.

25. Mechanic R, Perloff J, Litton T, Edwards K, Muhlestein D. The 2018 annual ACO survey: examining the risk contracting landscape. *Health Affairs* (blog). 10.1377/hblog20190422.181228. https://www.healthaffairs.org/do/10.1377/hblog20190422.181228/full.

26. A majority of physicians now take part in an ACO . . .

27. CMS. Primary Care First Model Options. https://innovation.cms.gov/initiatives/primary-care-first-model-options.

28. *Rx for Health Care Reform*, 172.

29. U.S. Census Bureau. Population estimates for July 1, 2018, New York and Spokane. https://www.census.gov/quickfacts/fact/table/newyorkcitynewyork,spokanecitywashington.

30. World Population Review. Spokane, Washington population 2019. http://worldpopulationreview.com/us-cities/spokane-population.

31. Center for Health Workforce Studies. New York physician supply and demand through 2030: Executive Summary. March 2009. https://www.albany.edu/news/images/PhysicianShortagereport.pdf.

32. Center for Health Workforce Studies. Washington State's Physician Workforce in 2014. http://depts.washington.edu/uwrhrc/uploads/CHWS_WA_Phys_Workforce_2014.pdf.

33. Here's how I calculated the number of PCP groups required under this model: The U.S. population in 2018 was 327.2 million people. According to one estimate, the average PCP panel size is 2,300 patients (Altschuler J, Margolius D, Bodenheimer T, Grumbach K. Estimating a reasonable patient panel size for primary care physicians with team-based task delegation. *Ann Fam Med*. 2012, 10;5:396-400. doi: 10.1370/afm.1400. http://www.annfammed.org/content/10/5/396.full). If the average group had 50 PCPs, each with 2,300 patients, they could care for 115,000 people. Dividing the U.S. population by that number yields 2,845 groups. However, as Altschuler *et al.* point out, PCPs cannot provide comprehensive care to patient panels this large. They argue for care teams taking some of the burden off doctors, so they'd only have to directly care for, say, 1,500 patients. Another study from 2016 (Raffoul M, Moore M, Kamerow D, Bazemore A. A primary care panel size of 2500 Is neither accurate nor reasonable. *J Am Board Fam Med* 2016;29:496–499. https://www.jabfm.org/content/jabfp/29/4/496.full.pdf) estimates that actual panel sizes range from 1,200 to 1,900 patients per PCP. Using 1,500 as an average panel size, a group of 50 physicians could care for 75,000 people. With that many patients per group, 4,363 primary care practices of this size would be needed to provide care to the U.S. population.

34. Brook RH, McGlynn EA, Shekelle PG, *et al.* Report cards for health care: is anyone checking them? *RAND Research Brief*. 2002. https://www.rand.org/pubs/research_briefs/RB4544.html.

35. Sinaiko AD, Eastman D, Rosenthal MB. How report cards on physicians, physician groups, and hospitals can have greater impact on consumer choices. *Health Aff.* 31(3):602-11. https://doi.org/10.1377/hlthaff.2011.1197.

36. Findlay SD. Consumers' interest in provider ratings grows, and improved report cards and other steps could accelerate their use. *Health Aff.* 35(4):688-96. https://doi.org/10.1377/hlthaff.2015.1654.

37. *Ibid.*

38. *Ibid.*

39. CMS. Performance Information and Physician Compare. https://www.cms.gov/Medicare/Quality-Initiatives-Patient-Assessment-Instruments/physician-compare-initiative/Quality-Data-and-Physician-Compare-.html#performance.

40. Consumers' interest in provider ratings grows . . .

41. California Office of the Patient Advocate. Health care quality report cards, 2018-19 edition. https://www.opa.ca.gov/reportcards/Pages/default.aspx.

42. CMS. Physician Compare Initiative. https://www.cms.gov/medicare/quality-initiatives-patient-assessment-instruments/physician-compare-initiative.

43. Wisconsin Collaborative for Healthcare Quality. Measure summary. https://reports.wchq.org/measure-summary.

44. MN Community Measurement. https://mncm.org.

45. How report cards on physicians, physician groups, and hospitals can have greater impact . . .

46. Consumers' interest in provider ratings grows . . .

47. How report cards on physicians, physician groups, and hospitals can have greater impact . . .

48. Jonas DE, Ferrari RM, *et al.* Evaluating evidence on intermediate outcomes: considerations for groups making healthcare recommendations. *Am J Prev Med.* 54(1S1):S38-S52. https://doi.org/10.1016/j.amepre.2017.08.033.

49. Weldring T, Smith SMS. Patient-reported outcomes (PROs) and patient-reported outcome measures (PROMs). *Health Serv Insights.* 2013;6:61-68. https://www.ncbi.nlm.nih.gov/pmc/articles/PMC4089835/

50. Wagle NW. Implementing patient-reported outcome measures. *NEJM Catalyst.* Oct. 12, 2017. https://catalyst.nejm.org/implementing-proms-patient-reported-outcome-measures.

51. *Ibid.*

52. Terry K. *Rx for Health Care Reform.* Nashville: Vanderbilt University Press;2007:185-191.

CHAPTER 9

1. Edwards K, Richards R, Muhlestein D. The 2018 ACO survey: unique paths to success. Leavitt Partners report. March 2019. https://cdn2.hubspot.net/hubfs/4795448/2018%20ACO%20Survey%20Report%20March%202019.pdf?utm_campaign=White%20Papers&utm_source=hs_automation&utm_medium=email&utm_content=71259667&_hsenc=p2ANqtz-9bSZvAZfdNG1gtrLgnUt-0hZ3QSZ5OVhxrF3xc9K6DtQti9ZPMSrUapg4lqeANI7yajy42OqwJtfgxAZUSay9_hwDQ3A&_hsmi=71259667.

2. Colla CH, Lewis VA, Shortell SM, Fisher ES. First national survey of ACOs finds that physicians are playing strong leadership and ownership roles. *Health Aff.* 33(6): 964-71. doi: 10.1377/hlthaff.2013.1463. https://www.healthaffairs.org/doi/pdf/10.1377/hlthaff.2013.1463.

3. Fleming NS, Culler SD, *et al.* The financial and nonfinancial costs of implementing electronic health records in primary care practices. *Health Aff.* 30(3):481-9. https://doi.org/10.1377/hlthaff.2010.0768.

4. National Association of Accountable Care Organizations (NAACOS). ACO cost and MACRA implementation survey. May 2016. https://www.naacos.com/aco-cost-and-macra-implementation-survey#investment.

5. Lemaire N, Singer SJ. Do independent physician-led ACOs have a future? *NEJM Catalyst.* Feb. 22, 2018 https://catalyst.nejm.org/do-independent-physician-led-acos-have-a-future.

6. Health Care Payment Learning & Action Network (HCP-LAN). Primary care payment models. 2017. https://hcp-lan.org/workproducts/pcpm-whitepaper-final.pdf.

7. Evolent Health. https://www.evolenthealth.com/ipa.

8. Lightbeam Health. https://www.lightbeamhealth.com.

9. Mark Foulke, Privia Health, personal communication.

10. Privia Health. http://www.priviahealth.com.

11. Aledade. https://www.aledade.com/our-solutions.

12. Lumeris. https://www.lumeris.com/improve-patient-outcomes.

13. Arcadia. https://www.arcadia.io.

14. Caravan Health. https://caravanhealth.com.

15. Partners in Care. https://www.piccorp.com/about.

16. Paul Keckley. Is Phycor 2.0 Ahead? *The Keckley Report.* July 11, 2016. https://www.paulkeckley.com/the-keckley-report/2016/7/11/is-phycor-20-ahead.

17. Centers for Medicare and Medicaid Services (CMS). Medicare Shared Savings Program & Medicare ACO Track 1+ Model repayment mechanism arrangements. April 2019. https://www.cms.gov/

Medicare/Medicare-Fee-for-Service-Payment/sharedsavingsprogram/Downloads/Repayment-Mechanism-Guidance.pdf

18. CMS. NHE Fact Sheet. https://www.cms.gov/research-statistics-data-and-systems/statistics-trends-and-reports/nationalhealthexpenddata/nhe-fact-sheet.html.

19. Sisko AM, Keehan SP, *et al.* National health expenditure projections, 2018-27: Economic and demographic trends drive spending and enrollment growth. Health Aff. 38(3):491-501. https://www.healthaffairs.org/doi/abs/10.1377/hlthaff.2018.05499.

20. Bipartisan Policy Center. Transitioning from volume to value: Accelerating the shift to alternative payment models. July 2015. https://bipartisanpolicy.org/wp-content/uploads/2019/03/BPC-Health-Alternative-Payment-Models.pdf.

21. CMS, Medicare Shared Savings Program: Shared savings and losses and assignment methodology. Feb. 2019. https://www.cms.gov/Medicare/Medicare-Fee-for-Service-Payment/sharedsavingsprogram/Downloads/Shared-Savings-Losses-Assignment-Spec-V7.pdf.

22. *Ibid.*

23. *Ibid.*

24. Niles J, Litton T, Mechanic R. An initial assessment of initiatives to improve care for high-need, high-cost individuals in accountable care organizations. *Health Affairs* (blog). April 11, 2019. 10.1377/hblog20190411.143015. https://www.healthaffairs.org/do/10.1377/hblog20190411.143015/full/?utm_campaign=HASU+4-14-19&utm_medium=email&utm_content=ACA+Litigation+Update%3B+Health+Equity+In+Cancer+Care%3B+Rx+Drug+Rebates%3B+Comparing+Medicare+Advantage+And+Traditional+Medicare+Enrollees&utm_source=Newsletter.

25. Altschuler J, Margolius D, Bodenheimer T, Grumbach K. Estimating a reasonable patient panel size for primary care physicians with team-based task delegation. *Ann Fam Med* 2012;10:396-400. doi:10.1370/afm.1400. http://www.annfammed.org/content/10/5/396.full.pdf.

26. Terry K. The promise of telemedicine: Providing curbside consults for chronic care, urgent care, and pain. *Chronic Pain Perspectives* 59;9:58-62. https://mdedge-files-live.s3.us-east-2.amazonaws.com/files/s3fs-public/Document/September-2017/CHPP001090S50.pdf

27. Robert Wood Johnson Foundation. Project ECHO: bridging the gap in health care for rural and underserved communities. April 24, 2014. https://www.rwjf.org/en/library/research/2014/04/project-echo--bridging-the-gap-in-health-care-for-rural-and-unde.html

28. *Ibid.*

29. *Ibid.*

30. Davy C, Bleasel J, Liu H, *et al.* Effectiveness of chronic care models: opportunities for improving healthcare practice and health outcomes: a systematic review. *BMC Health Serv Res.* 15:194. doi:10.1186/s12913-015-0854-8. https://bmchealthservres.biomedcentral.com/articles/10.1186/s12913-015-0854-8#citeas.

31. *Ibid.*

32. Stellefson M, Dipnarine K, Stopka C. The chronic care model and diabetes management in US primary care settings: a systematic review. *Prev Chronic Dis.* 2013;10:120180. http://dx.doi.org/10.5888/pcd10.120180.

33. Group Health Cooperative Institute. Reducing care fragmentation. Group Health Cooperative Institute http://www.improvingchroniccare.org/downloads/reducing_care_fragmentation.pdf.

34. Barnett ML, Song Z, Bitton A, Rose S, Landon BE. Gatekeeping and patterns of outpatient care post healthcare reform. *Am J Manag Care.* 24(10):e312-e316. https://www.ajmc.com/journals/issue/2018/2018-vol24-n10/gatekeeping-and-patterns-of-outpatient-care-post-healthcare-reform.

35. Wachter RM, Goldman L. Zero to 50,000—the 20th anniversary of the hospitalist. *N Engl J Med* 2016;375:1009-11. https://www.nejm.org/doi/full/10.1056/NEJMp1607958.

36. Palabindala V, Salim SA. Era of hospitalists. *J Community Hosp Intern Med Perspect.* 2018; 8(1):16-20. doi: 10.1080/20009666.2017.1415102.

37. Terry K. The changing face of hospital practice. *Medical Economics.* Aug. 23, 2002.

38. Livingston S. UnitedHealthcare outpatient surgery policy threatens hospital revenue. *Modern Healthcare.* Oct. 17, 2019. https://www.modernhealthcare.com/payment/unitedhealthcare-out-patient-surgery-policy-threatens-hospital-revenue.

39. Medicare Payment Advisory Commission. Ambulatory surgical center services. Chapter 5 of Report to the Congress: Medicare Payment Policy, 130. March 2019. http://www.medpac.gov/docs/default-source/reports/mar19_medpac_ch5_sec.pdf?sfvrsn=0.

CHAPTER 10

1. Day S, Seninger C, *et al.* Digital health consumer adoption report 2019. Stanford Medicine and Rock Health. https://rockhealth.docsend.com/view/i6j4ieu.

2. Sinsky C, Colligan L, Li L, Prgomet M, Reynolds S, *et al.* Allocation of physician time in ambulatory practice: a time and motion study in 4 specialties. *Ann Intern Med.*165(11):753-60. doi:10.7326/M16-0961. https://adfm.org/media/1476/ann-2016-time-study.pdf.

3. Arndt BG, Beasley JW, *et al.* Tethered to the EHR: Primary care physician workload assessment using EHR event log data and time-motion observations. *Ann Fam Med* 15;4:419-26. doi 10.1370/afm.2121. http://www.annfammed.org/content/15/5/419.full.

4. Cohen DJ, Dorr DA, Knierim K, DuBard , *et al.*, Challenges in using electronic health record data for quality improvement CA. *Health Aff.* 37(4):635-43. doi: 10.1377/hlthaff.2017.1254. https://www.healthaffairs.org/doi/pdf/10.1377/hlthaff.2017.1254.

5. Wachter R, Goldsmith J. To combat physician burnout and improve care, fix the electronic health record. *Harvard Business Review.* March 30, 2018. https://hbr.org/2018/03/to-combat-physician-burnout-and-improve-care-fix-the-electronic-health-record.

6. American Medical Association. Improving electronic health records. https://www.ama-assn.org/practice-management/digital/improving-electronic-health-records.

7. Terry K. Why electronic health records aren't more usable. *cio.com.* Dec. 3, 2015. https://www.cio.com/article/3011576/why-electronic-health-records-arent-more-usable.html.

8. Posnack S. API conditions of certification (and more!). Office of the National Coordinator for Health Information Technology. https://www.healthit.gov/sites/default/files/page/2019-02/PosnackAPICoCFeesIB.pdf.

9. Terry K. CMS aims to reduce physician EHR burden, provide more data. *Medscape Medical News.* Aug. 2, 2019. https://www.medscape.com/viewarticle/916422.

10. Hodach R, Grundy P, Jain A, Weiner M. *Provider-Led Population. Health Management: Key Strategies for Healthcare in the Cognitive Era, 2d ed.* Indianapolis: John Wiley & Sons;2016:225-227.

11. Terry K. Voice-enabled AI app may reduce EHR documentation time. *Medscape Medical News.* Nov. 20, 2019. https://www.medscape.com/viewarticle/921215.

12. Hsu W, Taira RK, *et al.* Context-based electronic health records: towards patient specific healthcare. *IEEE Trans Inf Technol Biomed.*16(2):228-34. doi: 10.1109/TITB.2012.2186149.

13. Lovett L. Google demos its EHR-like clinical documentation tool. *Mobihealthnews.* Nov. 21, 2019. https://www.mobihealthnews.com/news/north-america/google-demos-its-ehr-clinical-documentation-tool?mkt_tok=eyJpIjoiWXpNeVlqWXpOalJsTVRRRdyIsInQiOiJJdDgzQVo3ZWFaOHhPWm15VG9sMll6Z3Q1cVFJU2gzK1ZVbDJia0oozeFhmaTlWRkdkem1BbDA3eklUMmpJT

0VkUitMdlwvTEt3VDRcLzhTVmM5S0VGTUNjTjZyN3p6Z1FHZ0ZBaW9XRVVpamR4MFpy
RzV2YllBV3lqdVpaNlhvSnZZIn0%3D.

14. Patel V, Pylypchuk Y, *et al.* Interoperability among office-based physicians in 2015 and 2017. Office of the National Coordinator for Health Information (ONC) *Technology Data Brief.* May 2019. https://www.healthit.gov/sites/default/files/page/2019-05/ONC-Data-Brief-47-Interoperability-among-Office-Based-Physicians-in-2015-and-2017.pdf.

15. Pylypchuk Y, Johnson C, *et al.* Variation in interoperability among U.S. non-federal acute care hospitals in 2017. *ONC Technology Data Brief.* Nov. 2018. https://www.healthit.gov/sites/default/files/page/2018-11/Interop%20variation_0.pdf

16. Cohen JK. Hospitals lack CEO buy-in to invest in interoperability. *Modern Healthcare.* Aug. 19, 2019. https://www.modernhealthcare.com/information-technology/hospitals-lack-ceo-buy-invest-interoperability?utm_source=modern-healthcare-hits&utm_medium=email&utm_campaign=20190819&utm_content=article1-headline.

17. Landi H. DirectTrust hits milestone of 1B messages exchanged; developing instant messaging standard. *Fierce Healthcare.* Aug. 5, 2019. https://www.fiercehealthcare.com/tech/directtrust-hits-milestone-1b-messages-exchanged-developing-instant-messaging-standard.

18. David Kibbe, personal communication.

19. Terry K. What is FHIR? The eventual answer to healthcare interoperability. *cio.com.* July 10, 2019. https://www.cio.com/article/3407778/what-is-fhir-the-eventual-answer-to-healthcare-interoperability.html.

20. *Ibid.*

21. *Ibid.*

22. Terry K. New rule provides telemedicine opportunity. *Medical Economics.* May 1, 2019. https://www.medicaleconomics.com/article/new-rule-provides-telemedicine-opportunity.

23. Yang YT. Telehealth parity laws. *Health Affairs Health Policy Brief.* Aug. 15, 2016. doi: 10.1377/hpb20160815.244795. https://www.healthaffairs.org/do/10.1377/hpb20160815.244795/full.

24. Comstock J. CMS proposes new rule to boost telehealth payments. *Healthcare IT News.* July 12, 2018. https://www.healthcareitnews.com/news/cms-proposes-new-rule-boost-telehealth-payments.

25. CMS finalizes policies to bring innovative telehealth benefit to Medicare Advantage. Centers for Medicare and Medicaid Services (CMS) press release. April 5, 2019. https://www.cms.gov/newsroom/press-releases/cms-finalizes-policies-bring-innovative-telehealth-benefit-medicare-advantage.

26. Medicare telemedicine health care provider fact sheet. CMS. March 17, 2020. https://www.cms.gov/newsroom/fact-sheets/medicare-telemedicine-health-care-provider-fact-sheet

27. Terry K. Telehealth, urgent care, retail clinics getting more popular. *Medscape Medical News.* April 2, 2019. https://www.medscape.com/viewarticle/911252.

28. Landi H. Only 1 in 10 patients use telehealth as lack of awareness hinders adoption, J.D. Power survey finds. *FierceHealthcare.* July 31, 2019. https://www.fiercehealthcare.com/tech/only-1-10-patients-use-telehealth-as-lack-awareness-hinders-adoption-j-d-power-survey-finds?mkt_tok=eyJpIjo iTkRZd00yRTNPV0l6WVRKbSIsInQiOiJGVkMxNkNRSXgzZTRFYThtMDQwU0RqMExuVX drMyttV1BjSzc0YVdUbGUzcjFzTHk3RkdaYkY0NGE0V2ViWWQ3RktadnQxNTJITjhWRUN-BUG0rY3F3TTU4RlpSdHZiWDJHUzQ1dzJNN3lwZTMySTkrWm5mTlZ6a09IblZTaUhocSJ9& mrkid=629433.

29. McKinney B. Why is telemedicine utilization so low? *MedCity News.* Sept. 12, 2016. https://medcitynews.com/2016/09/telemedicine-utilization-low/?utm_source=hs_email&utm_medium=email&utm_content=34136600&_hsenc=p2ANqtz-_crjWr7QqP5vUtOiW3IzON98d MOp03gOVEBs-wH_tnbOQemPpZKXqU_PvvnoRaWGuDxDcdZZPkh4gPRtNMKuTJU0cjqA&_hsmi=34136600.

30. New rule provides telemedicine opportunity . . .

31. *Ibid.*

32. Wicklund E. Kaiser Permanente sees good results with video-based telehealth. Oct. 16, 2018. https://mhealthintelligence.com/news/kaiser-permanente-sees-good-results-with-video-based-telehealth.

33. New rule provides telemedicine opportunity . . .

34. Kvedar J, Coye MJ, Everett W. Connected health: a review of technologies and strategies to improve patient care with telemedicine and telehealth. *Health Aff.* 33(2):194-99. doi: 10.1377/hlthaff.2013.0992. https://www.healthaffairs.org/doi/pdf/10.1377/hlthaff.2013.0992.

35. California Healthcare Foundation. Evaluation of Provider Experiences with eConsults. Oct. 22, 2019. https://www.chcf.org/publication/evaluation-provider-experiences-econsults/#related-links-and-downloads.

36. Dorsey ER, Topol EJ. State of telehealth. *N Engl J Med.* 2016; 375:154-161. doi: 10.1056/NEJMra1601705. https://www.nejm.org/doi/full/10.1056/NEJMra1601705?query=TOC.

37. Terry K. How mobility, apps and BYOD will transform healthcare. *Information Week.* July 2012. https://dsimg.ubm-us.net/envelope/280742/481693/strategy-how-mobility-apps-and-byod-will-transform-healthcare_750049.pdf.

38. Connected health: a review of technologies and strategies . . .

39. The return on investment of patient-generated health data & remote patient monitoring. *eHealth Initiative issue brief.* July 2018. https://www.ehidc.org/sites/default/files/resources/files/ROIPGHD_7.26.18_final.pdf.

40. *Ibid.*

41. Trong K. Preliminary results are in from the massive Apple Heart Study. *MedCity News.* March 18, 2019. https://medcitynews.com/2019/03/preliminary-results-are-in-from-the-massive-apple-heart-study/?utm_campaign=MCN%20Daily%20Top%20Stories&utm_source=hs_email&utm_medium=email&utm_content=70908696&_hsenc=p2ANqtz-_0F8UM5THYQEXxqX-_HJeDOMBjh7UdcsT20dJ-wEsIy-_G9WcZAM89ojzfBMSpP-Pdmwl8wpg46k8xV-9E_n32exvAFg&_hsmi=70908696.

42. Terry K. Number of health apps soars, but use does not always follow. *Medscape.* Sept. 18, 2015. https://www.medscape.com/viewarticle/851226.

43. IMS digs deep into mHealth, finds $7B in value. *Klick Wire.* April 19, 2018. https://www.klick.com/health/news/blog/mhealth/ims-digs-deep-into-mhealth-finds-7b-in-value.

44. Number of health apps soars, but use does not always follow . . .

45. IMS digs deep into mHealth, finds $7B in value . . .

46. Comstock C. Scripps wired for health study results show no clinical or economic benefit from digital health monitoring. *Mobihealthnews.* Jan. 19, 2016. https://www.mobihealthnews.com/content/scripps-wired-health-study-results-show-no-clinical-or-economic-benefit-digital-health.

47. How mobility, apps and BYOD will transform healthcare . . .

48. IMS digs deep into mHealth, finds $7B in value . . .

49. Muoio D. Positive outcomes from WellDoc's BlueStar translate to cost savings, analysis finds. *Mobihealthnews.* Jan. 4, 2018. https://www.mobihealthnews.com/content/positive-outcomes-welldocs-bluestar-translate-cost-savings-analysis-finds.

50. Comstock J. Lilly-funded study shows Livongo diabetes program can save employers $20 to $50 per member per month. *Mobihealthnews.* May 9, 2019. https://www.mobihealthnews.com/content/north-america/lilly-funded-study-shows-livongo-diabetes-program-can-save-employers-20-50.

51. Lovett L, Rock Health, Stanford report: Consumerization of health reshaping doctor-patient relationships, data conversations. *Mobihealthnews.* Oct. 29, 2019. https://www.mobihealthnews.

com/news/north-america/rock-health-stanford-report-consumerization-health-reshaping-doctor-patient?mkt_tok=eyJpIjoiTUdKalpERTBOMll3T0RGaiIsInQiOiJYemtwUlZ1UWFxa05CNkR4OUZiRFZ4dFwvMjZaSU9JaE1WVUlEVUNPS3I2SkpuUXdIQ29ueGpVNXdcL0J2NmVoYnZZuY00zS05hOFJDXC91ZVRmaG5lVFlcL1dYSjRhcGVhSGdvZUjFDMTYwTlFBMGZFeDNkS3VNUEtzUDYwZVwvUStEeeFZ3In0%3D.

52. Terry K. Over a third of docs recommend mHealth apps, survey shows. *Medscape*. June 10, 2014. https://www.medscape.com/viewarticle/826460.

53. Topol E. Getting doctors in sync with patients and mHealth. *H&HN Daily*. Feb. 20, 2014. https://www.hhnmag.com/articles/5099-getting-doctors-in-sync-with-patients-and-mhealth?dcrPath=%2Ftemplatedata%2FHF_Common%2FNewsArticle%2Fdata%2FHHN%2FDaily%2F2014%2FFeb%2F022014-Topol-mHealth-Doctors.

54. State of telehealth . . .

55. Connected health: a review of technologies and strategies . . .

56. Chan MHM, Keung DTF, *et al.* A validation study of a smartphone application for functional mobility assessment of the elderly. *Hong Kong Physiother J*. 2016 Apr 12;35:1-4. https://www.sciencedirect.com/science/article/pii/S1013702515300051.

CHAPTER 11

1. Institute of Medicine. The healthcare imperative: lowering costs and improving outcomes. Workshop series summary. 2010. https://www.ncbi.nlm.nih.gov/books/NBK53942.

2. Shrank WH, Rogstad TL, Parekh N. Waste in the US health care system: estimated costs and potential for savings. *JAMA*. 2019;322(15):1501-09. doi:10.1001/jama.2019.13978. https://jamanetwork.com/journals/jama/fullarticle/2752664?guestAccessKey=bf8f9802-be69-4224-a67f-42bf2c53e027&utm_source=For_The_Media&utm_medium=referral&utm_campaign=ftm_links&utm_content=tfl&utm_term=100719.

3. Jha AK. Population health management: saving lives and saving money? *JAMA Forum*. June 26, 2019. https://newsatjama.jama.com/2019/06/26/jama-forum-population-health-management-saving-lives-and-saving-money/.

4. Russell LB. Preventing chronic disease: An important investment, but don't count on cost savings. *Health Aff*. 28(1): 42-45. https://doi.org/10.1377/hlthaff.28.1.42.

5. Aledade Medicare ACOs improve quality of care and health outcomes, save Medicare over $69 million in 2018. Aledade press release. Sept. 30, 2019. https://www.aledade.com/aledade-medicare-acos-improve-quality-care-and-health-outcomes-save-medicare-over-69-million-2018.

6. Altschuler J, Margolius D, Bodenheimer T, Grumbach K. Estimating a reasonable patient panel size for primary care physicians with team-based task delegation. *Ann Fam Med*. 2012;10:396-400. doi:10.1370/afm.1400. http://www.annfammed.org/content/10/5/396.full.pdf.

7. *Ibid.*

8. Laff M. Patient panel size uncertainty complicates workforce projections. *AAFP News*. July 20, 2016. https://www.aafp.org/news/practice-professional-issues/20160720rgc-panelsize.html.

9. Frellick M. Primary care appointment numbers dropping, despite ACA. *Medscape Medical News*. Nov. 18, 2019. https://www.medscape.com/viewarticle/921524.

10. Weiner JP, Yeh S, Blumenthal D. The impact of health information technology and e-health on the future demand for physician services. *Health Aff*. 32(11):1998-2004. doi: 10.1377/hlthaff.2013.0680.

11. Bynam J, Passow H, Carmichael D, Skinner J. Exnovation of low value care: a decade of prostate-specific antigen screening practices. J Am Geriatr Soc. 2019 Jan;67(1):29-36. doi: 10.1111/jgs.15591. https://onlinelibrary.wiley.com/doi/pdf/10.1111/jgs.15591.

12. Siwicki B. McLaren Health Care reduces lab tests per patient per day by $5.6%, saving $383,000. *Healthcare IT News.* Oct. 31, 2019. https://www.healthcareitnews.com/news/mclaren-health-care-reduces-lab-tests-patient-day-56-saving-383000?mkt_tok=eyJpIjoiTldaaE9USTNOekpsWWpKa SIsInQiOiJLUDJPd2ZoS011YWlQVDl4VE5cL2VxaGRKTWVYWVFXQmFoMEkxSVwvTUh kXC9EdDlWQmJsQzB4ckVLNTN6TVBFd0I4UEhmczZzOCtzV3lzVjUrTDF6RkVVRM1o2NX pqY3RcL2cwMURqamd2RGlnUDFmV0ZqZFJWbHppVlFBK3pCMFFF2MEcifQ%3D%3D.

13. Rothberg MB, Class J, Bishop TF, Friderici J, Kleppel R, Lindenauer PK. The cost of defensive medicine on three hospital medicine services, JAMA Intern Med. 2014 Nov 1; 174(11): 1867–1868. doi: 10.1001/jamainternmed.2014.4649. https://www.ncbi.nlm.nih.gov/pmc/articles/PMC4231873.

14. Wennberg JE, Fisher ES, Skinner JS. Geography and the debate over Medicare reform. *Health Aff. 2002 July-Dec;Suppl Web Exclusives W96-114.* https://doi.org/10.1377/hlthaff.w2.96.

15. Weinstein JN, Bronner KK, Morgan TS, Wennberg JE. Trends and geographic variations in major surgery for degenerative diseases of the hip, knee and spine, *Health Aff.* 2004;Suppl Variation:VAR81-9. https://www.ncbi.nlm.nih.gov/pubmed/15471768.

16. Institute of Medicine. *Crossing the Quality Chasm: A New Health System for the 21st Century.* Washington, DC: National Academy Press; 2001:186-188.

17. Bloche MG. *The Hippocratic Myth: Why Doctors Are Under Pressure to Ration Care, Practice Politics, and Compromise Their Promise to Heal.* London: Palgrave MacMillan; 2011:26.

18. Choosing Wisely. Choosing Wisely: a report on the first five years. http://www.choosingwisely.org/wp-content/uploads/2017/10/Choosing-Wisely-at-Five.pdf.

19. Clemens J, Gottlieb JD. In the shadow of a giant: Medicare's influence on private physician payments. *Journal of Political Economy* 125(1):9-10. http://users.nber.org/~jdgottl/ShadowOfAGiant.pdf.

20. Gillis KD. Physicians' patient mix—a snapshot from the 2016 benchmark survey and changes associated with the ACA. *AMA Policy Research Perspectives.* https://www.ama-assn.org/sites/ama-assn.org/files/corp/media-browser/public/health-policy/PRP-2017-physician-benchmark-survey-patient-mix.pdf.

21. Zuckerman S, Skopec L, Epstein M. Medicaid physician fees after the ACA primary care fee bump. Urban Institute. March 2017. https://www.urban.org/sites/default/files/publication/88836/2001180-medicaid-physician-fees-after-the-aca-primary-care-fee-bump_0.pdf

22. Luthi S. Medicaid buy-in proposals prompt similar worries as "Medicare for All." *Modern Healthcare.* Oct. 17, 2018. https://www.modernhealthcare.com/article/20181017/NEWS/181019897/medicaid-buy-in-proposals-prompt-similar-worries-as-medicare-for-all.

23. Stein J. What would Sanders's Medicare-for-all plan mean for doctor pay? *Washington Post.* Aug. 27, 2018. https://www.washingtonpost.com/business/2018/08/27/what-would-sanderss-medicare-for-all-plan-mean-doctor-pay.

24. Pollin R, Heintz J, Arno P, Wicks-Lim J, Ash M. Economic analysis of Medicare for All. Political Economy Research Institute (PERI). Nov. 2018. 103. https://www.peri.umass.edu/publication/item/download/805_42f6acc20a83c79049e68b270e30ee43.

25. Sisko AM, Keehan SP, *et al.* National health expenditure projections, 2018-27: economic and demographic trends drive spending and enrollment growth. *Health Aff.* 38(3): 491-501. https://www.healthaffairs.org/doi/abs/10.1377/hlthaff.2018.05499.

26. Medscape Physician Compensation Report 2019. *Medscape.* April 10, 2019. https://www.medscape.com/slideshow/2019-compensation-overview-6011286#1.

27. National health expenditure projections, 2018-27 . . .

CHAPTER 12

1. Olson J. Son's death pushes Minnesota mom into fight against high, rising drug prices. *Minneapolis StarTribune*. May 11, 2018. http://www.startribune.com/son-s-death-pushes-mom-into-drug-price-spotlight/482344871.

2. Magee M. *Code Blue: Inside America's Medical Industrial Complex*. New York: Grove Atlantic; 2019.

3. Cahill J. Price-fixing alleged in lawsuit against insulin makers. *Insulin Nation*. Feb. 1, 2017. https://insulinnation.com/living/price-fixing-alleged-in-lawsuit-against-insulin-makers/.

4. Palmer E. Price 'scheme' lawsuit targets CVS, Express Scripts as well as Novo, Lilly, Sanofi. *FiercePharma*. March 21, 2017. https://www.fiercepharma.com/pharma/price-scheme-lawsuit-targets-cvs-express-scripts-as-wells-as-novo-lilly-sanofi.

5. Sachs R. Prescription drug legislation in Congress: an update. *Health Affairs* (blog). Dec. 12, 2019. doi 10.1377/hblog20191211.802562. https://www.healthaffairs.org/do/10.1377/hblog20191211.802562/full/?utm_source=Newsletter&utm_medium=email&utm_content=%5BPresented+by+Harvard+Medical+School%5D+Prescription+Drug+Legislation+In+Congress%3B+Medicaid+Recipient+Awareness+Of+Work+Requirements%3B++Decline+In+Rural+Medical+Students&utm_campaign=HAT+12-11-19.

6. Firth S. House Dems pass Bill to lower drug prices. *MedPage Today*. Dec. 12, 2019. https://www.medpagetoday.com/publichealthpolicy/healthpolicy/83867?xid=nl_mpt_DHE_2019-12-13&eun=g1342670d0r&utm_source=Sailthru&utm_medium=email&utm_campaign=Daily%20Headlines%20Top%20Cat%20HeC%20%202019-12-13&utm_term=NL_Daily_DHE_dual-gmail-definition.

7. Waxman HA. Lower drug costs now. *Health Affairs* (blog). Oct. 4, 2019. 10.1377/hblog20191003.118206. https://www.healthaffairs.org/do/10.1377/hblog20191003.118206/full/?utm_source=Newsletter&utm_medium=email&utm_content=Tennessee+s+Block+Grant+Proposal%3B+Henry+Waxman+On+The+Lower+Drug+Costs+Now+Act%3B+CMS+Hospital+Ratings&utm_campaign=HAT+10-4-19.

8. Thomas K. Drug prices keep rising despite intensive criticism. *New York Times*. April 26, 2016. https://www.nytimes.com/2016/04/27/business/drug-prices-keep-rising-despite-intense-criticism.html?hp&action=click&pgtype=Homepage&clickSource=story-heading&module=first-column-region&region=top-news&WT.nav=top-news.

9. Garber AM, Sox HC. The role of costs in comparative effectiveness research. *Health Aff*. 29(10):1805-11, doi: 10.1377/hlthaff.2010.0647. https://www.healthaffairs.org/doi/pdf/10.1377/hlthaff.2010.0647.

10. Robinson JC, Ex P, Panteli D. Single-payer drug pricing in a multipayer health system: does Germany offer a model for the US? *Health Affairs* (blog). March 22, 2019. doi: 10.1377/hblog20190318.475434.

11. Ventola CL. Direct-to-consumer pharmaceutical advertising: therapeutic or toxic? *Pharmacy & Therapeutics*. 2011 Oct;36(10):669-74, 681-84. https://www.ncbi.nlm.nih.gov/pmc/articles/PMC3278148.

12. Endo reports fourth-quarter and full year 2018 financial results. Endo Pharmaceuticals press release. Feb. 28, 2019. http://investor.endo.com/news-releases/news-release-details/endo-reports-fourth-quarter-and-full-year-2018-financial-results.

13. Kantor ED, Rehm CD, Haas JS, Chan AT, Giovannucci EL. Trends in prescription drug use among adults in the United States from 1999-2012. *JAMA*. 2015;314(17):1818-30. doi:10.1001/jama.2015.13766. https://www.ncbi.nlm.nih.gov/entrez/eutils/elink.fcgi?dbfrom=pubmed&retmode=ref&cmd=prlinks&id=26529160.

14. Hartman M, Martin AB, Benson J, Catlin A, *et al.* National health care spending in 2018: growth driven by accelerations in Medicare and private insurance spending. *Health Aff.* 39(1):8-17. doi: 10.1377/hlthaff.2019.01451. https://www.healthaffairs.org/doi/pdf/10.1377/hlthaff.2019.01451.

15. Bloche G, Sukhatme N, Marshall JL. Health policy's Gordian Knot: rethinking cost control. *Health Affairs* (blog). April 26, 2017. https://www.healthaffairs.org/do/10.1377/hblog20170426.059805/full/.

16. Wineinger NE, Zhang Y, Topol EJ. Trends in prices of popular brand-name prescription drugs in the United States. *JAMA Netw Open.* 2019;2(5):e194791. doi:10.1001/jamanetworkopen.2019.4791. https://jamanetwork.com/journals/jamanetworkopen/fullarticle/2734804.

17. Institute for Clinical and Economic Review (ICER). Unsupported price increase report: 2019 assessment. Oct. 8, 2019. https://icer-review.org/wp-content/uploads/2019/01/ICER_UPI_Final_Report_and_Assessment_110619.pdf.

18. Dieguez G, Alston M, Tomicki S. A primer on prescription drug rebates: Insights into why rebates are a target for reducing prices. Milliman white paper. May 2018. http://www.milliman.com/uploadedFiles/insight/2018/Prescription-drug-rebates.pdf.

19. U.S. Government Accountability Office. Medicare Part D use of pharmacy benefit managers and efforts to manage drug expenditures and utilization. July 2019. https://www.gao.gov/assets/710/700259.pdf.

20. Pharmacy benefit managers and their role in drug spending. *To the Point.* Commonwealth Fund. April 22, 2019. https://www.commonwealthfund.org/publications/explainer/2019/apr/pharmacy-benefit-managers-and-their-role-drug-spending.

21. *Ibid.*

22. *Ibid.*

23. *Code Blue: Inside America's Medical Industrial Complex.*

24. Prescription drug costs trend update. Blue Cross and Blue Shield Association press release. Nov. 14, 2018. https://www.bcbs.com/the-health-of-america/reports/prescription-drug-costs-trend-update?utm_source=pressrelease&utm_medium=branded_content&utm_campaign=rxtrndupdt 2018.

25. Woolston C, Levine S. Generic drugs. *HealthDay* website (updated in Jan. 2019). https://consumer.healthday.com/encyclopedia/drug-center-16/misc-drugs-news-218/generic-drugs-646396.html.

26. Trends in prices of popular brand-name prescription drugs . . .

27. CVS Health. Current and new approaches to making drugs more affordable. Aug. 2018. https://cvshealth.com/sites/default/files/cvs-health-current-and-new-approaches-to-making-drugs-more-affordable.pdf.

28. Brennan T. Drug detailing works, but for whom? CVS Health briefing. May 3, 2017. https://payorsolutions.cvshealth.com/insights/drug-detailing-works-but-for-whom.

29. *Code Blue: Inside America's Medical Industrial Complex.*

30. Terry K. *Rx for Health Care Reform.* Nashville: Vanderbilt University Press;2007:154.

31. Keown A. Analysis shows Eli Lilly's half-price Humalog generic is not readily available across the U.S. *Biospace.* Aug. 29, 2019. https://www.biospace.com/article/analysis-shows-eli-lilly-s-half-price-humalog-generic-is-not-readily-available-across-the-u-s-/.

32. Pollack A. Drug goes from $13.50 a tablet to $750, overnight. *New York Times.* Sept. 20, 2015. https://www.nytimes.com/2015/09/21/business/a-huge-overnight-increase-in-a-drugs-price-raises-protests.html.

33. U.S. Government Accountability Office. Generic drugs under Medicare: Part D generic drug prices declined overall, but some had extraordinary price increases. USGAO. Aug. 2016. https://www.gao.gov/assets/680/679022.pdf.

34. Conti RM, Nguyen KH, Rosenthal MB. Generic prescription drug price increases: which products will be affected by proposed anti-gouging legislation? J Pharm Policy Pract. 2018;11:29. Published online Nov 21, 2018. doi: 10.1186/s40545-018-0156-8.

35. House Dems pass Bill to lower drug prices . . .

36. Sachs R. Prescription drug legislation in Congress: an update. *Health Affairs* (blog). Dec. 12, 2019. doi: 10.1377/hblog20191211.802562. https://www.healthaffairs.org/do/10.1377/hblog20191211.802562/full/?utm_source=Newsletter&utm_medium=email&utm_content=%5BPresented+by+Harvard+Medical+School%5D+Prescription+Drug+Legislation+In+Congress%3B+Medicaid+Recipient+Awareness+Of+Work+Requirements%3B++Decline+In+Rural+Medical+Students&utm_campaign=HAT+12-11-19.

37. *Ibid.*

38. O'Brien J. Senate Finance Committee passes bipartisan drug pricing bill. *HealthLeaders.* July 25, 2019. https://www.healthleadersmedia.com/finance/senate-finance-committee-passes-bipartisan-drug-pricing-bill.

39. Kerins J, Johnson DW. Commercializing breakthrough drugs in a value-based market. *4sightHealth Market Corner Commentary.* Dec. 10, 2019. https://gallery.mailchimp.com/8a4bf5d1617f86a90e5a909f0/files/939d355c-68af-4486-afdb-93d2bff19fa1/4sightHealth_Drug_Development.MCC.12_10_19.pdf?utm_source=4sight+Health+Readers&utm_campaign=a90126ee17-CMS+Misdirection_COPY_01&utm_medium=email&utm_term=0_96b6d85309-a90126ee17-147472109.

40. DiMasi JA, Grabowski HG, Hansen RA. Innovation in the pharmaceutical industry: new estimates of R&D costs. *J Health Econ.* 2016;47:20-33. https://doi.org/10.1016/j.jhealeco.2016.01.012.

41. U.S. Government Accountability Office. Drug industry profits, research and development spending and merger and acquisition deals. USGAO. Nov. 2017. https://www.gao.gov/assets/690/688472.pdf.

42. *Rx for Health Care Reform*: 144-45.

43. Mikulic M. U.S. pharmaceutical industry—statistics & facts. *Statista.* May 9, 2017. https://www.statista.com/topics/1719/pharmaceutical-industry/.

44. Conti RM, Kleutghen P. Is "competitive licensing" proposed in HR 1046 practical for lowering drug prices? *Health Affairs* (blog). July 29, 2019. https://www.healthaffairs.org/do/10.1377/hblog20190724.85223/full/?utm_source=Newsletter&utm_medium=email&utm_content=Competitive+Licensing+For+Prescription+Drugs%3B+Prices+And+Hospital+Quality%3B+Relationship+Between+State+Policies+And+Medicaid+Disenrollment&utm_campaign=HAT+7-29-19

45. Health Policy's Gordian Knot: Rethinking cost control . . .

46. Anderson GF, Reinhardt UE, Hussey PS, Petrosyan V. It's the prices, stupid: why the United States is so different from other countries. *Health Aff.* 22(3):89-105. https://doi.org/10.1377/hlthaff.22.3.89.

47. Anderson GF, Hussey P, Petrosyan V. It's still the prices, stupid: why the US spends so much on health care, and a tribute to Uwe Reinhardt. *Health Aff.* 38(1):87-95. https://doi.org/10.1377/hltaff.2018.05144.

48. *Ibid.*

49. Squires DA. Explaining high health care spending in the United States: An international comparison of supply, utilization, prices and quality. *Commonwealth Fund Issue Brief.* May 2012. https://www.commonwealthfund.org/sites/default/files/documents/___media_files_publications_issue_brief_2012_may_1595_squires_explaining_high_hlt_care_spending_intl_brief.pdf.

50. *Rx for Health Care Reform*: 283.

51. *Ibid.*

52. Hughes S. "Low value" care? More controversy for statins in primary prevention. *Medscape*. Oct. 30, 2019. https://www.medscape.com/viewarticle/920603.

53. The role of costs in comparative effectiveness research . . .

54. *Ibid.*

55. Paulden M. Recent amendments to NICE's value-based assessment of health technologies: implicitly inequitable? *Expert Review of Pharmacoeconomics & Outcomes Research* 17;3:239-42. https://doi.org/10.1080/14737167.2017.1330152.

56. Pizzi LT. The Institute for Clinical and Economic Review and its growing influence on US healthcare. Am Health Drug Benefits. 2016 Feb; 9(1): 9-10. https://www.ncbi.nlm.nih.gov/pmc/articles/PMC4822973.

57. Dranove D. *What's Your Life Worth?* Upper Saddle River, N.J.: Financial Times Prentice Hall; 2003:98-104.

58. Recent amendments to NICE's value-based assessment of health technologies . . .

59. Claxton K, Martin S, Soares M, Rice N, *et al.* Methods for the estimation of the National Institute for Health and Care Excellence cost-effectiveness threshold. *Health Technol Assess*. 2015 Feb; 19(14):1-503, v-vi. doi: 10.3310/hta19140. https://www.ncbi.nlm.nih.gov/pubmed/25692211

60. *Ibid.*

61. Cameron D, Ubels J, Norstrom F. On what basis are medical cost-effectiveness thresholds set? Clashing opinions and an absence of data: a systematic review. Glob Health Action. 2018; 11(1): 1447828. doi: 10.1080/16549716.2018.1447828.

62. *Ibid.*

63. Raferty J. Ever higher cancer drug prices—driven by US policies and genetic sequencing. *BMJ Opinion*. July 1, 2015. https://blogs.bmj.com/bmj/2015/07/01/james-raftery-ever-higher-cancer-drug-prices-driven-by-us-policies-and-genetic-sequencing/.

64. Recent amendments to NICE's value-based assessment of health technologies . . .

65. Kassam A. The serious flaw in Canada's healthcare system: prescription drugs aren't free. *The Guardian*. Oct. 20, 2017. https://www.theguardian.com/world/2017/oct/20/canada-national-pharmacare-prescription-drugs

66. Canada announces regulations to cut price of prescription drugs. *Reuters*. Aug. 9, 2019. https://www.theguardian.com/world/2019/aug/09/canada-prescription-drugs-cut-cost.

67. Canadian Agency for Drugs and Technology (CADTH). https://www.cadth.ca/about-cadth/what-we-do/products-services.

68. On what basis are medical cost-effectiveness thresholds set? . . .

69. CADTH Canadian Drug Expert Committee Recommendation for lanadelumab. https://www.cadth.ca/sites/default/files/cdr/complete/SR0618%20Takhzyro%20-%20CDEC%Decemer December20Final%20Recommendation%20November%2022%2C%202019_for%20posting.pdf.

70. Single-payer drug pricing in a multipayer health system . . .

71. Sieler S, Rudolph T, Brinkann-Sass C, Sear R. AMNOG revisited. McKinsey & Co. report. May 2015. https://www.mckinsey.com/~/media/McKinsey/Industries/Pharmaceuticals%20and%20Medical%20Products/Our%20Insights/AMNOG%20revisited/AMNOG_revisited.ashx.

72. Single-payer drug pricing in a multipayer health system . . .

73. ICER website. https://icer-review.org.

74. ICER. The QALY: Rewarding the care that most improves patients' lives. Dec. 2018. https://icer-review.org/wp-content/uploads/2019/04/QALY_evLYG_FINAL.pdf.

75. ICER. ICER comments on the FDA approval of Zolgensma for the treatment of spinal muscular atrophy. https://icer-review.org/announcements/icer_comment_on_zolgensma_approval/.

76. ICER. Oral semaglutide for type 2 diabetes: effectiveness and value. Sept. 11, 2019. https://icer-review.org/wp-content/uploads/2019/04/ICER_Diabetes_Draft-Evidence-Report_091119-1.pdf.

77. Roehrig C. The impact of new hepatitis C drugs on national health spending. *Health Affairs* (blog). Dec. 7, 2015. doi: 10.1377/hblog20151207.052128.

78. The Institute for Clinical and Economic Review and its growing influence on US healthcare . . .

79. ICON. Payers report that ICER analyses increasingly guide US price negotiations. ICON press release. Nov. 15, 2019. https://www.iconplc.com/insights/blog/2019/11/15/payers-report-that-icer-analyses-increasingly-guide-us-price-negotiations.

80. Taylor RS, Iglesias CP. Assessing the clinical and cost-effectiveness of medical devices and drugs: Are they that different? Value Health. 2009 Jun;12(4):404-6. doi: 10.1111/j.1524-4733.2008.00476_2.x. Epub 2008 Nov 19. https://www.valueinhealthjournal.com/article/S1098-3015(10)60779-6/pdf.

81. Iglesias CP. Does assessing the value for money of therapeutic medical devices require a flexible approach? *Expert Review of Pharmacoeconomics & Outcomes Research.* 15;1 (2015): 21-32. doi: 10.1586/14737167.2015.982098.

82. *Ibid.*

83. *Ibid.*

84. Neumann PJ, Chambers JD. Medicare's reset on "coverage with evidence development." *Health Affairs* (blog). April 1, 2013. 10.1377/hblog20130401.029345.

85. Centers for Medicare and Medicaid Services (CMS). Coverage with Evidence Development. https://www.cms.gov/Medicare/Coverage/Coverage-with-Evidence-Development/index. There are 23 technologies on the CED list, but others have dropped off, based on a comparison with the Neumann/Chambers list in 2013.

86. CMS proposes coverage with evidence development for chimeric antigen receptor (CAR) T-cell therapy. CMS press release. Feb. 15, 2019. https://www.cms.gov/newsroom/press-releases/cms-proposes-coverage-evidence-development-chimeric-antigen-receptor-car-t-cell-therapy.

87. Pear R. Medicare aims to expand coverage of cancer care. But is it enough? *New York Times.* April 13, 2019. https://www.nytimes.com/2019/04/13/us/politics/medicare-car-t-cancer.html.

88. CMS expands coverage of CAR T-Cell therapy for Medicare beneficiaries. *ASCO Post.* Sept. 25, 2019. https://ascopost.com/issues/september-25-2019/cms-expands-coverage-of-car-t-cell-therapy-for-medicare-beneficiaries.

89. Patient-Centered Outcomes Research Institute (PCORI). Highlights of PCORI-funded research results. https://www.pcori.org/research-results/explore-our-portfolio/highlights-pcori-funded-research-results.

90. PCORnet, https://pcornet.org.

91. Sukhatme NU, Bloche MG. Health care costs and the arc of innovation. *Minnesota Law Review* 104;2:955. https://scholarship.law.georgetown.edu/cgi/viewcontent.cgi?article=3171&context=facpub.

FINAL THOUGHTS

1. Thompson D. Health care just became the U.S.'s largest employer. *The Atlantic.* Jan. 9, 2018. https://www.theatlantic.com/business/archive/2018/01/health-care-america-jobs/550079/.

2. Turner A, Roehrig C, Hempstead K. What's behind 2.5 million new health jobs? *Health Care* (blog). March 17, 2017. https://www.healthaffairs.org/do/10.1377/hblog20170317.059235/full.

3. Herman B. Healthcare adds 474,700 jobs in 2015. *Modern Healthcare.* Jan. 8, 2016. http://www.modernhealthcare.com/article/20160108/NEWS/160109901.

4. Bannow T. Strong September healthcare hiring behind historically low unemployment rate. *Modern Healthcare*. Oct. 4, 2019. https://www.modernhealthcare.com/healthcare-economics/strong-september-healthcare-hiring-behind-historically-low-unemployment-rate?utm_source=modern-healthcare-hits-friday&utm_medium=email&utm_campaign=20191004&utm_content=article7-headline.

5. Bannow T. Hospitals continue to shed jobs in May as healthcare bounces back. *Modern Healthcare*. June 5, 2020. https://www.modernhealthcare.com/providers/hospitals-continue-shed-jobs-may-healthcare-bounces-back?utm_source=modern-healthcare-alert&utm_medium=email&utm_campaign=20200605&utm_content=hero-headline.

6. Kaiser Family Foundation. Health care employment as a percent of total employment. May 2017. https://www.kff.org/other/state-indicator/health-care-employment-as-total/?currentTimeframe=0&sortModel=%7B%22colId%22:%22Location%22,%22sort%22:%22asc%22%7D.

7. Weisbart S. Insurance industry employment trends: 1990-2018. Insurance Information Institute. March 9, 2018. https://www.iii.org/presentation/insurance-industry-employment-trends-1990-2018-january-2018-030918.

8. US biopharma industry: 854,000 jobs, $1.2 trillion in total economic output. *Pharmaceutical Commerce*. May 17, 2016. https://pharmaceuticalcommerce.com/business-and-finance/us-biopharma-industry-854000-jobs-1-2-trillion-total-economic-output/.

9. Diamond D. Bernie's health plan: Bad for health care workers? *Politico*. Feb. 24, 2016. https://www.politico.com/tipsheets/politico-pulse/2016/02/califf-poised-for-confirmation-who-and-white-house-both-ask-for-zika-dollars-212864.

10. Pollin R, Heintz J, Arno P, Wicks-Lim J, Ash M. Economic analysis of Medicare for All. Nov. 2018. https://www.peri.umass.edu/publication/item/download/805_42f6acc20a83c79049e68b270e30ee43.

11. Manjoo F. The American health care industry is killing people. *New York Times*. Dec. 4, 2019. https://www.nytimes.com/2019/12/04/opinion/healthcare-industry-medicare.html.

12. Economic analysis of Medicare for All . . .

13. Noack R, Kornfield M, Hawkins D, Armus T, Taylor A, Iati M. White House task force projects 100,000 to 240,000 deaths in U.S., even with mitigation efforts. Washington Post. April 1, 2020. https://www.washingtonpost.com/world/2020/03/31/coronavirus-latest-news/.

14. Terry K. Hard truths from infectious disease specialists. Medscape Medical News. April 4, 2020. https://www.medscape.com/viewarticle/928146

15. Terry K. Hospitals face cash crunch in 60-90 days due to COVID-19: report. Medscape Medical News. March 27, 2020. https://www.medscape.com/viewarticle/927612.

16. Medical Group Management Association. COVID-19 financial impact on medical practices. https://mgma.com/getattachment/9b8be0c2-0744-41bf-864f-04007d6adbd2/2004-G09621D-COVID-Financial-Impact-One-Pager-8-5x11-MW-2.pdf.aspx?lang=en-US&ext=.pdf

17. Terry K. CMS to front Medicare payments to physicians for 3 months. Medscape Medical News. March 30, 2020. https://www.medscape.com/viewarticle/927798

18. Livingston J. Immediate changes needed for physicians to stay in business during the pandemic. The Health Care Blog. March 31, 2020. https://thehealthcareblog.com/blog/2020/03/31/immediate-changes-needed-for-physicians-to-stay-in-business-during-the-pandemic/.

19. King R. Bon Secours, Boston Medical among hospitals forced to furlough workers due to COVID-19. FierceHealthcare. March 31, 2020. https://www.fiercehealthcare.com/hospitals-health-systems/hospitals-forced-to-furlough-workers-as-they-lose-money-from-low-patient?mkt_tok=eyJpIjoiWVdZZEE0yRmlNV0ptWm1FNSIsInQiOiJRblZxekkwKysrUnFIXC9BbCtkTytUYm9yU1p6VThmRmlZdjRhd0M3RzNxcUwzZkR6YzBOcEpxY1VxWGF0VFVxbUZrNDdOMmhsd2oyamRJZ3I2UHVtWWV1WldlCbjhPdGGVDUXp5RVB6MXJ0U3ZTQlRvN2VWUWVmb3NuUE5aVnVUdjkifQ%3D%3D&mrkid=629433.

20. Twachtman G. COVID-19 Spurs Telemedicine, Furloughs, Retirement. Medscape Medical News. April 29, 2020. https://www.medscape.com/viewarticle/929624

21. Covered California releases the first national projection of the coronavirus (COVID-19) pandemic's cost to millions of Americans with employer or individual insurance coverage. Covered California press release. March 24, 2020. https://www.coveredca.com/newsroom/news-releases/2020/03/24/covered-california-releases-the-first-national-projection-of-the-coronavirus-covid-19-pandemics-cost/.

22. Simmons-Duffin S. Some insurers waive patients' share of costs for COVID-19 treatment. NPR. March 30, 2020. https://www.npr.org/sections/health-shots/2020/03/30/824075753/good-news-with-caveats-some-insurers-waive-costs-to-patients-for-covid-19-treatm.

23. Blues plans to waive patient costs for COVID-19 treatment. Modern Healthcare. April 3, 2020. https://www.modernhealthcare.com/safety-quality/coronavirus-outbreak-live-updates-covid-19?utm_source=modern-healthcare-covid-19-coverage&utm_medium=email&utm_campaign=20200402&utm_content=article5-headline.

24. Gangopadhyaya A, Garrett B. Unemployment, health insurance, and the COVID-19 recession. Urban Institute Brief. April 1, 2020. https://www.rwjf.org/en/library/research/2020/03/unemployment-health-insurance-and-the-covid-19-recession.html.

25. Goldberg M. New estimate: 3.5 million workers likely lost their employer-sponsored health insurance in the past two weeks. State of Reform. April 2, 2020. https://stateofreform.com/covid-19/2020/04/new-estimate-3-5-million-workers-likely-lost-their-employer-sponsored-health-insurance-in-the-past-two-weeks/.

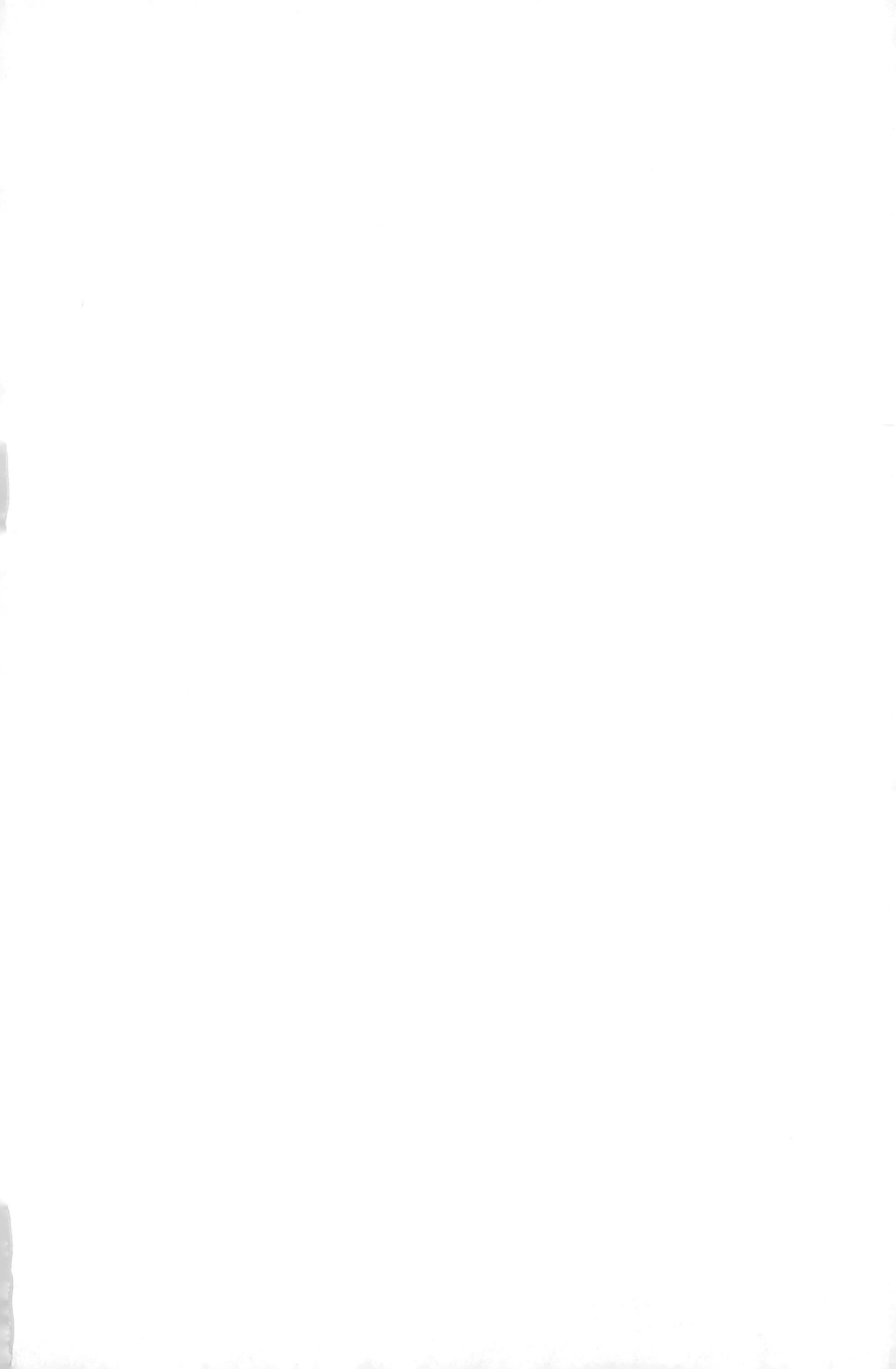

www.ingramcontent.com/pod-product-compliance
Lightning Source LLC
Chambersburg PA
CBHW080518220326
41599CB00032B/6127